PROGRESS IN CLINICAL AND BIOLOGICAL RESEARCH

RECENT TITLES

Vol 311: **Molecular and Cytogenetic Studies of Non-Disjunction,** Terry J. Hassold, Charles J. Epstein, *Editors*

Vol 312: **The Ocular Effects of Prostaglandins and Other Eicosanoids,** Laszlo Z. Bito, Johan Stjernschantz, *Editors*

Vol 313: **Malaria and the Red Cell: 2,** John W. Eaton, Steven R. Meshnick, George J. Brewer, *Editors*

Vol 314: **Inherited and Environmentally Induced Retinal Degenerations,** Matthew M. LaVail, Robert E. Anderson, Joe G. Hollyfield, *Editors*

Vol 315: **Muscle Energetics,** Richard J. Paul, Gijs Elzinga, Kazuhiro Yamada, *Editors*

Vol 316: **Hemoglobin Switching,** George Stamatoyannopoulos, Arthur W. Nienhuis, *Editors.* Published in two volumes: Part A: *Transcriptional Regulation.* Part B: *Cellular and Molecular Mechanisms.*

Vol 317: **Alzheimer's Disease and Related Disorders,** Khalid Iqbal, Henryk M. Wisniewski, Bengt Winblad, *Editors*

Vol 318: **Mechanisms of Chromosome Distribution and Aneuploidy,** Michael A. Resnick, Baldev K. Vig, *Editors*

Vol 319: **The Red Cell: Seventh Ann Arbor Conference,** George J. Brewer, *Editor*

Vol 320: **Menopause: Evaluation, Treatment, and Health Concerns,** Charles B. Hammond, Florence P. Haseltine, Isaac Schiff, *Editors*

Vol 321: **Fatty Acid Oxidation: Clinical, Biochemical, and Molecular Aspects,** Kay Tanaka, Paul M. Coates, *Editors*

Vol 322: **Molecular Endocrinology and Steroid Hormone Action,** Gordon H. Sato, James L. Stevens, *Editors*

Vol 323: **Current Concepts in Endometriosis,** Dev R. Chadha, Veasy C. Buttram, Jr., *Editors*

Vol 324: **Recent Advances in Hemophilia Care,** Carol K. Kasper, *Editor*

Vol 325: **Alcohol, Immunomodulation, and AIDS,** Daniela Seminara, Ronald Ross Watson, Albert Pawlowski, *Editors*

Vol 326: **Nutrition and Aging,** Derek M. Prinsley, Harold H. Sandstead, *Editors*

Vol 327: **Frontiers in Smooth Muscle Research,** Nicholas Sperelakis, Jackie D. Wood, *Editors*

Vol 328: **The International Narcotics Research Conference (INRC) '89,** Rémi Quirion, Khem Jhamandas, Christina Gianoulakis, *Editors*

Vol 329: **Multipoint Mapping and Linkage Based Upon Affected Pedigree Members: Genetic Analysis Workshop 6,** Robert C. Elston, M. Anne Spence, Susan E. Hodge, Jean W. MacCluer, *Editors*

Vol 330: **Verocytotoxin-Producing** *Escherichia coli* **Infections,** Martin Petric, Charles R. Smith, Clifford A. Lingwood, James L. Brunton, Mohamed A. Karmali, *Editors*

Vol 331: **Mouse Liver Carcinogenesis: Mechanisms and Species Comparisons,** Donald E. Stevenson, R. Michael McClain, James A. Popp, Thomas J. Slaga, Jerrold M. Ward, Henry C. Pitot, *Editors*

Vol 332: **Molecular and Cellular Regulation of Calcium and Phosphate Metabolism,** Meinrad Peterlik, Felix Bronner, *Editors*

Vol 333: **Bone Marrow Purging and Processing,** Samuel Gross, Adrian P. Gee, Diana A. Worthington-White, *Editors*

Vol 334: **Potassium Channels: Basic Function and Therapeutic Aspects,** Thomas J. Colatsky, *Editor*

Please contact publisher for information about previous titles in this series.

URO-ONCOLOGY: CURRENT STATUS AND FUTURE TRENDS

URO-ONCOLOGY: CURRENT STATUS AND FUTURE TRENDS

Proceedings of a Uro-Oncological Workshop, Held in Würzburg, Federal Republic of Germany, June 22–25, 1988

Editors

Hubert G.W. Frohmüller
Manfred P. Wirth
Department of Urology
University of Würzburg
Würzburg, Federal Republic of Germany

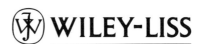

WILEY-LISS

A JOHN WILEY & SONS, INC., PUBLICATION
NEW YORK • CHICHESTER • BRISBANE • TORONTO • SINGAPORE

Address all Inquiries to the Publisher
Wiley-Liss, Inc., 41 East 11th Street, New York, NY 10003

Copyright © 1990 Wiley-Liss, Inc.

Printed in United States of America

The publication of this volume was facilitated by the authors and editors who submitted the text in a form suitable for direct reproduction without subsequent editing or proofreading by the publisher.

Library of Congress Cataloging-in-Publication Data

Uro-Oncological Workshop (1988 : Würzburg, Germany)
    Uro-oncology : current status and futures trends : proceedings of a Uro-Oncological Workshop, held in Würzburg, Federal Republic of Germany, June 22-25, 1988 / editors, H.G.W. Frohmüller, Manfred Wirth.
        p.   cm. -- (Progress in clinical and biological research ; v. 350)
    Includes index.
    ISBN 0-471-56816-3
    1. Genitourinary organs--Cancer--Congresses.   I. Frohmüller, H. G. W. (Hubert George W.), 1928-   . II. Wirth, Manfred.
III. Title.   IV. Series.
    [DNLM: 1. Bladder Neoplasms--therapy--congresses.   2. Carcinoma, Renal Cell--therapy--congresses.   3. Prostatic Neoplasms--therapy--congresses.   4. Testicular Neoplasms--therapy--congresses.   W1 PR668E v. 350 / WJ 504 U78u 1988]
RC280.G4U75   1988
616.99'46--dc20
DNLM/DLC
for Library of Congress   90-12322
                                                              CIP

Contents

Contributors

Rüdiger Arndt, Department of Urology, University of Hamburg, 2000 Hamburg 20, Federal Republic of Germany **[35]**

Anton J.M.C. Beniers, Department of Urology, Urological Research Laboratory, University Hospital Nijmegen, 6525 GA Nijmegen, The Netherlands **[243]**

J. Blom, Departments of Urology and Pathology, University of Rotterdam, Rotterdam, The Netherlands **[41]**

C.G.D. Boeken Krueger, Departments of Urology and Pathology, University of Rotterdam, Rotterdam, The Netherlands **[41]**

Michael Boyer, Urological Cancer Research Unit and Department of Clinical Oncology, Royal Prince Alfred Hospital, Sydney, N.S.W., Australia **[309]**

Konrad Burk, Department of Medical Oncology, Farmitalia Carlo Erba, D-7800 Freiburg, Federal Republic of Germany **[187]**

M. Cacciatore, Institute of Urology and Interdepartment Center for Research in Clinical Oncology, University of Palermo Polyclinic Hospital ''P. Giaccone'', 90127 Palermo, Italy **[149]**

P.J. Carpentier, Departments of Urology and Pathology, University of Rotterdam, Rotterdam, The Netherlands **[41]**

H. Ballentine Carter, Department of Urology, The James Buchanan Brady Urological Institute, The Johns Hopkins University School of Medicine, Baltimore, MD 21205 **[129]**

G. Casanova, Department of Urology, University of Bern, Inselspital, 3010 Bern, Switzerland **[81]**

N. Cavallo, Institute of Urology and Interdepartment Center for Research in Clinical Oncology, University of Palermo Polyclinic Hospital ''P. Giaccone'', 90127 Palermo, Italy **[149]**

Clayton Chong, Department of Medical Oncology, Section of Genitourinary Oncology, The University of Texas M.D. Anderson Cancer Center, Houston, TX 77030 **[107,301]**

Stefan Conrad, Department of Urology, University of Hamburg, 2000 Hamburg 20, Federal Republic of Germany **[275]**

G. Daricello, Institute of Urology and Interdepartment Center for Research in Clinical Oncology, University of Palermo Polyclinic Hospital "P. Giaccone", 90127 Palermo, Italy [149]

Frans M.J. Debruyne, Department of Urology, University Hospital Nijmegen, 6525 GA Nijmegen, The Netherlands [243]

Pieter H.M. de Mulder, Department of Medical Oncology, University Hospital Nijmegen, 6525 GA Nijmegen, The Netherlands [243]

F.-J. Deutz, Department of Urology, RWTH Aachen, Federal Republic of Germany [61]

Francisco H. Dexeus, Department of Medical Oncology, Section of Genitourinary Oncology, The University of Texas M.D. Anderson Cancer Center, Houston, TX 77030 [107,301]

John P. Donohue, Department of Urology, Indiana University Medical Center, Indianapolis, IN 46223 [283]

Mart P.H. Franssen, Department of Urology, University Hospital Nijmegen, 6525 GA Nijmegen, The Netherlands [243]

Fuad Freiha, Divisions of Oncology and Urology, Stanford University Medical Center, Stanford, CA 94305 [171]

H.G.W. Frohmüller, Department of Urology, School of Medicine, University of Würzburg, 8700 Würzburg, Federal Republic of Germany [257]

J.M. Groen, Departments of Urology and Pathology, University of Rotterdam, Rotterdam, The Netherlands [41]

J.W. Grups, Department of Urology, School of Medicine, University of Würzburg, 8700 Würzburg, Federal Republic of Germany [257]

V. Harvey, Department of Oncology, University of Auckland, Auckland, New Zealand [319]

Harry W. Herr, Urologic Service, Department of Surgery, Memorial Sloan-Kettering Cancer Center, New York, NY 10021 [295]

F. Hofstädter, Department of Pathology, RWTH Aachen, Federal Republic of Germany [61]

Edith Huland, Department of Urology, University of Steglitz, D-1000 Berlin 45, Federal Republic of Germany [35]

Hartwig Huland, Department of Urology, University of Steglitz, D-1000 Berlin 45, Federal Republic of Germany [35]

John T. Isaacs, Department of Urology, The James Buchanan Brady Urological Institute, The Johns Hopkins University School of Medicine, Baltimore, MD 21205 [129]

Stephen C. Jacobs, Department of Urology, Medical College of Wisconsin, Milwaukee, WI [13,101]

Herbert Klosterhalfen, Department of Urology, University of Hamburg, 2000 Hamburg 20, Federal Republic of Germany [275]

R. Kraft, Division of Diagnostic Cytology Institute of Pathology, University of Bern, Inselspital, 3010 Bern, Switzerland [81]

K.H. Kurth, Department of Urology, University of Amsterdam, Amsterdam, The Netherlands [41]

J. Levi, Department of Clinical Oncology, Royal North Shore Hospital, Sydney 2065, N.S.W., Australia [319]

Christopher J. Logothetis, Department of Medical Oncology, Section of Genitourinary Oncology, The University of Texas M.D. Anderson Cancer Center, Houston, TX 77030 **[107,301]**

Ken Marumo, Department of Urology, School of Medicine, Keio University, Tokyo, 160 Japan **[263]**

David S. Menashe, Department of Urology, Medical College of Wisconsin, Milwaukee, WI **[101]**

W. Meyers, Documentation and Statistics Med. Faculty, RWTH Aachen, Federal Republic of Germany **[61]**

Alvaro Morales, Department of Urology, Queen's University, Kingston, Ontario, Canada **[25]**

K. Mross, Department of Oncology, Free University, Amsterdam, The Netherlands **[41]**

D.W.W. Newling, Department of Urology, Princess Royal Hospital, Hull, HU8 9HE, England **[115]**

Sheryl Ogden, Department of Medical Oncology, Section of Genitourinary Oncology, The University of Texas M.D. Anderson Cancer Center, Houston, TX 77030 **[107,301]**

Ullrich Otto, Department of Urology, University of Hamburg, 2000 Hamburg 20, Federal Republic of Germany **[275]**

C. Pavone, Institute of Urology and Interdepartment Center for Research in Clinical Oncology, University of Palermo, Polyclinic Hospital ''P. Giaccone'', 90127 Palermo, Italy **[149]**

M. Pavone-Macaluso, Institute of Urology and Interdepartment Center for Research in Clinical Oncology, University of Palermo, Polyclinic Hospital ''P. Giaccone'', 90127 Palermo, Italy **[149]**

Derek Raghavan, Urological Cancer Research Unit and Department of Clinical Oncology, Royal Prince Alfred Hospital, Sydney 2050, N.S.W., Australia **[309,319]**

Jeffery Reese, Division of Urology, Stanford University Medical Center, Stanford, CA 94305, and Veterans Administration Medical Center, Palo Alto, CA 94304 **[171]**

C. Romano, Institute of Urology and Interdepartment Center for Research in Clinical Oncology, University of Palermo, Polyclinic Hospital ''P. Giaccone'', 90127 Palermo, Italy **[149]**

H. Rübben, Department of Urology, Knappschaftskrankenhaus Bardenberg, Urologische University, D-4300 Essen 7, Federal Republic of Germany **[61]**

Jack A. Schalken, Department of Urology, Urological Research Laboratory, University Hospital Nijmegen, 6525 GA Nijmegen, The Netherlands **[243]**

Andreas W. Schneider, Department of Urology, University of Hamburg, 2000 Hamburg 20, Federal Republic of Germany **[35,275]**

Avishay Sella, Department of Medical Oncology, Section of Genitourinary Oncology, The University of Texas M.D. Anderson Cancer Center, Houston, TX 77030 **[107,301]**

V. Serretta, Institute of Urology and Interdepartment Center for Research in Clinical Oncology, University of Palermo, Polyclinic Hospital ''P. Giaccone'', 90127, Palermo, Italy **[149]**

Mark S. Soloway, Department of Urology, University of Tennessee, Memphis, Baptist Memorial and VA Hospitals, Memphis, TN 38163 **[71, 141]**

U.E. Studer, Department of Urology and Institute of Pathology, University of Bern, Inselspital, 3010 Bern, Switzerland [81]

David A. Swanson, Department of Urology, The University of Texas M.D. Anderson Cancer Center, Houston, TX 77030 [201]

Hiroshi Tazaki, Department of Urology, School of Medicine, Keio University, Tokyo, 160 Japan [263]

F. ten Kate, Departments of Urology and Pathology, Erasmus University of Rotterdam, Rotterdam, The Netherlands [41]

D. Thomson, Department of Medical Oncology, Princess Alexandra Hospital, Brisbane, Queensland, Australia [319]

Frank M. Torti, Department of Medicine, Division of Oncology, Stanford University Medical Center, Stanford, CA 94305, and Veterans Administration Medical Center, Palo Alto, CA 94304 [171]

O. van Aubel, Gouda, Roosendaal, Haarlem, The Netherlands [41]

R.D. van Caubergh, Departments of Urology and Pathology, University of Rotterdam, Rotterdam, The Netherlands [41]

I. van Reyswoud, Departments of Urology and Pathology, Erasmus University of Rotterdam, Rotterdam, The Netherlands [41]

G. Weissglas, Departments of Urology and Pathology, Erasmus University of Rotterdam, Rotterdam, The Netherlands [41]

Willet F. Whitmore, Jr., Urology Service, Department of Surgery, Memorial Sloan-Kettering Cancer Center, New York, NY 10021 [1]

M.P. Wirth, Department of Urology, School of Medicine, University of Würzburg, 8700 Würzburg, Federal Republic of Germany [159]

Alan Yagoda, Solid Tumor Service, Department of Medicine, Memorial Sloan-Kettering Cancer Center, New York, NY 10021 [87,227]

E.J. Zingg, Department of Urology, University of Bern, Inselspital, 3010 Bern, Switzerland [81]

Preface

At the Uro-oncological workshop held June 22–25, 1988, in Würzburg, Federal Republic of Germany, internationally known experts presented their research data and views on their respective fields concerning bladder cancer, prostate cancer, renal cell carcinoma, and testicular tumors. The names of the participants stand for the high quality of the papers collected in these proceedings.

The rationale for locally applied adjuvant treatment of superficial bladder cancer with BCG or chemotherapeutic agents was extensively discussed, and a review of systemic treatment of advanced carcinoma of the bladder was presented. In the field of prostate cancer, emphasis was placed on hormonal therapy and on the question of chemotherapeutic treatment of advanced stages of this tumor. Systemic treatment modalities of renal cell cancer with biological response modifiers was another interesting topic of discussion. The disappointing results of chemotherapy in this type of tumor were reviewed. In testicular cancer, main subjects included the different concepts of a "wait and see" policy in stage I disease as well as the nerve-preserving modification of retroperitoneal lymphadenectomy. Finally, an overview of systemic chemotherapy in advanced cancer of the testis was presented.

In our time, with its quick turnover of scientific knowledge, meetings like this are of particular value because they permit a personal exchange of the newest research data available. This fact and the opportunity for direct communication make workshops such as this exciting and worthwhile events.

We want to take the opportunity to thank all the participants of this symposium for their traveling to Würzburg as well as for their excellent presentations. We are grateful to Farmitalia Carlo Erba GmbH, Federal Republic of Germany, who made this meeting possible by generous support. The assistance of Priv.-Doz. Dr. K. Burk (Farmitalia Carlo Erba GmbH) in organizing this workshop is especially appreciated. The close collaboration of Wiley-Liss, Inc., in publishing these proceedings is gratefully acknowledged.

H.G.W. Frohmüller
M.P. Wirth

Uro-Oncology: Current Status
and Future Trends, pages 1–12
© 1990 Wiley-Liss, Inc.

THE EVOLUTION OF UROLOGIC ONCOLOGY:
A PERSONAL PERSPECTIVE

Willet F. Whitmore, JR.

Urology Service, Department of Surgery

Memorial Sloan-Kettering Cancer Center, NY, NY, 10021

Although one may trace contributions to urologic oncology back into antiquity, it is over the past 40-50 years that the concentration of interest and a sufficient body of knowledge have fostered the emergence of urologic oncology as a "subspecialty". More than 40 years as a urologist at the Memorial Sloan-Kettering Cancer Center have given me a relatively unique opportunity to observe this evolution and it is this personal perspective which forms the basis for my remarks.

Although the foundations of anatomy and physiology had been reasonably well established by the end of the 18th century, medicine remained largely an art and a craft until the middle of the 19th century when science became progressively more and more the new religion. Urology developed as a surgical specialty during the last quarter of the 19th century, aided by Nitze's invention of the cystoscope in 1877. Although the American Urologic Association was founded in 1902, some 13 years after the founding of the French Urologic Association, not until 1935 was the status of urology as a surgical specialty formally solidified in the U.S.A. by the creation of the American Board of Urology.

The explosion of medical knowledge that occurred in the decade 1940-1950, doubtless stimulated in part by the exigencies of World War II, provided a fertile soil for the evolution of urologic oncology. Among the notable major advances in medicine that occurred in the 1940-1950 decade were the development of antimicrobial agents beginning with the sulfonamides and following with penicillin and later antibiotics; new techniques and agents for anesthesia; greater availability and understanding of blood, fluid and electrolyte replacement; advances in surgical physiology and perioperative care; and improvements in both diagnostic and therapeutic technology. Specifically impacting favorably on the evolution of urologic oncology were the development of megavoltage irradiation, the introduction of modern chemotherapy resulting in part from the study of the pharmacologic properties of nitrogen mustard as a potential war gas, and an influx of risk takers, both patients and physicians, ready to explore the potential usefulness of a variety of new tools for the treatment of neoplasms. The energetic and innovative intellectual climate that followed WWII served as an atmospheric catalyst.

Since it is impossible within a reasonable time frame to provide a comprehensive account, my intent is to give some personal perceptions of representative events eventuating in current concepts of the treatment of the principal urologic neoplasms.

KIDNEY NEOPLASMS: Although urologic surgeons had for some time appreciated the possibilities of perirenal extension, venous involvement and regional lymph node metastases from kidney cancers and had variously included removal of the perinephric fat with the kidney (Thompson & Douglas, 1954), the observations of Beer (1937) and of McDonald and Priestley (1943) relative to major vein involvement, of Beare and McDonald (1949) relative to perinephric fat invasion, and of Chute et al. (1959), Robson (1963), Angervall et al. (1969) and Hulten et al. (1969) relative to regional lymph node metastases provided the logical basis for formal efforts at systematic radical nephrectomy. The requirements of adequate exposure imposed by the latter procedure contributed to the use of new surgical approaches. Although Kocher in 1876 had utilized a transabdominal approach to the kidney, the lumbar incision was the most commonly employed incision for nephrectomy at that time. In 1947 Sweetser introduced an extended oblique lumbar incision. In 1948 Mortensen utilized a thoracoabdominal approach, modifying an incision advocated in 1930 by Constantini and Bernasconi. In 1950 Nagamatsu introduced a dorsolumbar incision. Reports of the use of radical nephrectomy by Chute et al. (1949), Foley (1952), Robson et al. (1969), Wahlqvist (1969) and Skinner et al. (1971) followed. Although no randomized trial of simple versus radical nephrectomy for kidney cancer has been performed, the available data suggest that radical nephrectomy has had little impact either on apparent cure rates or on local recurrence rates compared to simple nephrectomy. A logical explanation resides in the possibilities that perirenal extension and/or regional lymph node involvement imply a high probability of preexisting distant metastases and that local recurrences are too difficult to detect and too slow in growth rate to become clinically manifest in a setting wherein distant metastases is the major cause of treatment failure.

At the present time radical nephrectomy is the standard procedure for the treatment of renal cell cancer. It does not add to the operative mortality or morbidity or detract from the quality of life to any greater extent than does simple nephrectomy. Partial nephrectomy for selected tumors or extended nephrectomy for neoplasms with thrombotic extensions into the lumen of renal vein and inferior vena cava yield survival and local control rates similar to those achieved by radical nephrectomy in the usual setting. Renal transplantation or chronic dialysis remains for the patient in whom the sacrifice in renal function involved with treatment of the cancer leaves too little renal function to support life. The absence of reasonable alternatives to surgery in the treatment of kidney cancer has extended the limits of surgical ingenuity in its treatment. Since neither radiation therapy nor chemotherapy has proved effective and since there has long been circumstantial evidence that immune mechanisms may influence the course of the disease, immunotherapy has been a major area of investigation in patients for whom surgical treatment has nothing to offer.

BLADDER NEOPLASMS: It is now difficult to appreciate the enormous impact on our understanding of bladder tumors that was afforded by the work of Jewett and Strong. Their 1946 report of the autopsy findings in a group of patients who had died with but not necessarily of bladder cancer yielded insights into the behavior, established a basis for the current staging classification, and provided a logical basis for treatment of such neoplasms. Although Broders in 1922 had devised a system of grading for cancers and Aschner in 1928 had indicated the relevance of tumor infiltration to prognosis, it was the work of Jewett and Strong which crystallized relationships between tumor infiltration and prognosis. Assessing theoretical curability by cystectomy on the basis of autopsy findings in over 100 patients with bladder cancer, they demonstrated that extravesical tumor was uncommon in patients with superficial lesions and increased in incidence as tumors became more infiltrative. They furthermore showed that a proportion of patients with deeply infiltrating tumors had extravesical disease apparently confined to the perivesical fat and/or regional lymph nodes, an observation which lead directly to the evolution of radical cystectomy with pelvic lymph node dissection. As with radical versus simple nephrectomy, any survival advantage achieved by radical cystectomy with pelvic lymph node dissection over simple cystectomy is probably small: in patients with superficial tumors, the more radical operation may be unnecessary whereas in patients with muscle infiltrating tumors, it may be insufficient. Nevertheless, a small proportion of patients with limited pelvic lymph node metastases are apparently cured by the more radical excision.

A renewed interest in cystectomy restimulated interest in urinary diversion. Simon in 1852 had first performed ureterointestinal diversion in a patient with bladder extrophy and by 1936 Hinman and Weyrauch identified more than 60 different techniques of ureterointestinal diversion reported by more then 50 different surgeons involving one or more of 11 surgical principles. In 1950 Ferris and Odel published a classic paper on hyperchloremic acidosis following ureterointestinal anastomosis stimulating a host of further studies which have illuminated the pathophysiology of intestinal urinary diversion. In the same year Bricker (1950) reported the use of a ureteroileal conduit with the Rutzen bag as a collecting device for the abdominal stoma. Although Seiffert in 1935 had reported a similar technique, the absence of suitable collecting devices may have contributed to the apparent lack of immediate interest in the procedure. In any event, Bricker deserves the credit for introducing the technique into the practical armamentarium. Since that time many more surgeons have developed further techniques of diversion using additional surgical principles. At the present time there is widespread interest in continent urinary diversion achieved by the use of continent abdominal stomas amenable to catherization or by the use of internal intestinal urinary reservoirs anastomosed above an intact external sphincter in the male. These techniques represent laudable efforts to improve quality of live for patients requiring urinary diversion but it will be some years before the various methods can be fully evaluated.

Megavoltage irradiation for bladder cancer received wide exploration after WWII, particularly in Europe. Although there is little doubt that some patients with muscle infiltrating tumors of the bladder may be cured thereby, the local failure rate of 50 % or more far exceeds that following radical cystectomy. The prospects of potential bladder preservation, however, have encouraged the use of megavoltage irradiation as initial therapy employing salvage cystectomy in those with persistent or recurrent tumor 3 months or more after such irradiation.

Chemotherapy emerged as a new discipline immediately after WWII but it was not until the initiation of Phase II disease-site oriented studies of bladder cancer in 1972 that real progress in the chemotherapy of this disease became apparent. Such studies are epitomized by those of Yagoda (1987) are defined the single agent activity of cisplatin, adriamycin, methotrexate and vinblastine, and leading to the development of combination regimens which are being widely explored not only in patients with metastatic disease but also in a variety of adjuvant and neoadjuvant settings.

In 1961 Jones and Swinney and Veenema et al. simultaneously reported the use of intravesical thiotepa in the management of superficial bladder tumors. Since then an enormous experience with a variety of intravesical agents has accumulated. Most studies have been empiric with relatively little pharmacodynamic or pharmacokinetic basis and there is still much uncertainty regarding the how, when and what of intravesical therapy. In 1976 Morales et al. reported the usefulness of intravesical BCG in the management of superficial bladder tumors and this experience has been widely confirmed and extended.

At the present time endoscopic destruction and intravesical therapy or prophylaxis are the usual basis for management of superficial tumors. For patients with muscle infiltrating tumors, the spectrum of treatment possibilities is large. Surgical treatment may vary from transurethral resection to radical cystectomy although the latter procedure is the standard by which the effectiveness of alternative treatments are judged. Megavoltage irradiation controls some such tumors and salvage cystectomy rescues some of the radiation failures. Chemotherapy alone or combined with irradiation and/or surgery is also under exploration. A major problem is to define amongst this array of variously successful treatments the optimal management for a particular patient and his particular tumor. Control of metastatic disease in patients with bladder cancer has been addressed with various regimens of combination chemotherapy but randomized Phase III studies of different chemotherapeutic regimens have been few.

PROSTATE CANCER: The last 50 years have seen enormous progress in the treatment of prostate cancer. In 1941 Huggins and Hodges established the rational basis for endocrine therapy and this remains the best means of palliation of patients with metastatic disease.

Although Hugh Young in 1904 first utilized radical prostatectomy for the treatment of prostatic cancer, the operation was never widely utilized. In 1945 Millin developed the retropubic approach to benign prostatic enlargements and this was subsequently adapted to the performance of radical prostatectomy. However, it was not until after Walsh and Donker (1982) defined the anatomical basis for the impotence which generally followed radical prostatectomy that Walsh et al. (1983) devised the nerve sparing technique of radical prostatectomy that has placed the surgical treatment of early prostatic cancer firmly in the treatment armamentarium.

The exploration of megavoltage radiation therapy for prostatic cancer was pioneered by Bagshaw and Kaplan in 1962 and by Budhraja and Anderson in 1964, opening Pandora's box relative to the treatment of prostatic cancer.

At present the polemic between radiation therapists and surgeons relative to the optimal treatment of prostatic cancer has crystallized the need for standardization of criteria of grading, staging, response criteria and data reporting. The optimal therapy of early prostatic cancer remains debatable although it is evident that each method is effective in some patients. Although a large scale randomized trial might well establish the superiority of one method of treatment over another, the historical data suggest that the differences will at best be small and the results, in any event are unlikely to determine the optimal treatment for the individual patient.

In spite of the enormous amount of clinical and laboratory investigation that has followed the observations of Huggins and Hodges relative to the endocrine responsiveness of prostatic cancers, there remains no convincing evidence that anything other then an abrogation of the effects of testosterone on the tumor is responsible for the favorable effects. Furthermore, although a variety of methods induces such abrogation, no one method appears superior to any other relative to effects on the tumor per se. Whether endocrine therapy prolongs life in patients with advanced prostatic cancer remains uncertain. Although it has become ethically impossible for this question to be answered convincingly, it is hard for those of us who witnessed the often dramatic effects of endocrine therapy on patients terminally ill with prostatic cancer 40 years ago to escape the conviction that such treatment does prolong survival in some patients. A further important and unanswered question is whether endocrine therapy applied to early stage prostatic cancer may have beneficial effects exceeding those when it is applied later in the course of the disease.

TESTIS TUMORS: Prior to WWII the relative roles of retroperitoneal lymph node dissection and retroperitoneal radiation therapy in the management of non-seminomatous germ cell tumors were uncertain on both sides of the Atlantic.   During WWII a large experience with testis tumors in the military population was assembled at the Walter Reed Army Hospital in Washington, D.C. There, the presence of pathologists Nathan Friedman (1946), Frank Dixon and Robert Moore (1953), of the radiation therapist Milton

Friedman (1913), and of surgeons John Kimbrough (1952) and Lloyd Lewis (1953) led to the characterization of the pathology and pathogenesis of testis tumors, the not undisputed concept that nonseminomatous germ cell tumors were radioresistant, and the demonstration of the feasibility and potential effectiveness of retroperitoneal lymph node dissection. Simultaneously, on the other side of the Atlantic and especially in England, experience with megavoltage irradiation, epitomized by Sir Stanford Cade (1940), Gordon Taylor and Wyndham (1947) , and Boden and Gibb (1951) led to emergence of radiation therapy as the standard management of the retroperitoneal lymph nodes in patients with germ cell tumors of all types.

Explorations of chemotherapy in metastatic germ cell tumors began soon after WWII but it was the regimen of Li et al. (1960) combining actinomycin D, chlorambucil and methotrexate which first provided a basis for cautious optimism. Approximately 40% of patients experienced objective response, 20% had complete remissions and 5-10% were apparently cured. In 1972 Samuels and Howe identified vinblastine, in 1974 Yagoda et al. and the EORTC reported bleomycin, and in 1978 Higby, Wallace and Holland characterized cisplatin as active agents against germ cell tumors. Thereafter, a variety of cisplatin based regimens revolutionized the treatment of germ cell tumors, significantly modifying both the use of retroperitoneal lymph node dissection and of radiation therapy.

At the present time the thrust of clinical studies is towards reducing the burden of therapy in good risk patients without compromising the currently excellent cure rates and attempting to increase the effectiveness of treatment in poor risk patients. To these ends risk factors in various settings are being progressively better defined and treatment in specific situations appropriately modified.

GENERALIZATIONS: Using various "appropriate" methods of treatment roughly 90 % of urologic tumors can be controlled locally and most treatment failures result from metastases. Selection for optimal local control with maximal preservation of function and quality of life is the goal. In contrast to 40 years ago when treatment options were relatively limited, the multiplicity of current potentially effective treatments poses problems in treatment selection which remain to be resolved.

Empiricism has dominated past therapeutic approaches, the endocrine therapy of prostatic cancer being one of the more notable exceptions. Yet, empiricism has yielded notable advances, well illustrated by chemotherapy.

Advances in knowledge of tumor biology have tempered expectations from treatment. Limitations of the concept that if a small operation will cure a little cancer, a big operation will cure a large cancer are better recognized.

Quality of life issues have become progressively more important as illustrated by the revival of radical prostatectomy fostered by the development of a potency sparing procedure and by the interest in continent urinary diversions.

FUTURE PROSPECTS: As the molecular basis for neoplasia becomes better understood, new markers in the form of oncogenes, growth factors and cell surface antigens are being defined. These offer prospects for use in diagnosis and also as specific targets for therapy.

Clinical characterization of tumor heterogeneity is becoming progressively more important. Why some tumors respond to a particular treatment and other apparently similar lesions do not remains obscure. With an increasing multiplicity of treatments, selection of the optimal management becomes of increasing practical importance. Some of the molecular markers alluded to above may provide a basis for a more sophisticated stratification of tumors than is possible with conventional methods of histologic grading and clinical staging and such stratifications may have pertinence to treatment response.

The possibility that cancers may best be regarded as disorders of growth and differentiation promotes the rational concept that treatment strategies may be designed not to destroy the cancer cell but to redirect it (Pierce and Speers, 1988).

Although the future poses formidable problems for urologic oncology, progress over the past 40-50 years has exposed many promising avenues for potentially fruitful investigation.

REFERENCES:

Angervall L, Carlstrom E, Wahlqvist L, et al. (1969). Effects of clinical and morphological variables on spread of renal carcinoma in an operative series. Scand. J. Urol.Nephrol. 3:134-140.

Aschner PW (1928). The pathology of vesical neoplasms. Its evaluation in diagnosis and prognosis. J.A.M.A. 91:1697- 1704.

Bagshaw MA, Kaplan HS (1962). Radical external radiation therapy of localized prostatic carcinoma. Presented at the 10th International Congress of Radiology, Montreal, PQ, Canada.

Beare JB and McDonald JR (1949). Involvement of the renal capsule in surgically removed hypernephroma. A gross and histopathologic study. J. Urol. 61:857-861.

Beer E (1937). Some aspects of malignant tumors of the kidney. Surg. Gyn. & Obst. 65:433-446.

Boden G, Gibb R (1951). Radiotherapy and testicular neoplasms. Lancet 2:1195-1197.

Bricker EH (1950). Bladder substitution after pelvic evisceration. Surg. Clin. N. Amer. 30:1511-1521.

Broders AC (1922). Epithelioma of the genitourinary organs. Ann.Surg.574-580.

Budhraja SN, Anderson JD (1964). An assessment of the value of radiotherapy in the management of carcinoma of the prostate. Br. J. Urol. 36:535-540.

Cade Sir S (1940). Malignant disease and its treatment by radium. Bristol: John Wright & Sons.

Chute R, Soutter L & Kerr WS Jr (1949). Value of thoraco-abdominal incision in removal of kidney tumors. New England J. Med. 241:951-960.

Clinical Screening Co-operative Group of the European Organization for Research on the Treatment of Cancer. Study of clinical efficiency of bleomycin (1970). Brit. Med. J. 2:643.

Constantine & Bernasconi (1933). Kidney Surgery, In History of Urology (Ballenger EG, Frontz WA, Hamer HG, Lewis B [Eds]). Baltimore, Williams and Wilkins, Vol 1, pp.

Dixon FJ, Moore RA (1953). Testicular tumors: clinicopathological study. Cancer 6:427-454.

Ferris DO and Odel HM (1950) Electrolyte pattern of the blood after bilateral ureterosigmoidostomy. J.A.M.A. 634- 641.

Foley FEB, Mulvaney WP, Richardson EJ & Victor I (1952). Radical nephrectomy for neoplasms. J. Urol. 68:39-42.

Friedman M, Di Rienzo AJ (1963). Treatment of tropocarcinoma (embryonal carcinoma) of the testis. Radiology 80:550-565.

Friedman NB, Moore RA (1946). Tumors of the testis. Report on 922 cases. Mil. Surgeon 99:573-593.

Gordon-Taylor G and Wyndham NR (1947). On malignant tumours of testic. Brit. J. Surg. 35:6-17.

Higby DJ, Wallace J, Holland JF (1973). Cis-diamminedi-chloroplatinum (NSC-119875). Cancer Chemotherapy Ret. Part 1, 57:459-463.

Hinman F and Weyrauch HM Jr (1937). Collective review: A critical study of the different principles of surgery which have been used in ureterointestinal implantation. Surg. Gyn. & Obst. 64:313-303.

Huggins C, Hodges CV (1941). Studies on prostatic cancer. I. The effect of castration, of estrogen, and of androgen injection on serum phosphatase in metastatic carcinoma of the prostate. Cancer Res. 1:293-297.

Hulten L, Rosencrantz M, Seeman T, Wahlqvist L & Ahren C (1969). Occurrence and localization of lymphnode metastases in renal carcinoma. Scand. J. Urol. Nephrol. 3:973-977.

Jewett HJ and Strong GH (1946). Infiltrating carcinoma of the bladder: relation of depth of penetration of the bladder wall to incidence of local extension and metastases. J. Urol. 55:366-372.

Jones HC and Swinney J (1961). Thiotepa in the treatment of tumours of the bladder. Lancet ii 615-618.

Kimbrough JC (1952). Tumors of the testicle. Surg. Gyn. Obstet. 94:535-538.

Kocher cited in Herbst RH and Polkey HJ. Kidney surgery, In History of Urology (Ballenger EG, Frontz WA, Hamer HG, Lewis B [Eds.]). Baltimore, Williams and Wilkins, 1933, Vol 1, pp 279-385.

Lewis LG (1953). Radioresistant testis tumors: results in 133 cases; five-year follow-up. J.Urol.69:841-844.

Li MC, Whitmore WF Jr, Golbey RB, Grabstald H (1960). Effects of combined drug therapy on metastatic cancer of the testis. J. Amer. Med. Ass. 174:1291-1299.

McDonald JR and Priestley JT (1943). Malignant tumors of the kidney: surgical and prognostic significance of tumor thrombosis of the renal veins. Surg. Gyn.Obst.77:295-306.

Millin T (1945). Retropubic prostatectomy, new extravesical technique: Report on 20 cases. Lancet 2:693-696.

Morales A, Eidinger D, Bruce AW (1976). Intracavitary bacillus Calmette-Guerin in the treatment of superficial bladder tumors. J. Urol. 116:180-183.

Mortenson H (1948). Transthoracic nephrectomy. J. Urol. 60:855-858.

Nagamatsu G (1950). Dorso-lumbar approach to the kidney and adrenal with osteoplastic flap. J.Urol.63:569.

Nitze cited by Ernest G Mark. Cystoscopy and Urethroscopy, in History of Urology (Ballenger EG, Frontz WA,Hamer HG, Lewis B [Eds]). Baltimore, Williams and Wilkins, 1933, Vol I, pp 160-172.

Robson CJ (1963). Radical nephrectomy for renal cell carcinoma. J. Urol. 89:37-42.

Robson CJ, Churchill BM, Anderson W (1969). The results of radical nephrectomy for renal cell carcinoma. J Urol 101:297-301.

Samuels ML and Howe CD (1970). Vinblastine in the management of testicular cancer. Cancer 25:1009.

Seiffert L (1935). Die "Darm-Siphonblase". Arch. klin. Chir. 183:569-574.

Simon J 1852 (Lancet) cited in Herbst RH and Polkey HJ. Surgery of the ureter, in History of Urology (Ballenger EG, Frontz WA, Hamer HG, Lewis [Eds]). Baltimore, Williams and Wilkins, 1933, Vol II, pp 321-343.

Skinner DG, Colvin RB, Vermillion CD, Pfister RC, Leadbetter WF (1971). Diagnosis and management of renal cell carcinoma. A clinical and pathologic study of 309 cases. Cancer 28:1165-1177.

Sweetser TH (1947). The surgical approach to renal and other retroperitoneal tumors. J. Urol. 57: 651-659.

Thompson HT and Douglas E (1954). Radical surgery in renal neoplasm. J. Urol. 72:777-782.

Veenema RJ, Dean AL, Roberts M, Fingerhut B, Chowhury BK (1962). Bladder carcinoma treated by direct instillation of thiotepa. J. Urol. 88:60-63.

Wahlqvist L (1969). Factors of importance for primary surgical therapy in renal carcinoma. Nephrectomy and kidney resection. Scand. J. Urol. Nephrol. 4:suppl.

Walsh PC, Donker PJ (1982). Impotence following radical prostatectomy: Insight into etiology and prevention. J. Urol. 128:492-497.

Walsh PC, Lepor H, Eggleston JC (1983). Radical prostatectomy with preservation of sexual function. Anatomical and pathological considerations. Prostate 4:473-485.

Yagoda A (1987). Chemotherapy of urothelial tract tumors. Cancer 60:574-585.

Yagoda A, Mukherji B, Young C, Etcubanas E, Lamonte C, Smith JR, Tan CTC, Krakoff IH (1972). Bleomycin, an antitumor antibiotic. Ann. Intern. Med. 77:861.

Young HH (1905). The early diagnosis and radical cure of carcinoma of the prostate - Being a study of 40 cases and presentation of a radical operation which was carried out in four cases. Johns Hopkins Hosp. Bull. 16:315-321.

Uro-Oncology: Current Status
and Future Trends, pages 13–23
© 1990 Wiley-Liss, Inc.

GROWTH FACTORS AND GENITOURINARY CANCER

Stephen C. Jacobs, M.D.

Department of Urology, Medical College of
Wisconsin

Milwaukee, Wisconsin, USA

Growth factors are hormone-like proteins that are
recognized by their target cells through specific high
affinity plasma membrane receptors and through that
interaction mediate cell growth or cell proliferation,
but do not actually take part in cellular biosynthesis,
metabolism, or catabolism. There have been a great
number of growth factors identified, primarily in cell
culture model systems. As their primary structures
become elucidated, it is becoming apparent that most of
these will prove to be identical or closely related to
just a few growth factors. Growth factors are
cellularly synthesized and released for reception by
the target cells in the following manners: 1. Autocrine
– the growth factor receptor is on the same cell that
synthesizes the growth factor. This autoregulation of
the cell's own growth basically defines transformation.[1]
2. Endocrine – the growth factor receptor receives the
growth factor from the blood stream. 3. Paracrine –
the growth factor receptor receives the growth factor
from a nearby growth factor producing cell. 4.
Exocrine – the growth factor receptor receives the
growth factor from an exocrine body secretion. There is
no clear-cut guideline as to where paracrine and
exocrine separate. Certainly when the growth factor
acts on receptors in a different organ or even organism,
then paracrine can no longer describe the action.
5. Storage – growth factors can be synthesized and
stored in extracellular locations for future use by
receptor containing cells. The "stormones"[2] produced

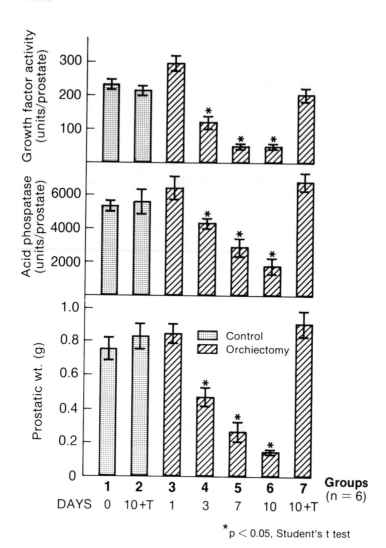

FIGURE 1: The effect of orchiectomy on rat ventral prostatic weight, tissue acid phosphatase, and total growth factor activity, as measured by the incorporation of ^{3}H-thymidine by human foreskin fibroblasts.[29] Animals were 300g 6 month old Sprague-Dawley rats with orchiectomy day 0 and prostate removal as indicated by days. T = 10mg/kg IM Testosterone days 0,5.

require a further action to release their potential to act as growth factors.

This presentation will discuss two growth factors – EGF and bFGF – found in genitourinary tissues and neoplasms as prototypes for systems that are much more complex. EGF is the best characterized of all the growth factors and, yet, its true physiological role remains unestablished. EGF is a 53 amino acid single polypeptide chain with a molecular weight of 6045. The protein has 3 intramolecular disulfide linkages that are essential for biological activity. The tertiary structure of the molecule is very stable to acid and boiling. The mRNA encoding the EGF precursor predicts a high molecular weight prepro form of the EGF molecule. A 9000MW pre-EGF form is then produced by enzymatic digestion. In tissue a tetrameric complex of two molecules of EGF and two carrier molecules is found. Free EGF interacts with a complex receptor molecule which crosses the cell membrane. Part of the extracellular portion of the receptor binds avidly with EGF molecule and this reaction causes the cell to bring both the receptor and the EGF into the cell. EGF is then degraded. The transmembrane domain of the EGF receptor is essentially passive. The intracellular portion of the EGF receptor phosphorylates tyrosine and starts a cascade of action leading to mitosis about 12 hours later. Mutant receptor molecules that do not require EGF for activation are possible: the erb B oncogene is homologous to the protein kinase domain of the EGF receptor. Removal of the EGF binding domain appears essential to remove a restraining influence on the protein tyrosine kinase activity. Deletion of the regulatory region results in an oncogene that expresses tyrosine protein kinase constituitively and results in transformation.

However, the most common EGF associated abnormality in malignancy is an increased expression of the EGF receptor. There appears to be a causal relationship between increased receptor concentration and tumor growth in vivo.[3]

EGF is normally found in the kidney and the prostate and has been demonstrated in renal and prostatic malignancies. In the kidney and salivary gland, EGF precursor mRNA is 3 orders of magnitude

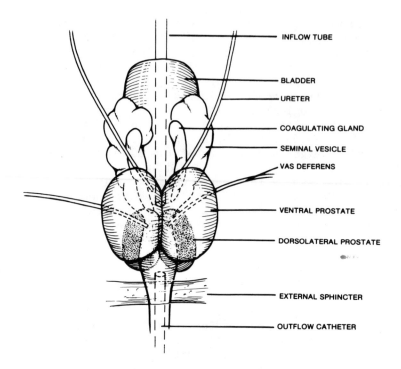

Isolated perfusion of the rat prostatic urethra

FIGURE 2: Surgical preparation for collection of rat prostatic fluid.

higher than other tissues.[4] EGF is secreted into the urine and saliva and its synthesis appears to be under androgen control in both the kidney and the salivary glands. The abundance of EGF in urine makes its downstream action on urothelium potentially tumor promoting. Messing et al[5] showed that EGF could stimulate normal urothelial cells as well as bladder tumor cell lines. Neal et al[6] reported that invasive bladder cancers are more likely to display EGF receptors than non-invasive tumors and that normal transitional epithelium does not contain EGF receptors.

We have looked at growth factor activity in the prostate gland. Total mitogenic activity in the prostate depends on androgen dependent cells for its synthesis. Figure 1 shows that following castration prostatic weight and tissue acid phosphatase fall in parallel to the fall in growth factor activity. Testosterone replacement restores growth factor activity.

In the rat prostate, EGF and bFGF account for the majority of growth factor activity.[7] EGF appears as both a 25kd form[8] and a free 6000mw form that accounts for about one half of the growth factor activity found in the rat prostate. Li et al[9] have recently confirmed the presence of rat prostatic EGF and gone on to detect the presence of EGF mRNA in rat prostate. In the human prostate, EGF has not yet been identified: there it is not as major a portion of the total growth factor.[10,11] However, EGF does appear in human prostatic fluid and, therefore, must be synthesized or concentrated in the human prostate.

We have developed an in vivo isolated perfusion model of the rat prostatic urethra in order to explore the prostatic exocrine secretion of EGF.[12] Figure 2 diagrams the surgical preparation. The vasa deferentia, coagulating glands, and seminal vesicles are ligated to prevent their contents from entering the urethra. An inflow tube is placed at the bladder neck so as to exclude any urine from entering the prostatic urethra. An outflow urethral catheter is placed at the external sphincter level. Tris buffered saline with added protease inhibitors is pumped in at the bladder and the effluent collected via the urethral catheter. Agents affecting the secretion of EGF are administered IV or

IP. The cholingeric agonist pilocarpine causes the secretion of EGF and this can be blocked with atropine. The α-adrenergic agonist phenylephrine causes significant secretion of EGF and this can be blocked with the α_1 blocker prazosin, but not the α_2 blocker yohimbine. β adrenergic agonists do not stimulate any EGF secretion. Vasoactive intestinal peptide does not augment either α_1 adrenergic or cholinergic stimulation of EGF secretion. Thus, EGF secretion into prostatic fluid is under both α_1 adrenergic and cholinergic control.

This control of EGF secretion into rat exocrine prostatic fluid implies that the growth factor may be physiologically important downstream from its site of synthesis. A local prostatic target for the secreted EGF is one alternative. EGF receptors are found in prostatic cell membranes and androgen down-regulates these receptors.[13] Traish and Wotiz proposed that androgen deprivation might allow EGF receptor induction and, therefore, promote cell growth and prevent complete prostatic regression with castration.[13] Other possible functions for EGF within the prostate gland include control of smooth muscle contraction, pH maintenance, and membrane ion flux. However, the fact that EGF appears in the prostatic fluid forces consideration of the possibility that the substance may interact with receptors in the female genital tract. The uterus contains high affinity EGF receptors whose numbers are regulated by estrogen.[14,15,16]

With EGF appearing in the prostatic fluid, its role in carcinogenesis or tumor promotion must be considered. Issacs reviewed the relationship between prostatic secretory function and prostatic carcinoma and proposed that "the initiation and/promotion of prostatic carcinogenesis may well involve the chronic modulation/interaction of the prostatic glandular cells with their lumenal fluid."[17] EGF needs to now be included in those endogenous components that are secreted into prostatic fluid and may be involved in malignant transformation.

The second prototype growth factor to be addressed is bFGF, a 146 amino acid protein which is also found in several truncated forms that remain biologically active.[18,19] This growth factor also interacts with a high affinity plasma membrane receptor. Though these receptors have not, as yet, been purified, there appear to be approximately $10^3 - 10^5$ receptors per target cell. Tissue localization studies show that most embryonic tissues as well as cell lines have FGF receptors present. The unique aspect of bFGF is its ability to bind to heparin. This heparin binding site is at a location on the molecule different from the biologically active site needed to bind to its high affinity receptor. This trait bFGF of binding to heparin allowed for the purification of the protein by heparin sepharose chromatography. Story et al[20] purified a 16kd growth factor from benign or malignant prostatic tissue and termed it prostatic growth factor. Using antibodies to synthetic peptides identical to portions of the bFGF molecule, western blot analysis showed the prostatic growth factor to be identical or nearly identical to bFGF. In the rat prostate, we have also shown that bFGF represents approximately 1/3 of the total growth factor activity.[7] By similiar methods, bFGF has also been demonstrated to be present in the testis.[21]

It appears that the mitogenic signal of bFGF is transmitted to the receptor cell in quite a different manner. As cells are laying down extracellular matrix and basement membrane, they secrete heparan sulfate which makes up a large part of the tissue glycosaminoglycans. Bound to the heparan sulfate and secreted at the same time is bFGF. Later, should an injury occur, the bFGF could be released and interact with a nearby membrane receptor.

It has been established that bFGF is an important angiogenesis factor and is responsible for new capillary growth in vivo.[2,22] As such, tumors may depend on its liberation from extracellular matrix in order to stimulate their own capillary blood supply. The mechanism for the release of bFGF from the heparan sulfate may be enzymatic. Baird and Ling[23] proposed that the neovascular response induced by tumors may be mediated by the initial release of heparinase-like enzymes which would mobilize a secondary local release

of FGF from the extracellular matrix and induce a
proliferative vascular response.

Heparinase-like enzymes are produced by cancer
cells,[24,25] platelets,[26] liver microsomes and
flavobacteria.[27] When initially described, these
enzymes were felt to explain how tumor cells could
extravasate into interstitium. Now, however, the
enzymes may help explain how tumors induce angiogenesis.

Because tumors grow as cylinders around new
capillary tufts, interference with the release or action
of bFGF may prove to have great therapeutic importance.
Tumor angiogenesis inhibitors are being aggressively
investigated. Four types of compounds are known to
interfere with bFGF functions: 1. Angiostatic
steroids,[28] 2. fungal peptides, 3. synthetic peptide
analogues, 4. heparin derivatives or inhibitors of
heparan degradation. Any of these compounds may be
useful in forcing tumors to grow to only a size that
they receive their oxygen by diffusion from the nearest
established vessel.

REFERENCES

1. Sporn, M.B., Todaro, G.J (1980). Autocrine
    Secretion and Malignant Transformation of cells.
    New Engl. J. Med. 303:878-880.
2. Folkman, J., Klagsbrun, M. Sasse. J., Wadzinski, M.,
    Ingber, D., Vlodavsky, I (1988). A
    Heparin-binding Angiogenic Protein - Basic
    Fibroblast Growth Factor - is Stored Within
    Basement Membrane. Am. J. Pathol. 130:393-400.
3. Gill, G.N., Santon, J.B., Bertics, P.J (1987)
    RegulatoryFeatures of The Epidermal Growth Factor
    Receptor. J. Cell. Physiol. Suppl. 5:35-41.
4. Rall, L.B., Scott, J., Bell, G.I., Crawford, R.J.,
    Penshow, J.D., Niall, H.D., Coughlan, J.P (1985)
    Nature 313:228-230.
5. Messing, E.M., Bubbers, J.E., DeKernion, J.B.,
    Fahey, J.L (1984) Growth Stimulating Activity
    Produced by Human Bladder Cancer Cells. J. Urol.
    132: 1230-1234.

6. Neal, D.E., Bennett, M.K., Hall, R.R., Marsh, C., Abel, P.D., Sainsburg, J.R.C., Harris, A.L (1985) Epidermal Growth Factor Receptors in Human Bladder Cancer: Comparison of Invasive and Superficial Tumors. Lancet i :366-368.

7. Jacobs, S.C., Story, M.T., Sasse, J., Lawson, R.K (1988) Characterization of Growth Factors Derived From the Rat Ventral Prostate. J. Urol. 139:1106-1110.

8. Li, D., Nanri, H., Chu, M., Deuel, T.F (1988) Isolation of EGF-like Peptides in Rat Prostates. J. Cell. Biochem. Suppl 12A: 134.

9. Story, M.T., Jacobs, S.C., Lawson, R.K (1983) Epidermal Growth Factor is Not The Major Growth Promoting Agent in Extracts of Prostate Tissue. J. Urol. 130:175-179.

10. Elson, S.D., Browne, C.A., Thorburn, G.D (1984) Identification of Epidermal Growth Factor-like Activity in Human male Reproductive Tissue and Fluids. J. Clin. Endocrinol. Metab. 58: 589-594.

11. Gregory, H., Willshire, I.R., Kavanagh, J.P., Blacklock, N.J., Chowdury, S., Richards, R.C (1986) Urogastrone-Epidermal Growth Factor Concentration in Prostatic Fluid of Normal Individuals and Patients with Benign Prostatic Hypertrophy. Clin. Sci. 70:359-363.

12. Jacobs, S.C., Story, M.T: Exocrine Secretion of Epidermal Growth Factor by the Rat Prostate: Effect of Adrenergic Agents, Cholinergic agents, and Vasoactive Intestinal Peptide. Prostate (in press).

13. Traish, A.M., Wotiz, H.H (1987) Prostatic Epidermal Growth Factor Receptors and Their Regulation by Androgen. Endocrinology 121: 1461-1467.

14. Chegini, N., Rao, C.V., Wakim, N., Sanfilippo (1986) Binding of ^{125}I-epidermal Growth Factor in Human Uterus. Cell Tiss. Res. 246: 543-548.

15. Mukku, V.R., Stancel, G.M (1985) Regulation of Epidermal Growth Factor by Estrogen. J. Biol. Chem. 260: 9820-9824.

16. Gardner, R.M., Lingham, R.B., Stancel, G.M (1987) Contraction of the Isolated Uterus Stimulated by Epidermal Growth Factor. FASEB J. 1:224-228.

17. Isaacs, J.T (1983) Prostatic Structure and Function in Relation to The Etiology of Prostatic Cancer. Prostate 4:351-366.
18. Gospodarowicz, D., Neufeld, G., Schweigerer (1987) Fibroblast Growth Factor: Structural and Biological Properties. J. Cell. Physiol. Suppl. 5:15-26.
19. Thomas, K.A (1987) Fibroblast Growth Factors. FASEB J., 1:434-440.
20. Story, M.T., Sasse, J., Jacobs, S.C., Lawson, R.K: Prostatic Growth Factor (1987) Purification and Structural Relationship to Basic Fibroblast Growth Factor. Biochemistry 26: 3843-3849.
21. Story, M.T., Sasse, J., Kakuska, D., Jacobs, S.C., Lawson, R.K (In Press) A Growth Factor in Bovine and Human Testis Structurally Related to Basic Fibroblast Growth Factor. J. Urol.
22. Hayek, A., Culler, F.L., Beattie, G.M., Lopez, A.D., Cuevas, P., Baird, A (1987) An In Vivo Model for Study of The Angiogenic Effects of Basic Fibroblast Growth Factor. Biochem. Biophys. Res. Comm. 147:876-880.
23. Baird, A., Ling, N (1987) Fibroblast Growth Factors are Present in the Extracellular Matrix Produced by Endothelial Cells In Vitro: Implications For a Role of Heparinase-Like Enzymes in The Neovascular Response. Biochem. Biophys. Res. Comm. 142:428-435.
24. Kramer, R.H., Vogel, K.G., Nicolson, G.L (1982) Solubilization and Degradation of Subendothelial Matrix Glycoproteins an Proteoglycans by Metastatic Tumor Cells. J. Biol. Chem. 257:2678-2686.
25. Vlodavsky, I., Fuks, Z., Bar-Ner, M., Ariav, Y., Schirrmacher, V (1983) Lymphoma Cell-Mediated Degradation of Sulfated Proteoglycans in The Subendothelial Extracellular Matrix: Relationship to Tumor Cell Metastatis. Cancer Res. 43:2704-2711.
26. Oosta, G.M., Faureau, L.V., Beeler, D.L., Rosenberg, R.D: Purification and Properties of Human Platelet Heparitinase.
27. Lindhardt, R.J., Fitzgerald, G.L., Cooney, C.L., Cooney, C.L., Langer, R (1982) Mode of Action of Heparin Lyase on Heparin. Biochem. Biophys. Acta 702:197-203.

28. Folkman, J., Ingber, D.E (1987) Angiostatic
    Steroids. Ann. Surg. 206:374-383.
29. Story, M.T., Jacobs, S.C., Lawson, R.K (1984)
    Partial Purfication of a Prostate-Associated
    Growth Factor. J. Urol. 122:1212.

Uro-Oncology: Current Status
and Future Trends, pages 25–33
© 1990 Wiley-Liss, Inc.

IMMUNE MODIFIERS IN THE TREATMENT OF BLADDER CANCER

Alvaro Morales, M.D.

Professor & Chairman, Department of Urology
Queen's University, Kingston, Ontario, CANADA

A sound approach to the clinical immunotherapy of malignant disease must be based on experimental studies of the immunobiology of cancer in general and, of course, on the immune responsiveness of the organ of origin of the neoplasm under study. In the case of bladder cancer, two experimental studies are of special significance in the planning and development of immune modulation strategies for therapeutic gain.

Two decades ago, Coe and Feldman (1) clearly demonstrated in elegant experiments that the bladder is an ideal organ for the development of delayed hypersensitivity reactions. Their studies showed that previously immunized guinea pigs exposed to an antigenic challenge exhibited particularly strong delayed hypersensitivity reactions in the skin and in the bladder, while responses were much less significant in kidney, muscle or testes. These important observations were largely ignored, however, during the immunotherapy renaissance of the late 1960s.

Equally important and of crucial significance was the series of experiments of Zbar and his group (2) which conclusively established the basis for successful non-specific active immunotherapy, principles that can be applied in all probability to all forms of clinical and experimental immunotherapy (active, passive and adoptive).

These investigators, employing a hepatoma model in guinea pigs and immune modulation with Mycobacterium bovis established the following basic principles for optimal results with biological response modifiers:

- Tumors respond better when confined to the parent organ or when their microscopic spread is limited to the regional lymph nodes.

- The tumor burden must be small; the diameter and mass of the tumor appear to be critical factors in response.

- Direct contact between tumor cells and vaccine is essential.

- The dose of the immunizing agent must be adequate. In the case of M. bovis, effectiveness was confined in a range of 10 - 10 viable organisms injected into the transplanted tumor.

BLADDER CANCER ANIMAL MODELS

Bladder cancer can be produced consistently in a variety of experimental animals by feeding N-[4-{5-nitro-2-furyl}-2-thiazolyl] formamide (FANFT). Studies using chemically-induced tumors may help in the understanding of the biological behavior of their human counterparts because of the similarities they share: chemical etiology, prolonged latent period and histological appearance. The use of various carcinogens, particularly FANFT, has permitted the development of autochthonous and transplantable bladder tumors which have been useful in the development of clinical immunotherapy protocols.

A bladder tumor induced by FANFT administration into C3H mice produced the MBT-2 cell line initially employed at the American National Cancer Institute (3). The development of a tumor cell line and the availability of tissue culture cells from this tumor proved to be a major advance in immunological studies of bladder cancer. Initial studies with the in vivo line had demonstrated the MBT-2 tumor to be immunogenic (4). The availability of an in vitro cell line provided a fairly uniform cell population, a relatively abundant source of cells free of overt microbiological contamination and necrotic material and permitted the extraction of antigens on repeated occasions (5).

A wealth of information on the immunobiology of bladder cancer has been obtained by detailed studies of the MBT-2 tumor and immunotherapy protocols have been refined and improved by observations made on the biological behavior of this experimental neoplasm. However, important data in the context of developing immunotherapy for bladder cancer were obtained without the use of an experimental bladder tumor.

The MBT-2 tumor has permitted comparative studies of various non-specific immune modifiers (5,6). Data obtained from this and other chemically-induced tumors will aid in improving the effectiveness and decreasing the side effects of currently available agents.

The interesting studies of Shapiro et al (7) showing the effectiveness of intravesical bacillus Calmette-Guerin (BCG) vaccine in preventing tumor takes in the disrupted mucosa of mice receiving live MBT-2 cells are a case in point. It is believed that such tumor implants occur clinically after transurethral resection and it appears that this occurrence may be eliminated by post-operative instillations of the vaccine.

It is appropriate to mention here that a variety of immune modifiers have been tried in the treatment of superficial bladder cancer. Keyhole limpet hemocyanin (KLH) has been used for many years in the assessment of immune reactivity by delayed cutaneous hypersensitivity. Over a decade ago, Olsson et al (8) found decreased cutaneous responses in patients with bladder cancer and later used KLH in an attempt to prevent recurrence of superficial tumors. Although they found a significant reduction in the number of recurrences in those patients receiving and reacting to KLH, conclusive evidence was not presented in the study. Additional investigations with KLH, unfortunately, were not pursued by this or any other group of investigators.

Further compounds used as immune modifiers include levamisole and polyinosinic and polycyticylic acids (poly I:C). Levamisole was reported to be ineffective in the prevention of recurrences in a randomized trial of patients with various stages of superficial and invasive bladder cancer (9). Poly I:C is an interferon inducer and it was hoped that it would, indirectly, promote and enhance immune responses in humans. Although evidence was found for the effectiveness of poly I:C as an interferon inducer, its systemic administration proved to be ineffective in the treatment of transitional cell carcinoma (10). It is possible that regional instead of systemic administration of poly I:C may be more effective if higher local levels of interferon are produced. Other compounds such as transfer factor and bacterial preparations, including Corynebacterium parvum have been used with little success (11).

INTRAVESICAL BCG IMMUNOTHERAPY

The notable exception to the disappointing role of immunotherapy in urological malignancies has been the effectiveness of BCG in superficial bladder cancer. Successful destruction of a metastatic vesical melanoma by intratumoral transurethral injection of BCG in a patient previously immunized with the vaccine has been reported (12). This single observation was in keeping with the experimental data indicating that the bladder responds promptly and strongly to antigenic challenge. Furthermore, it provided clinical support to the observations of Bloomberg et al (13) and the model for BCG immunotherapy of Zbar et al (2). Our group (14) reported preliminary experience with systemic and intravesical administration of BCG in patients with superficial bladder cancer. The results showed that the vaccine exhibited significant activity against non-infiltrating transitional cell carcinoma of the bladder. Further non-randomized studies by the same group also showed that BCG was effective in the treatment of residual tumors (15) and of carcinoma in situ (16).

Experience at Queen's University affiliated hospitals with the use of intravesical BCG includes the prevention of superficial recurrence, the treatment of residual papillary lesions not amenable to endoscopic surgery and the treatment of carcinoma in situ. The results of our studies are summarized in Tables 2, 3 and 4.

The effectiveness of BCG in the prophylaxis and treatment of superficial bladder cancer has now been conclusively established. Controlled studies (17-19) have clearly shown that the vaccine prevents the number and frequency of recurrences after endoscopic treatment. The anti-tumor activity of the vaccine has also been clearly established in independent studies (17,18) showing that residual lesions are amenable to treatment with intravesical BCG.

Perhaps the most dramatic results have been observed in the treatment of carcinoma in situ (16, 18-22). Our earlier results indicated a response rate of 77% with a mean follow-up period of almost 4 years (23). Brosman (17), however, has reported an astonishing 94% complete response rate with a protocol which differs from ours in the strain of the vaccine and duration of treatment. These results cannot be ignored but very clearly point to the need for fine tuning and improvement of the current treatment protocols.

Investigations in various countries have supported the concept that intravesical administration of BCG has a significant anti-neoplastic potential. Recent studies have been aimed at determining better schedules of administration. Our initial experience indicates that reduced doses of the vaccine are effective but do not carry the annoying side effects of the full doses currently used (120 mg). Kavoussi et. al (26) have found that 2 courses of immunizations offer better results than a single 6 week series. Our own expereince does not support this concept and it is evident that further assessment of the vaccine in regard to length of administration is required.

There is a further need to establish the value of BCG in relation to other agents used intravesically. In addition, salvage of chemotherapy failures by BCG has been rarely used but a response rate of about 50% has been documented.

Despite the effectiveness of the vaccine, a great deal of concern has been expressed because of potential side effects which may result. However, recent review of over 1000 patients (24) has shown that BCG is well tolerated and produces only self-limiting complications. Another drawback of the vaccine is the difficulty in quantifying the amount administered and the potential for bacterial growth which may produce "BCG-osis" with involvement of other organs.

An assessment of the safety and effectiveness of BCG was recently conducted (25). In both categories the vaccine scored very highly. It is anticipated that in the United States, it will be approved for clinical use in the near future.

Work is currently being done at our institution to isolate extracellular capsular components of live BCG. Preliminary in vitro and animal studies are encouraging. The possibility of administering a substance of a defined composition, not subject to the vagaries of culturing, preservation and reconstitution would be a significant step forward in the use of this particular immune modifer.

TABLE 1

RESPONSE TO PROPHYLACTIC THERAPY

N = 62

Complete* : 36 (58%)
18 – 108 mos. (mean: 47)

Partial** : 9 (15%)
16 – 63 mos. (mean: 35)

Failure : 17 (27%)

* No recurrence during follow-up
** Decrease of more than 50% in the number of recurrences and over 100% increase in disease-free intervals

TABLE 2

RESPONSE TO RESIDUAL TUMORS

N = 36

Complete : 19 (53%)
14 – 43 mos. (mean: 34)

Failure : 17 (47%)

TABLE 3

RESPONSE TO TREATMENT – CIS

N = 43

Complete : 32 (73%)
14 – 88 mos. (mean: 47)

Failure : 11 (26%)

REFERENCES

1.   Coe, J.E. and Feldman, J.D.: Extracutaneous delayed hypersensitivity, particularly in the guinea pig bladder. Immunology 10:127, 1966.
2.   Zbar, B., Bernstein, I.D., Bartlett, G.L., Hannah, M.G., Rapp, H.J.: Immunotherapy of cancer: regression of intradermal tumors and prevention of growth of lymph node metastases after intralesional injection of living Mycobacterium bovis. N. Natl. Cancer Inst. 49:119, 1972.
3.   Soloway, M.S.: Intravesical and systemic chemotherapy of murine bladder cancer. Cancer Res. 37:2918, 1977.

4.   Javadpour, N., Hyatt, C.L., Soaries, T.: Immunologic features of a carcinogen induced murine bladder cancer: in vivo and in vitro studies. J. Surg. Oncol. 11:153, 1979.

5.   Morales, A., Djeu, J., Herberman, R.B.: Immunization by irradiated whole cells or cell extracts against an experimental bladder tumor. Invest. Urol. 17:310, 1980.

6.   Pang, A.S.D., Morales, A.: Chemoimmunoprophylaxis of an experimental bladder cancer with retinoids and BCG. J. Urol. 130:166, 1985.

7.   Shapiro, A., Ratliff, T.L., Oakley, D.M., Catalona, W.J.: Reduction of bladder tumor growth in mice treated with intravesical BCG and its correlation with BCG viability and natural killer cell activity. Cancer Res. 43:1611, 1983.

8.   Olsson, C.A., Chute, R., Rao, C.N.: Immunological reduction of bladder cancer recurrence rate. J. Urol. 111:173, 1974.

9.   Smith, R.B., deKernion, J., Lincoln, B., Skinner, D.G., Kaufman, J.J.: Preliminary report of the use of levamisole in the treatment of bladder cancer. Cancer Treat. Rep. 62:1709, 1978.

10.   Herr, H.W.: Carcinoma in situ of the bladder. Sem. Urol. 1:15, 1983.

11.   Shapiro, A., Kadmon, D., Catalona, W.J., Ratliff, T.L.: Immunotherapy of superficial bladder cancer. J. Urol. 128:891, 1982.

12.   deKernion, J.B., Golub, S.H., Gupta, R.K., Silverstein, M., Morton, D.L.: Successful transurethral intralesional BCG therapy of bladder melanoma. Cancer 36:1662, 1975.

13.   Bloomberg, S.D., Brosman, S.A., Hausman, M.S., Cohen, A., Battenberg, J.D.: The effect of BCG on the dog bladder. Invest. Urol. 12:423, 1975.

14.   Morales, A., Eidinger, D., Bruce, A.W.: Intracavitary bacillus Calmette-Guerin in the treatment of superficial bladder tumors. J. Urol. 116:10, 1976.

15.   Morales, A., Ottenhof, P., Emerson, L.: Treatment of residual non-infiltrating bladder cancer with bacillus Calmette-Guerin. J. Urol. 125:649, 1981.

16.   Morales, A.: Treatment of carcinoma in situ of the bladder with BCG. A phase II trial. Cancer Immunol. Immunother. 9:69, 1980.

17.   Brosman, S.A.: Experience with bacillus Calmette-

Guerin in patients with superficial bladder carcinoma. J. Urol. 128:27, 1982.

18. deKernion, J.B., Huang, M., Lindner, A., Smith, R.B., Kaufman, J.J.: The management of superficial bladder tumors and carcinoma in situ with intravesical bacillus Calmette-Guerin. J. Urol. 133:598, 1985.

19. Lamm, D.L.: Bacillus Calmette-Guerin immunotherapy for bladder cancer. J. Urol. 134:40, 1985.

20. Lamm, D.L., Crawford, D.E., Montie, J.D., Scardino, P.T., Stanisic, D.H., Grossman, H.D.: BCG vs. adriamycin in the treatment of transitional cell carcinoma in situ. A Southwest Oncology Group Study. J. Urol. 133:184A, 1985.

21. Herr, H.W., Pinsky, C.W., Whitmore, W.F. et al: Long term effect of intravesical BCG on flat carcinoma in situ of the bladder. J. Urol. 135:265, 1986.

22. Kelley, D.R., Haat, E.O., Becich, M. et al: Prognostic value of PPD skin test and granuloma formation in patients treated with intravesical BCG. J. Urol. 135:268, 1986.

23. Morales, A.: Long-term results of BCG therapy for bladder cancer. J. Urol. 132:457, 1984.

24. Lamm, D.L., Stogdill, V.D., Stogdill, B.J., Crispen, R.G.: Complications of BCG immunotherapy in 1,278 patients with bladder cancer. J. Urol. 135:272, 1986.

25. Diagnostic and Therapeutic Technology Assessment (DATTA). J.A.M.A. 259:2153, 1988.

26. Kavoussi, L.R., Torrence, R.J., Gillen, D.P., M'Liss, A.H., Haaff, E.O., Dressner, S.M. Ratlitt, T.L., Catalona, W.J.: Results of 6 weeks intravesical BCG on the treatment of superficial bladder tumors. J. Urol. 139:935, 1988.

Uro-Oncology: Current Status
and Future Trends, pages 35–39
© 1990 Wiley-Liss, Inc.

IMMUNOCYTOLOGY AS A POSSIBLE MARKER TO IDENTIFY PATIENTS WHO REQUIRE PROPHYLAXIS

Hartwig Huland, Andreas Schneider, Edith
Huland and Rüdiger Arndt, Department of
Urology, University, Steglitz, Berlin (H.H.,
E.H.) University of Hamburg (A.S., R.A.)

INTRODUCTION

Many studies have already proved that prophylaxis can influence the natural course of patients who have had a complete transurethral resection (TUR) due to a superficial bladder carcinoma. Our interest was focused on the use of mitomycin C bladder installations after TUR. In a prospective, randomized unicenter controlled study as well as in a multicenter study including 425 patients, we have shown that it is possible to a) reduce the recurrence rate from 60 percent to 15 percent, b) reduce the progression rate from 25 percent to 4 percent and c) influence the survival time of patients. One specific point of our study was that we included all consecutive patients, and our results show that in our hospital overtreatment – or better, overprophylaxis – is common. Data from our control group has shown that at least 40 percent of the patients who were prescribed prophylactic treatment will not develop recurrent tumors even without prophylaxis. Thus, the most important issue of our own as well as of many other studies was: Can those patients who will not develop a recurrent bladder tumor and who therefore do not need prophylactic therapy be reliably identified?

Most physicians use two information sources to decide whether or not a patient should receive prophylaxis after complete TUR, namely the patient's medical history and the analysis of the removed tumor. Prophylaxis is commonly prescribed for patients who have already had tumor recurrences in the past and for those who presently have T1, grade II and grade III lesions. Prophylaxis is generally not recommended for patients with a first-time occurrence of a small, solitary TA grade I lesion. This common practice is based on data from numerous studies which have demonstrated that recurrence and progression rates correlate with size, grade, stage and other parameters of these tumors. Such an approach is, in our opinion, not precise enough to predict the course of an individual patient. Studies with a longer follow-up of patients with superficial bladder carcinomas have shown that there is only a gradual difference with respect to recurrence and progression rates among patients who have tumors of different stage and grade. This hints that there might be a small group of so-called TA Grade 0 tumors that actually pose no real risk of recurrence or progression. Our group therefore concentrated on improving diagnosis in order to accurately identify those patients with a superficial bladder carcinoma who are at no risk of recurrent and progressive disease and who therefore need no prophylactic treatment.

We developed several monoclonal antibodies (MAB) directed against tumor-associated antigens in transitional cell carcinomas of the bladder. We named one of them 486P according to the cell line used for immunization. MAB 486P is an IgM antibody which detects glycoprotein in the cell membrane and has a high molecular weight of 200,000 dalton. In immune histological tests it reacts with 90 percent of the superficial bladder carcinomas. This MAB 486P was extremely helpful in identifying cells in the urine of patients with bladder carcinoma. Using indirect immune cytology with the help of an alkaline phosphatase reaction, this monoclonal antibody stained all malignant transitional cells in some patients. In most urine specimens of patients with bladder carcinoma, heterogenous cell staining occurs however, i.e., some morphologically similar malignant cells react with this MAB but some do not. Due to this heterogenous reaction and to the fact, in some normal patients, benign cells occasionally react with this MAB, we did a quantitative analysis of urine specimens whereby at least 100 transitional cells were counted in a given urine sample and the percentage of cells that reacted with our MAB was calculated. We thus could see in a control group that

about 50 percent of patients with BPH or UTI do not react
with the MAB at all, yet 50 percent have positive cells
but never more than 30 percent. We took this as a baseline dividing positive and negative quatitative immune
cytology. In our first study we were thus able to show
that, of 40 patients with superficial bladder carcinomas,
36 = 90 percent had a positive quantitative immunocytology according to the MAB 486P. The high rate of 90
percent sensitivity was much better than the 50 percent
which we obtained by using standard cytology. The reason
why quantitative immunocytology is so much better than
standard cytology was shown in a follow-up study on 69
patients with a superficial bladder carcinoma. In this
prospective study we compare the results of standard cytology, flow cytometry and quantitative immunocytology.
The analyses of this study show that the right positive
rate in grade I tumors was as good as in grade II and
grade III tumors according to our MAB 486P. The right
positive rate of standard cytology was no better than 34
percent in patients with grade I tumors. In patients
with grade I transitional cells of the bladder, we very
often observe a great number of benign looking cells
which stain intensively with our monoclonal antibody.
This means that the MAB 486P reacts with cells which
still are benign according to classic morphological
criteria but which have already undergone malignant
transformation.

To prove this thesis, we did extensive immune histological mapping studies of 6 bladders removed because of
a T-2 transitional cell carcinoma and compared the results with two normal bladders taken from kidney donors.
We specifically examined the morphologically normal areas
of the bladder distant from the tumor. In these areas we
find extensive fields reacting positively to the 486P
MAB. We also studied those areas which were morphologically benign but which stained with our MAB. Most of
these specific regions already showed loss of blood group
antigen, expression of T antigen and loss of T crypt
antigen. We therefore have indirect evidence of malignant transformation in those specimens that look morphologically benign but are 486P positive. From this study
we conclude that the monoclonal antibody 486P is a good
marker for detecting malignant transformation at a very
early stage, i.e., even before visible lesions can be
seen by morphology or endoscopy. Assuming this is true,

quantitative immunocytology should be an excellent marker in the follow-up of patients with superficial bladder carcinomas.

In order to prove this assumption, we started a prospective study 2-1/2 years ago. All patients with superficial bladder carciomas TA, T1, grade I to Grade III were included. The tumor was removed by transurethral resection, which was repeated in those with T1 lesions. Four weeks later cystoscopy and cytology were done to confirm completeness of surgical removal of the tumor. No prophylaxis was given. Urine samples were taken every four weeks from all patients. Cystoscopy was done every three months.

I now give a preliminary report on this on-going study. We now supervise 36 patients (28 males, 8 females) whose mean age is 65.8 years. There were: 15 TA lesions, 21 T1 lesions, 13 grade I lesions, 21 grade II lesions and 2 grade III lesions. We have examined 486 bladder specimens for cytology and immunocytology, which equates to 13.5 urinary examinations per patient. The follow-up period was 2 to 38 months with a mean of 18.5 months. The preliminary results show that, of 15 patients who never had a positive immunocytological test, 14 have not yet developed a recurrent tumor. Immune histological examination of the tumor of the single patient who had recurrent tumor showed that this specific tumor was 486P negative. In summary: about 40 percent of our patients had negative immunocytology and did not develop a recurrent tumor. It appears that quantitative immunocytology (486P) can reliably identify those 40 percent of patients who will not develop a recurrent tumor.

Twenty-one of the patients had more than one positive immunocytological test in the follow-up. Twelve of them have already developed a recurrent tumor 3 to 6 months after immunocytological tests became positive. A longer follow-up is needed to see whether the other 9 patients will have tumor recurrence. Assuming our results can be confirmed, quantitative immunocytology can be used as a marker to identify those who require prophylaxis.

We also plan to perform another study to test quantitative immunocytology as a marker to determine the required duration of prophylaxis. We will attempt to answer the question: Can quantitative immunocytology (specifically MAB 486P) be a marker to determine the duration and type of prophylaxis required in patients with a superficial transitional cell carcinoma of the bladder? The goal is to use quantitative immunocytology as a marker to perform more individualized prophylaxis in patients with superficial bladder carcinoma rather than performing merely schematic prophylaxis.

Uro-Oncology: Current Status
and Future Trends, pages 41–59
© 1990 Wiley-Liss, Inc.

PHASE I/II STUDY OF INTRAVESICAL EPIRUBICIN IN
PATIENTS WITH CARCINOMA IN SITU OF THE BLADDER

K. H. Kurth, K. Mross, F. ten Kate, G. Weissglas,
P. J. Carpentier, C. G. D. Boeken Krueger, J. Blom,
J. M. Groen, R. D. van Caubergh, O. van Aubel, I.
van Reyswoud.

Dept. of Urology, University of Amsterdam; Dept. of
Urology and Dept. of Pathology, University of
Rotterdam; Dept. of Urology, Aalst, Belgium; Gouda,
Roosendaal, Haarlem; Dept. of Oncology, Free
University, Amsterdam, The Netherlands.

Carcinoma in situ of the bladder is defined as an
anaplasia of the surface epithelium without
formation of papillary structure and without
infiltration (UICC). The histological criteria are
not clear cut and different pathologists do not
necessarily agree. However, consensus is achieved
that only $TiSG_3$ lesions are to be called true
carcinoma in situ and all other atypical cellular
patterns of the epithelial cells are interpreted
as atypia (or dysplasia) (Farrow et al., 1986).
Obviously this does not exclude report of severe
dysplasia by one pathologist whereas another
pathologist may report the same slide to show
carcinoma in situ. Carcinoma in situ without
exophytic bladder tumor is classified as primary
carcinoma in situ. Carcinoma in situ with
exophytic bladder tumor or a history of exophytic
tumor are classified as secondary carcinoma in
situ (De Voogt, 1977, Jakse, 1980, Consensus
Meeting, Hakone, 1987). Symptomatic and asymptoma-
tic carcinoma in situ describe clinical features,
the first seems to be prognostically worse
(Riddle, 1976). Carcinoma in situ is considered to

be the principal source of invasive carcinoma
(Koss, 1979, Kulatilake et al., 1970, Farrow,
1976, Yates-Bell, 1979). The time for progression
from in situ to invasive carcinoma has been
reported to be between 18 and 77 months (Melamed,
1964, Koss, 1969, Farrow, 1977). The hope is, that
early treatment could alter the neoplastic
potential of the urothelium either by retarding
the cascade of changes or by reversing the
carcinogenic changes (Hargreave, 1985). Generally
a patient may have a biopsy taken because of
symptoms such as urgency dysuria or frequency,
without obvious pathological changes during
endoscopy or at the presence of an overt bladder
tumor of either normal or abnormal looking mucosa.
There is accordance that symptomatic carcinoma in
situ is a highly malignant condition with the
potency of progressing to invasive and metastatic
carcinoma. Early radical treatment may be
indicated. Specially if the prostate is involved.
When carcinoma in situ is associated with an
exophytic tumor, generally local treatment
measures are applied first.
A trial of intravesical chemotherapy is justified
in symptomatic primary or secondary carcinoma in
situ, provided that the response is carefully and
critically evaluated. Promising results have been
reported following intracavitary treatment with
Adriamycin (Jakse, 1981, 1984, Glashan, 1982, Edsmyr, 1984), Mitomycin C (Soloway, 1983, Jauhiainen
1986), and BCG (Herr, 1986, Brosman, 1985, De
Kernion, 1985). Results with BCG were superior to
Adriamycin in a randomized study executed by Lamm
(1988). However, the frequency of local side
effects after local BCG treatment reach 93% and
systemic side effects are more frequent and
serious than after intracavitary chemotherapy
(Orihuela, 1987). Thus, there is still need for
well tolerated and effective intracavitary
chemotherapy.

Epirubicin is one of the series of new derivatives of Adriamycin synthesized with the aim of finding anthracyclin analogues with an improved spectrum of antitumor activity or lower toxicity. It appears to have similar antitumoral activity as the parent drug in experimental and human tumors, but with lower toxicity. An excellent overview of the preclinical and clinical data was published by Ganzina (1983).

The drug has also been evaluated by the EORTC clinical screening group confirming the general statements above (Hurteloup, 1983). Because of the similarity with Adriamycin, Epirubicin may be equally or even more effective than this drug. There is as yet no published information as to its effectiveness in carcinoma in situ of the bladder. However, the drug is therapeutically active in superficial papillary bladder tumor as shown by Denis, 1988. Complete remission of marker lesions was achieved in 38%. Therefore, a study was designed with the objectives to determine in three different dose levels of Epirubicin administered intravesically

1. the absorption- and recovery rate,
2. the rate of antitumor activity: response rate (complete remission) and duration of response,
3. the kind and frequency of local side effects.

The selected doses were 30 mg (1), 50 mg (2), 80 mg (3).

The purpose of the phase-I-part of the trial was to screen for toxicity and to determine a safe dose for further studies for therapeutic activity associated with the compound. In the phase-II-part of the trial the rate of complete remission and duration of remission after intracavitary treatment are evaluated.

METHODS OF THE STUDY

All patients with carcinoma in situ of the bladder (TiSG$_3$) proven by biopsy were considered eligible. Tissue samples were evaluated by a referee pathologist (J. t. K.). Patients with primary and secondary carcinoma in situ were considered for the protocol, provided that all papillary tumors were resected before entering the protocol.

Invasion of the prostatic mass by carcinoma in
situ had to be excluded by transrectal, perineal
or transurethral prostatic biopsy. Iso-osmotic
irrigating fluid was used for bladder biopsy, as
water causes the surface umbrella cells to
desquamate and results in poorer histological
preparations. A small portion of mucosa and muscle
was grasped by a means of a cup biopsy forceps.
Biopsies were taken from any area of abnormal
looking mucosa or at random if urine cytology
showed malignant cells in the absence of any
exophytic tumor anywhere in the urinary tract.
Biopsies were repeated two weeks after completed
intracavitary treatment and whenever urine
cytology showed malignant cells. Previous
intravesical treatment with cystostatic drugs was
allowed provided that the interval between the end
of the previous treatment and the entry of the
patient in the study was at least three months.
Patients with positive cytology (Papanicolau IV or
V) and/or positive biopsy after treatment course
with 30 mg (or 50 mg) could re-enter the protocol
and be treated with the higher dose (50 mg or 80
mg) provided that there were no signs of progression or carcinoma in situ outside of the bladder.
Patients with previous local radiotherapy within
twelve months prior to entry or with a bladder
capacity below 250 ml were considered ineligible.
Likewise patients with severe recurrent bacterial
cystitis. Any urinary tract infection had to be
treated before intracavitary therapy was started.
Patients went off study if recurrent severe drug-
induced cystitis occurred or when severe systemic
side effects were observed (white blood counts
below $3000/mm^3$ and/or platelets counts below
$100.000/m^{m3}$).

THERAPEUTIC REGIMENT
Epirubicin was delivered in vials of 10 and 50 mg
by Farmitalia Carlo Erba, Rotterdam, The Netherlands.
30 mg Epirubicin (or 50 mg or 80 mg) diluted in 50
ml normal saline was instilled into the bladder
through a urethral catheter the day after biopsy.

The catheter was clamped for 60 minutes. Thereafter the urine was collected and the bladder
irrigated by 100 ml normal saline. Saline and
first spontaneously produced urine were collected.
Aliquots of the instillation fluid (U1), the
content of the bladder after 1 hour (U2), irrigated
saline (U3) and spontaneous urine after
intracavitary treatment (U4) were kept for drug
analysis after measurement of the volumes. The
samples were stored in polypropylene at -20° C
until the assays were carried out.
During 8 courses with 30 mg of Epirubicin and 5
courses with 50 mg of Epirubicin and 3 courses with
80 mg Epirubicin, blood samples were collected in
heparinized tubes in 0, 30, 45, 60, 75, 90, 120,
150, 210 and 270 minutes after instillation of the
drug. These samples were immediately centrifuged at
4000 g for 10 minutes. The plasma was transferred
to polypropylene tubes. Epirubicin levels in plasma
samples were measured, based upon a previously
described anthracycline assay (Weenen et al., in
press). The instillation was repeated weekly during
8 weeks. Nitrofurantoin (3 times 100 mg a day) was
given for 3 days after each instillation (or
another urinary antiseptic if the patient was
allergic to Nitrofurantoin). Urine cytology and
urine analysis were repeated before each
instillation of Epirubicin. Bladder biopsy was
repeated at the end of the instillation treatment.
Biopsy could be done in the outpatient clinic (cold
cup biopsy).

The instillation was delayed if the patient had
chemical cystitis. After drug-induced cystitis, the
next instillation was given, if the symptoms
decreased or disappeared, in a total solution
volume of 100 cc normal saline. If drug-induced
cystitis could not be controlled or reappeared
after each instillation, the patient went off
study.

Blood controls during instillation treatment were
repeated biweekly. If the clinical and anamnestic
data suggested any signs of hematological or other
toxicity, immediate control was mandatory. When WBC
was under 3000 m^3 and when blood urea or creatinine
raised more than 100%, instillation was delayed
until recovery and further investigation performed.
Instillation was delayed if urinary tract infection
occurred. Possible late effects on the bladder wall
were controlled by measurement of bladder capacity
at the time of cystoscopy. The total maximal volume
was recorded in ml.

FOLLOW-UP
After instillation treatment, urine cytology was
controlled monthly in the first 3 months, thereafter 3-monthly together with cystoscopy. Whenever
positive cytology was seen on 2 successive
controls, a biopsy was done. If recurrent carcinoma
in situ of the bladder was proven by urine cytology
(at least two) or by bladder biopsy after completion of the instillation treatment, further
treatment was at the local investigator's discretion. A patient with a proven recurrent Tis lesion
after completion of the instillation treatment
could re-enter the study in the higher dose regime
(50 or 80 mg). All patients were followed until
progression or death.

STATISTICAL METHODS
Curves representing probability failure free (all
patients) and probability recurrence free (only
patients with complete remission) have been
estimated by the Kaplan-Meier method.

ETHICS
Each patient was informed about the objectives of
the trial, about the drug and about the possible
benefits and risks inherent in the trial. The
patient's consent was obtained before inclusion in
the trial.

EVALUATION OF RESPONSE

Conversion from positive to negative cytology after completion of the instillation treatment and bladder biopsies not showing carcinoma in situ were evaluated as complete remission. Twice positive cytology at any time after completion of instillation treatment was evaluated as failure. Any new bioptic proven flat lesion (Tis) or papillary lesion (Ta/T1) was evaluated as failure. Any increase in the T-category above T1 was evaluated as progression. The duration of complete remission was recorded in months.

MATERIAL

Thirty-four patients entered the trial. Patient characteristics are listed in table 1. Twenty-two patients were evaluable for report of treatment results. Reasons for ineligibility of 11 patients are listed in table 2.

(table 1)

Patients characteristics	No. of pts.
Patients registered	34
Inevaluable for treatment activity	1
(Systemic side effects (3rd instillation))	-
Ineligible	11
Evaluable for treatment activity	22
Evaluable for toxicity (local)	33

Age: (yrs) mean (range): 70.0 (58 - 80)

Sex:	
Male	18
Female	4
Primary carcinoma in situ	7
Secondary carcinoma in situ	15

(table 2)
Reason for ineligibility

Atypia (not TiSG$_3$)	8
T$_1$G$_2$ papillary lesion	1
Small bladder capacity (< 100 ml)	1
Tumor of the upper urinary tract	1

RESULTS
Overall 16/22 patients (73%) responded with
complete remission on intracavitary chemotherapy
with Epirubicin (table 3).
13/22 Patients showed a favourable response on the
first treatment course whereas 3/5 patients
responded only after a second treatment period
with a higher dose (table 4 and 5).

Six out of 7 patients (85%) with primary carcinoma
in situ G$_3$ and 10/15 patients (67%) with secondary
carcinoma in situ showed complete remission (Table
6).
Best results were achieved with the highest dose as
7/10 patients treated with 80 mg responded with
complete remission after a first treatment period.
Treatment with 30 mg led to complete remission in
3/7 patients and with 50 mg in 3/5 patients
respectively after a first treatment period.
Although patients showing complete remission after
a second treatment period were all, except one,
treated with a higher dose, it is unclear whether
this result is due to the higher dose or to the
second treatment period. In 4 non-responding
patients after the primary treatment course, the
responsible physician decided for an alternative
treatment because of failure in 3 cases (BCG in
case no. 20 and 29; cystectomy in case no. 21 in
Table 3) and because of progression in 1 case. All
other 5 non-responding patients had a second
treatment period with a favourable result in 3
cases.
From the 16 patients responding with complete
remission, 1 patient died, still in complete
remission, after myocardial infarct; 3 recurred

with carcinoma in situ G_3 and had cystectomy (1 case) and photoirradiation (1 case). In 2 patients with papillary recurrent tumor T_aG_2 and T_1G_2 the tumor was resected and patients remained in follow-up without additional treatment. Mucosal biopsy did not deliver recurrent carcinoma in situ G_3, urine cytology was negative after TUR. In 1 patient with recurrence 13 months after completion of intracavitary treatment, the tumor grew infiltrating into the muscle (T_2). Cystectomy was done with lymph node dissection. Histologically, the nodes were free of tumor, tumor infiltration was limited to the inner part of the bladder wall (pT_2). Median duration of complete remission is 21.7 months (range 3+ - 43+).

table 3
Characteristics and results of 22 evaluable patients

Patient	No.	Age	Sex	CR	Duration CR (in months)	Failure	Further Treatment	Total Follow-up (in months)
vdV	1	70	M	+	8	papillary tumor T_aG_2	Mitomycin C	18 (alive)
vdB	2	74	M	+	43	-	-	49 (alive)
vE	3	67	M	+	23	recurrent papillary tumor T_1G2	TUR	38 (alive)
vO	6	71	M	+	12	-	-	17 (alive)
M	7	74	M	+	17	-	-	17 (alive)
vdV	13	64	M	+	13	progression T_2	cystectomy	26 (alive)
S	16	59	M	+	30	recurrence $TiSG_3$	photo-irradiation	35 (alive)
LJ	17	66	M	+	18	-	-	18 (alive)
Sch	18	72	M	+	3	-	-	14 (refused control, died myocardial infarction)
B	22	74	M	+	18	-	-	23 (alive)
G	23	61	M	+	18	-	-	19 (alive)
L	25	67	F	+	11	recurrence $TiSG_3$	cystectomy	47 (alive)
L	28	80	F	+	6	-	-	15 (alive)
vdM	30	74	F	+	14	-	-	15 (alive)
K	31	77	F	+	11	-	-	18 (alive)
V	33	71	M	+	7	pos. cytol. $TiSG_3$	cystectomy planned	17 (alive)
vG	8	70	M	-	-	pos. cytol.	cystectomy	22 (alive)
O	12	76	M	-	-	$T_{4a}N_4$	chemotherapy	42 (alive)
L	20	67	M	-	-	pos. cytol.	BCG	25 (alive)
T	21	75	M	-	-	pos. cytol.	cystectomy	17 (alive)
M	29	72	M	-	-	pos. cytol	BCG	15 (alive)
LJ	32	58	M	-	-	T_2G_3	cystectomy	17 (alive)

```
-----------------------------------------------------
(table 4)
Distribution of patients according to dose
received and results of primary and secondary
treatment

Dose      No. of pts.    CR                Failure

30 mg         7          3      43%        4
50 mg         5          3 (1)  60%        2 (1)
80 mg        10          7 (2)  70%        3 (1)


             22         13 (3)             9 (2)


() Patients receiving a second treatment period
with a higher or the same Epirubicin-dose.
-----------------------------------------------------
```

```
-----------------------------------------------------
(table 5)
Treatment results in 5 patients after dose-
escalation

Patients treated with escalating dose

Patient no.   2     12     16      31      8
Dose/mg      30     30     30
             50     50     50      50
                           80      80      80
                                           80

Results      CR     NC     CR      CR      NC
```

5/22 showing NC (failure) after a first course
with Epirubicin received a second course with a
higher dose (4/5) or a second course with the same
dose (1/5, 80 mg).
3/5 responded with CR lasting 43+, 30, and 11+
months respectively.
+: still in CR
```
-----------------------------------------------------
```

(table 6)
Response of 22 evaluable patients in relation to
type of carcinoma in situ and Epirubicin-dose

| | primary TiS | | secondary TiS | |
	CR /	Failure	CR /	Failure
30 mg	1		2	1
50 mg	2		2	2
80 mg	3	1	6	2
	6	1	10	5

TOXICITY
Local side effects were minor. In 33 patients
evaluated the occurrence of chemical cystitis
after 313 instillations was 2,9% (9/313) and
required stop of further instillations in one
patient. The occurrence of chemical cystitis was
not clearly related to the dose of Epirubicin
applied, the percentage of chemical cystitis was
5.4% with 30 mg, 2.2% with 50 mg, and 1.2% with 80
mg respectively (related to the number of
instillations) (table 7).

Systemic side effects were reported in two
patients finally leading to stop of further
instillations after the third instillation in one
patient. This patient demonstrated dizziness,
nausea and hypotension one hour after application
of the drug. Most likely the symptoms developed
due to an allergic reaction.

ABSORPTION OF EPIRUBICIN AFTER INTRAVESICAL
ADMINISTRATION
Results for the plasma concentration of Epirubicin
following intravesical administration of 30, 50
and 80 mg of the drug are given in table 8 and
recovery in table 9.

(table 7)
Side effects observed in 33 patients evaluable for toxicity who received a total of 40 complete treatment periods

() patients who received a second treatment period with an escalating or same dose of Epirubicin

	No side effects	Bacterial cystitis			Chemical cystitis			Bact. + chem. cystitis			Other side effects		
		Not req. delay	req. delay	STOP	Not req. delay	req. delay	STOP	Not req. delay	req. delay	STOP	Not req. delay	req. delay	STOP
33 (7) eval. patients	20 (6) (65.0%)	8 (-)	-	-	2 (1)	-	-	1 (-)	-	-	1 (-)	-	1 (-)
313 evaluable instillations	285 (91.0%)	15 (4.8%)	-	-	8 (2.6%)	-	1 (0.3%)	-	-	-	3 (1.0%)	-	1 (0.3%)

(table 8)

Plasma concentrations of Epirubicin in ng/ml at 0 - 270 minutes following intravesical administration of 30, 50 and 80 mg of the drug

Pts. no.	Dose (mg)	0 (min.)	30	45	60	75	90	120	150	210	270
1	30	<2.0	<2.0	<2.0	<2.0	<2.0	<2.0	<2.0	<2.0	<2.0	<2.0
2	30	<2.0	<2.0	<2.0	<2.0	<2.0	<2.0	<2.0	<2.0	<2.0	<2.0
3	30	<2.0	<2.0	<2.0	<2.0	<2.0	<2.0	<2.0	<2.0	<2.0	<2.0
4	30	<1.0	1.2	<1.0	<1.0	1.8	1.1	1.8	1.2	*	*
5	30	<1.0	<1.0	<1.0	<1.0	1.9	1.4	<1.0	<1.1	*	*
6	30	<1.0	<1.0	<1.0	0.9	6.0	3.6	4.4	3.1	4.1	7.2
7	30	<0.5	11	24	34	16	262	<0.5	<0.5	<0.5	60
8	30	<0.5	4.8	1.0	1.0	1.6	<0.5	2.9	<0.5	1.6	<0.5
9	50	<2.0	<2.0	<2.0	<2.0	<2.0	<2.0	<2.0	<2.0	<2.0	<2.0
10	50	<1.0	<1.0	<1.0	<1.0	<1.0	<1.0	<1.0	<1.0	*	*
11	50	<0.5	3.2	3.2	<0.5	<0.5	<0.5	<0.5	<0.5	<0.5	3.2
12	50	<0.5	1.5	2.9	3.7	2.2	2.2	1.5	2.2	1.8	1.8
13	50	<0.5	5.7	<0.5	<0.5	<0.5	5.7	<0.5	2.9	<0.5	5.7
14	80	<0.5	*	*	0.6	*	*	<0.5	*	*	*
15	80	<0.5	*	*	0.8	*	*	<0.5	*	*	*
16	80	<0.5	*	*	1.9	*	*	<0.5	*	0.2	*

* Not sampled.

(table 9) Epirubicine concentrations (mean ±S. D. and range) in samples following 30 and 50 mg dosages

Dose of Epirubicin	Instillation fluid U1 (mg)	Recovered instillation fluid U2 (mg)	Irrigation fluid U3 (mg)	Initial urine voided U4 (mg)
30 mg (n=17)	26.7 ± 2.3 21.4 - 31.2	20.8 ± 4.9 8.5 - 31.0	1.4 ± 0.2 0.1 - 6.75	0.03 ± 0.04 0.002 - 0.14
50 mg (n=15)	45.8 ± 5.8 37.0 -56.6	36.6 ± 5.8 22.8 -45.4	1.4 ± 0.8 0.31- 3.54	0.29 ± 0.37 0.004 - 1.97

Penetration of Epirubicin into the blood during and following intravesical instillation was low. The plasma concentrations were close to the detection limit of the assay except for one patient in whom higher levels were observed.

Results of the amount of drug recovered in the instillations fluid, irrigation fluid and in the initial urine voided are given in table 9. (results of this part of the study were published earlier by Mross et al, 1987).

DISCUSSION

The likelihood of detecting early carcinoma in situ of the bladder has been considerably increased by cytological examination of the urinary sediment and transurethral multiple mucosal biopsies. The clinical management, however, remains a problem. Secondary carcinoma in situ seems to have a rather good prognosis, probably due to the early detection of TiS and early application of intravesical chemotherapy whereas primary CiS behaves less favourable (Fukui et al., 1987). It has been documented that CiS can be eradicated by TUR alone (Utz et al., 1970) and that CiS can remain 'quiet' for a long period without treatment (Weinstein et al., 1980). On the other hand radical cystectomy and urinary diversion on initial diagnosis is recommended in patients with multifocal or diffuse TiS and in patients with prostatic involvement (Utz and Farrow, 1984). In patients with negative biopsy of the bladder neck and prostatic urethra promptly started intravesical chemotherapy may cure the disease or may at least arrest the disease and delay cystectomy. Long-term benefit of intravesical chemotherapy for TiS has been reported (Jakse, 1984). Thus, bladder carcinoma in situ per se does not require cystectomy (Soloway, 1984). Possible progress must be strictly monitored by cystoscopic assessment at 3-month intervals and urinary cytology determination every month after intracavitary treatment for 6 months, thereafter, in case of negative cytology every three months together with cystoscopy.
BCG (Bacille Calmette-Guérin) has been found to be most effective for the treatment of TiS of the bladder. The complete response rate of 83 per cent in a combined experience with 180 patients with TiS TCC of the bladder treated with different BCG-strains (Armand-Frappier, Connaught and Tice) is higher than that reported with any other intravesical agent (table 10).

table 10
BCG Therapy for Carcinoma In Situ

Primary Author	Number	Complete Response	Percent
Morales	7	5	71
Lamm	23	22	96
Herr	47	34	72
Brosman	33	31	94
deKernion	19	13	68
Schellhammer	6	6	100
S. W. O. G. *	64	51	80
Total	180	149	83

* Current data from ongoing studies.
(Adopted from D. L. Lamm, 1988)

BCG treatment is burdened with a rate of local (93%) and systemic (40%) side effects (Orihuela et al., 1987). Severe side effects like arthralgia (5%), liver toxicity (3%) and lung infiltrate (2%) are unknown for the intravesically used cytostatic agents (Doxorubicin, Mitomycin-C).
Epirubicin in the present study led to complete remission in 73% (16/22). After a median follow-up of 22 evaluable patients (see table 3) of 18 months (range 14-49 months) only one patient recurred with invasive disease (pT_2), whereas two patients recurred with a lower grade papillary lesion without concurrent carcinoma in situ and three with TiS G_3. No patient developped metastatic disease. Local side effects were mild, one patient required stop of treatment because of hypotension, most probably due to an allergic reaction.
Plasma concentrations of Epirubicin after intravesical instillation were close to the detection limit of the essay (0.5 ng/ml plasma) except for one patient (262 ng/ml 90 minutes after

instillation). Epirubicin therefore can be safely
applied intravesically as long as there is not an
extended area of denuded mucosal bladder wall
after surgery and there is some delay between
surgery and first instillation (7 days).
Epirubicin is a therapeutically active drug for
the treatment of carcinoma in situ of the bladder
and leads to complete remission in a rate comparable to BCG without the high incidence of local
side effects reported for immunotherapy with BCG.
Epirubicin may be used as an alternative to BCG
for the treatment of carcinoma in situ of the
bladder. Because of the proven therapeutic
efficacy of the drug, studies to examine the
efficacy of the drug as an adjuvant after TUR of
papillary lesions of the bladder (T_a/T_1) are
indicated.

Acknowledgement:
This work was supported in part by SUWO (Foundation for Research in Urology, Rotterdam).

LITERATURE:

1. Farrow GM, Barlebo H, Enjoji M, Chisholm G,
    Friedell GH, Jakse G, Kakizoe T, Koss LG,
    Kotake T, Vahlensieck W: Transitional cell
    carcinoma in situ. Denis L, Niijima T, Prout
    G, Schröder FH (eds.) In: Progress in Clinical
    and Biological Research Vol 221: Developments
    in Bladder Cancer, Alan R. Liss, New York: 85-
    96, 1986
2. De Voogt HJ, Rathert P, Beyer-Boon ME:
    Carcinoma in situ. In: De Voogt HJ, Rathert P,
    Beyer-Boon ME (eds.): Urinary cytology.
    Springer Verlag, Berlin-Heidelberg-New York:
    127-133, 1977
3. Jakse G, Hofstädter F, Leither G, Marberger H:
    Carcinoma in situ of the urinary bladder. A
    diagnostic and therapeutic challenge. Urologe
    (A) 19: 93-99, 1980

4. Second International Consensus Development Conference on Guidelines for Clinical Research in Bladder Cancer, Hakone, Japan, September 28-30, 1987

5. Riddle PR, Chisholm GD, Trott PA, Pugh RCB: Flat carcinoma in situ of the bladder. Br. J. Urol 47: 829-833, 1976

6. Koss LG: Mapping of the urinary bladder: its impact on the concepts of bladder cancer. Hum. Pathol. 10: 533-54, 1979

7. Kulatilake AE, Chisholm GD, Olsen EGJ: In situ carcinoma of the urinary bladder. Proc. R. Soc. Med. 63: 95-97, 1970

8. Farrow GM, Utz DC, Rife CC: Morphological and clinical observations of patients with early bladder cancer treated with total cystectomy. Cancer Res. 36: 2495-2501, 1976

9. Yates-Bell AJ: Carcinoma in situ of the bladder. Br. J. Surg. 58: 359-364, 1979

10. Melamed MR, Voutsa NG, Grabstald H: Natural history and clinical behaviour of in situ carcinoma of the human urinary bladder. Cancer 17: 1533-1545, 1964

11. Koss LG, Melamed MR, Kelly RE: Further cytologic and histologic studies of bladder lesions in workers exposed to para-aminophenyl; progress report. J. Natl. Cancer Inst. 43: 233-234, 1969

12. Farrow GM, Utz DC, Rife CC, Greene LF: Clinical observations on sixty-nine cases of in situ carcinoma of the urinary bladder. Cancer Res. 37: 2794-2798, 1977

13. Hargreave TB: Carcinoma in situ. In: Zingg EJ and Wallace DMA (eds.) Bladder Cancer, Springer Verlag, Berlin-Heidelberg-New York-Tokio: 141-159, 1985

14. Jakse G, Hofstädter F, Marberger H: Intracavitary Doxorubicin hydrochloride therapy for carcinoma in situ of the bladder. J. Urol. 125: 185-190, 1981

15. Glashan RW: Intravesical therapy with Adriamycin in urothelial dysplasia and early carcinoma in situ. Can. J. Surg. 25: 30-32, 1982

16. Edsmyr F, Andersson L, Esposti PL: Intravesical chemotherapy of carcinoma in situ in bladder cancer. Urology Suppl. 23, 3: 37-39, 1984

17. Soloway MS, Ford KS: Subsequent tumor analysis of 36 patients who have received intravesical Mitomycin-C for superficial bladder cancer. J. Urol. 130: 74-78, 1983

18. Jauhiainen K, Sotarauta M, Permi J, Alfthan O: Effect of Mitomycin-C and Doxorubicin instillation on carcinoma in situ of the urinary bladder. Eur. Urol. 12: 32-27, 1986

20. Herr HW, Pinsky CM, Whitmore WF Jr, Sogani PC, Oettgen JF, Melamed MF: Long-term effect of intravesical Bacillus Calmette-Guérin in flat carcinoma in situ of the bladder. J. Urol 135: 265-267, 1985

21. Brosman SA: The use of Bacillus Calmette-Guérin in the therapy of bladder carcinoma in situ. J. Urol. 134: 36-39, 1985

22. deKernion JB, Huang MY, Lindner A, Smith RB, Kaufman JJ: The management of superficial bladder tumors and carcinoma in situ with intravesical Bacillus Calmette-Guérin. J. Urol. 133: 598-601, 1985

23. Lamm DL: BCG in carcinoma in situ and superficial bladder tumors. In: Schröder FH, Klijn JGM, Kurth KH, Pinedo HM, Splinter TAW, De Voogt HJ (eds.) EORTC GU Group Monograph 5: Progress and Controversies in Oncological Urology, Alan R. Liss, New York: 497-507, 1988

24. Orihuela E, Herr HW, Pinsky CM, Whitmore WF Jr: Toxicity of intravesical BCG and its management in patients with superficial bladder tumors. Cancer 60: 326-333, 1987

25. Ganzina F: 4' Epi-doxorubicin, ε new analogue of Doxorubicin: a preliminary overview of preclinical and clinical data. Cancer Treat. Rev. 10: 1-22, 1983

26. Hurteloup P, Cappelaere P, Mathé G, and EORTC Clinical Screening Group: Phase-II clinical evaluation of 4' Epi-doxorubicin. Cancer Treat. Rep. 67, 4: 337-341, 1982

27. Denis L, Bouffioux C, Bultinck J, Van Cangh P, Bono A, Bollack C, Calais da Silva F: Epirubicina: phase II chemoresection study. Acta Medica: 183-188, 1988

28. Weenen H, Osterop APRM, VAn der Poort SEJM, Lankelma J, Van der Vijgh WJF, Pinedo HM: Analysis of Doxorubicin, 4-Epi-doxorubicin and their metabolites by high pressure liquid chromatography. J. Pharm Sci (in press)

29. Mross K, Maessen, Van der Vijgh WJF, Bogdanowicz JF, Kurth KH, Pinedo HM: Absorption of Epi-doxorubicin after intravesical administration in patients with in situ transitional cell carcinoma of the bladder. Eur J. Cancer Clin. Oncol. 23, 5: 505-508, 1987

30. Morales A, Eidinger D, Bruce AW: Intracavitary Bacillus Calmette-Guérin in the treatment of superficial bladder tumors. J. Urol. 116: 180-183, 1976

31. Schellhammer PF, Ladaga LE: Bacillus Calmette-Guérin for therapy of superficial transitional cell carcinoma of the bladder. J. Urol 135: 261-264, 1986

32. Fukui I, Yokokawa M, Sekine H, Yamada Y, Hosoda K, Ishiwata D, Oka K, Sarada T, Tohma T, Yamada T, Oshima H: Carcinoma in situ of the urinary bladder: Effect of associated neoplastic lesions on clinical course and treatment. Cancer 59, 1: 164-173, 1987

33. Utz DC, Hanash KA, Farrow GM: The plight of the patients with carcinoma in situ of the bladder. J. Urol. 103: 160-164, 1970

34. Weinstein RS, Miller AW III, Pauli BU: Carcinoma in situ: Comments on the pathobiology of a paradox. Urol. Clin. North. Am. 7: 523-231, 1980

35. Utz DC, Farrow GM: Carcinoma in situ of the urinary tract. Urol. Clin. North. Am. 11, 4: 735-740, 1984

36. Jakse G, Hofstädter F, Marberger H: Topical Doxorubicin hydrochloride therapy for carcinoma in situ of the bladder: a follow-up. J. Urol. 131: 41-42, 1984

37. Soloway MS: Editorial comment, J. Urol. 131: 42, 1984

38. Lamm DL: BCG Immunotherapy in Bladder Cancer. Urology Annual, Vol 1: 69-86, 1985

Uro-Oncology: Current Status
and Future Trends, pages 61–70
© 1990 Wiley-Liss, Inc.

TREATMENT OF LOW AND HIGH RISK SUPERFICIAL BLADDER TUMORS (SBT)

H. Rübben, F.-J. Deutz*, F. Hofstädter**, W. Meyers***, Members of the RUTTAC****

Dept. Urology, Knappschaftskrankenhaus Bardenberg, *Dept. Urology, **Pathology, ***Documentation and Statistics Med. Faculty, RWTH Aachen, FRG ****Knappschaftskrankenhaus Bardenberg: R. Ostwald, St.- Elisabeth-Krankenhaus Neuwied: B. Opelt, Elisabeth-Krankenhaus Straubing: K. Naber, Marienhospital Marl: H. Möllhoff, Kreiskrankenhaus Deggendorf: P. Carl, Allg. Krankenhaus GmbH Viersen: J.E. Wildberger, St.-Elisabeth-Krankenhaus Köln Hohenlind: H.J. Peters, Städt. Krankenhaus Pforzheim: G. Leusch

After complete transurethral resection (TUR) of SBT 50 to 70% of the tumors recur and up to 25 % show a tumor progression of stage or grade (UICC 1978, HENEY et al. 1982, LUTZEYER et al. 1982, DALESIO et al. 1983).

There are three explanations for this high incidence of recurrences under discussion:

-multifocal dysplasia or carcinoma in situ beside the visible tumor,

-intraoperative tumor spread and implantation,

-continuous exposition of carcinogens.

Intravesical instillation of cytotoxic or immunotherapeutic agents is able to treat on carcinoma in situ and to destroy floating tumors cells as demonstrated in clinical trials and animal experiments (JAKSE et HOFSTÄDTER 1980, SOLOWAY et MARTINO 1976).

Aim of a study of the Registry for Urinary Tract Tumors (RUTTAC) was to analyse the prophylactic effect of intravesical application of adriamycin after TUR and to answer the question, whether adjuvant intravesical therapy is necessary in all cases of SBT, or is depending on the stage and the grade of the disease.

Study design: 268 consecutive patients with SBT entered the study between July 1979 and August 1981. All patients received 50 mg per 50 ml saline two hours before complete TUR of all visible tumors. After histological confirmation of the diagnosis and stratification in primary and recurrent disease patients were devided at random into three groups:

Group A: no further treatment after TUR,

Group B: adriamycin 50 mg/50 ml for two hours twice weekly for six weeks,

Group C: adriamycin twice weekly for six weeks, twice monthly for 4.5 months and after that once monthly for a total of one year.

Criteria for exclusion were: no histological slides being available for reclassification by the pathologist of the registry, palpable tumor after TUR by bimanual palpation, previous radiotherapy of a bladder tumor, intravesical chemotherapy in the last six months before entering the study and another malignant tumor beside the SBT.

All patients underwent random biopsies and cytological examination of a bladder wash out at the time of TUR. The follow up included cystoscopy every three months in the first two years and every six months thereafter. All visible lesions seen at cystoscopy were resected and examined by light microscopy.

Results: Age and sex of the 220 evaluable patients separated by treatment are listed in table 1.

Table 1: Age and sex separated by treatment
(pat. (1) = patients entered the trial
pat. (2) = patients evaluable after 5 years)

Group	pat.(1) (n)	pat.(2) (n)	mean age (y)	male (%)
A	89	82	67.5	77.2
B	91	79	64.2	78.6
C	88	59	64.1	79.4
total	268	220	65.3	78.3

About 20 % of the tumors invaded the lamina propria (T1), only less than 7 % of the tumors were poorly differentiated and about one fourth were recurrent tumors (s. table 2).

Table 2: Initial stage, grade, as well as primary and recurrent tumors separated by treatment.

Group	Ta (%)	G1 (%)	G2 (%)	G3 (%)	primary (%)
A	77	59	34	7	74
B	84	60	36	4	75
C	81	65	28	7	67
total	80	61	33	6	72

About 11 % of the patients in all treatment groups showed concomitant moderate or severe dysplasia in random biopsies and 17 % moderately well or poorly differentiated tumor cells by cytological examination of the bladder wash out after TUR of the tumor. 82 % of the tumors were less than 3 cm in largest diameter and 30 % showed multifocal growth pattern. The frequency of recurrences after 5 years is not reduced by short or long term chemoprophylaxis. The recurrence rate (HENEY et al. 1982, DALESIO et al. 1983), the tumor progression-rate (13.1 %) and the corrected and uncorrected 5 year-survival rate (5.1 % and 7.9 % respectively) remains unchanged by adjuvant therapy as well (s. table 3).

Table 3: Frequency recurrences (fr), recurrence rate (rr) (number of recurrences per 100 patients-months), tumor progression (pr) and survival rate (DOD) within 5 years after TUR (fr: curves are estimated by Kaplan Meier method and compared by using the Mantel Cox test; rr, pr, dod: chisquare test of homogeneity for contingency tables: $p > 0.35$).

Group	fr (%)	rr (%)	pr (%)	DOD (%)
A	61	2.7	12.0	7.2
B	55	2.5	16.0	5.3
C	57	2.3	10.7	1.8
total	59	2.5	13.1	5.1

There are no different results regarding selected subgroups of the study-population.
Systemic side effects could not be observed. Chemical cystitis was the most common local side effect in 38 % of the cases, but could be treated sufficiently by spasmoanalgetics in more than 90 % of the cases. Local side effects influenced on the completion of the adjuvant treatment. 11 % did not follow the study design in group A and B respectively, but 33 % in group C.

Discussion: Intravesical chemoprophylaxis has become accepted worldwide to reduce the high frequency of recurrences after TUR of SBT. Up to now prospective randomized studies including a sufficient number of patients did not clearly demonstrate the value of this adjuvant therapy with regard to the frequency of recurrences (s. table 4).

Tab. 4: Results of phase III studies on intravesical therapy after TUR (rec = recurrences)

substances	n	rec (%)	months follow up	authors
Adriamycin	86	52		KURTH
Epodyl	85	30	24	et al., 1984
TUR only	69	54		
Thiotepa	105	74		SCHULMAN
VM26	99	76	24	et al., 1982
TUR only	104	65		
Thiotepa	38	56		BYAR et
Pyridoxin	33	65	48	BLACKARD,
TUR only	50	72		1977
TUR only	27	52	18	LAMM, 1985
BCG Pasteur	30	20		
TUR only	123	36		
Thiotepa x 1	124	45	24	MRC, 1985
Thiotepa x 5	120	37		
Thiotepa	30	55	24	KOONTZ
TUR only	27	78		et al., 1981
Mitomycin	28	7	21	HULAND et
TUR only	32	75		OTTO, 1983
TUR only	29	48	60	KURTH et al.,
Epodyl	31	35		1983
TUR only	31	80	60	PROUT et al.,
Thiotepa	30	79		1983
Thiotepa		65		
Adriamycin	184	75	48	LLOPIS et al.,
Cisplatin		60		1985
Adriamycin	73	55	16	MORI et al.,
BCG-Pasteur	88	14		1986
BCG-Pasteur	43	75	24	PINSKY et
TUR only	43	95		al., 1985

The reported data concerning progression and metastases are very limited and the effectiveness of intravesical therapy cannot be demonstrated by these results. The progression rate of 20 % within 21 months in HULAND's study in the controlgroup is higher than expected in other protocols; most of the patients in this group showed a low risk SBT (s. table 5).

Table 5: Tumorprogression (progr.) and survival (DOD) after intravesical therapy in phase III studies

substances	n	progr. (%)	DOD (%)	months follow up	authors
TUR	31	10	19		GREEN et
Thiotepa	25	8	4	46	al., 1984
VM26	33	15	3		
Adriamycin x12	79	12	7		RÜBBEN et
Adriamycin x27	59	16	5	60	al., 1988
TUR	82	11	2		
TUR	45	7	2	60	PROUT et
Thiotepa	45	9	4		al., 1983
TUR	30	20	3	21	HULAND et
Mitomycin	28	4	-		OTTO, 1983

Therefore it is advisable to select those patients in advance who are at risk to get a recurrence or tumor progression and may profit from adjuvant therapy. In a retrospective study of the Registry for Urinay Tract Tumors of the RWTH Aachen (RUTTAC 1986/15) 2779 primary SBT (no recurrences) have been analysed after TUR. Depth of infiltration and grade of differentiation are essential prognostic parameters concerning the survival rate. After stratification according to these factors no other prognostic parameter like sex, age, tumorsize, location, multiplicity, growth pattern and concomitant anomalies (WHO 1973) could be shown to affect the survival function significantly. Only concomitant carcinoma in situ has some effect on the survival of patients treated by TUR ($p = 0.02$ logrank test). According to the T- and G-category at least three different prognostic groups of patients with SBT could be selected. The corrected five year survival for Ta and T1 G1-2 tumors after TUR alone is observed between 81 and 95 % of the cases. Patients with T1 G3-4 carcinomas show a significantly worse prognosis (s. table 6).

Tab. 6: Corrected 5 year survival depending on stage and grade (RUTTAC 1987)

stage	n	5-y. survival
Ta	1746	95 %
T1 G1-2	596	81 %
T1 G3-4	437	64 %

Survival of patients with superficial bladder tumors is determined by local progression of the disease or distant metastases deriving from the primary bladder tumor. An analysis of patients without local progression shows that Ta tumors metastasize in less than 1 %: In contrast T1 G3-4 tumors metastasize without local progression in more than 20 % of the cases (s. table 7).

Tab. 7: Frequency of metastases of patients with recurrent Ta-1 tumors without local progression

stage	n	metastases
Ta	196	0.7 %
T1 G1-2	59	13.9 %
T1 G3-4	31	22.1 %

These data show that topical therapy is unnecessary in the majority of patients with low risk tumors with respect to the rate of metastases and local tumorprogression. But if performed in high risk tumor patients, it has to be very effective (s. table 8).

Tab. 8: Tumor progression after TUR depending on stage and grade of the tumor (RUTTAC 1987)

stage	n	progression
Ta	1746	4.4 %
T1 G1-2	569	18.8 %
T1 G3-4	437	31.4 %

Survival is influenced significantly by the local progression as demonstrated in table 9.

Tab. 9: 5 year survival depending on tumor progression (RUTTAC 1987).

stage	n	progression (%)	
		yes	no
Ta	1746	77.7	95.3
T1 G1-2	485	78.6	82.9
T1 G3-4	365	38.7	67.6

Therefore any form of therapy after TUR should reduce the frequency of recurrences; but it is more important, that it is effective to control local progression and prevent metastases.

Concerning these results the following therapeutic regimen may be advisable:

-Ta G1, primary, no carcinoma in situ: The frequency of recurrences is low (less than 50 %) and in case of a recurrence the tumor becomes invasive in less than 5 % of the cases. Therefore we see no indication for adjuvant therapy after TUR in this selected group of patients (RUTTAC, 1986).

-Ta G2-3, T1 G1-2, recurrent, concomitant carcinoma in situ: The frequency of recurrences ranges between 50 and 70 % and up to 20 % of the tumor progression can be observed. In this group of patients adjuvant therapy after TUR may be indicated, especially in those cases with carcinoma in situ (ALTHAUSEN et al., 1976, SOLOWAY, 1978, JAKSE, 1981).

-T1 G3, concomitant carcinoma in situ: The clinical course of 129 patients was reevaluated by the RUTTAC: 31 underwent cystectomy and 98 were treated by TUR. Only 40 to 60 % of the patients survived five years regard less the therapy. This observation indicates, that not the intravesical recurrence but micrometastases, already present at the time of first treatment, are decisive for the poor prognosis (POCOCK ET AL., 1982, RÜBBEN et al., 1981, RUTTAC, 1985). Therefore a pilot study was initiated in 1982 to analyse the effect of an adjuvant systemic chemotherapy after TUR of T1 G3 tumors (FAGG et al., 1984, SOLOWAY et al, 1981, RHAGAVAN et al., 1985).

45 patients with T1 G3 and T2 transitional cell carcinoma entered the trial. After complete TUR of the tumor patients received three courses of cisplatinum 70 mg/qm or methotrexate 40 mg/qm plus cisplatinum 60 mg/qm plus vinblastine 3 mg/qm plus adriamycin 30

mg/qm in a monthly interval. After follow-up of 30 months 3 patients died; the death was related neither to the tumor progression, nor to the therapy. 2 patients died from tumor progression. Another 4 patients showed tumor progression and radical cystectomy has been performed. Three patients showed a T1 G3 tumor again and cystectomy was suggested but refused by two patients. After another three cycles of cisplatinum these patients were histologically free of disease. 9 patients got a noninvasive and well differentiated recurrence and were treated by TUR (s. table 10).

Tab. 10 Adjuvant systemic chemotherapy after complete TUR of T1 G3 and T2 bladder carcinomas after a follow up of 30 months

follow up	n
recurrences	18
progression	6
cystectomy	5
dead of disease	2
dead overall	5
total number of patients	45

If these preliminary results can be confirmed in a randomized trial, it might be possible to improve survival and avoid radical cystectomy in selected patients with high risk superficial bladder tumors.

To conclude our results we feel that with regard to progno stic parameters (stage, grade, carcinoma in situ) the appro priate use of "wait and see", adjuvant intravesical therapy and more aggressive treatment after TUR of SBT is rather indicated than general practice of chemoprophylaxis.

Literatur

ALTHAUSEN, A.F., G.R. PROUT, J.J. DALY (1976). Non-invasive papillary carcinoma of the bladder associated with carcinoma in situ. J. Urol. 116: 575

DALESIO, O., C.C. SCHULMAN, R. SILVESTER, M. DEPAUW, M. ROBINSON, L. DENIS, P. SMITH, G. VIGGIANO (1983). Prognostic factors in superficial bladder tumors. J. Urol. 129: 730

FRAGG, S.L., P. DAWSON-EDWARDS, M.A. HUGHES, T.N. LATIEF, E.B. ROLFE, J.W.FIELDING (1984). Cis-diamminedichloroplatinum (DDP) as initial treatment of invasive bladder cancer. Brit. J. Urol. 56: 296

HENEY, N.M., B.N. NOCKS, J.J. DALY, G.R. PROUT JR., J.B. NEWALL, P.P. GRIFFIN, T.L. PERRONE, W.A. SZYFELBEIN (1982). Ta and T1 bladder cancer: Location, recurrence and progression. Brit. J. Urol. 54: 152

JAKSE, G., F. HOFSTÄDTER (1980). Intravesical doxorubicin hydrochloride in the management of carcinoma in situ of the bladder. Eur. Urol. 6: 103

JAKSE, G. (1981). Intracavitary doxorubicin hydrochloride treatment for carcinoma in situ of the urinary bladder. Eur. Urol. 7: 68

LUTZEYER, W., H. RÜBBEN, H.H. DAHM (1982). Prognostic parameters in superficial bladder cancer - an analysis of 315 cases. J. Urol. 127: 250

PINSKY, C.M., F.J. CAMACHO, D. KERR, N.L. GELLER, F.A. KLEIN, H.A. HERR, W.F. WHITMORE jr., H.F. OETTGEN (1985). Intravesical administration of bacillus Calmette-Guerin in patients with recurrent carcinoma of the urinary bladder: Report of a prospective, randomized trial cancer treatment. Report 69:1

POCOCK, R.D., B.A.J. PONDER, J.P. O'SULLIVAN, S.K. IBRAHIM, D.F. EASTON, F.J. SHEARER (1982). Prognostic factors in noninfiltrating carcinoma of the bladder: a preliminary report. Brit. J. Urol. 54: 711

RAGHAVAN D., B. PEARSON, P. DUVAL, J. ROGERS, M. MEAGHER, R. WINES, H. MAMEGHAN, J. BOULAS, D. GREEN (1985). Initial intravenous cis-platinum therapy: improved management for invasive high risk bladder cancer? J. Urol. 133: 399

RUTTAC, Registry for Urinary Tract Tumors RWTH Aachen (1985). 9. Arbeitssitzung, Verh. Dtsch. Ges. Urol. 9

RUTTAC, Registry for Urinary Tract Tumors RWTH Aachen, FISCHER, N., H. RÜBBEN, W. LUTZEYER (1986). Intravesikale Chemorezidivprophylaxe superfizialer Blasenkarzinome mit Adriamycin. Verh. Dtsch. Ges. Urol. 9

RÜBBEN, H., H.H. DAHM, W. LUTZEYER (1981). Rezidivhäufigkeit und Tumorprogression superfizialer Harnblasenkarzinome. Urologe A 20: 211

SOLOWAY, M.S., C. MARTINO (1976). Prophylaxis of bladder tumor implantation. Urol. 7: 29

SOLOWAY, M.S. (1978). Cis-diamminedichloroplatinum (II) (DDP) in advanced urothelial cancer. J. Urol. 120: 716

SOLOWAY, M.S., M. IKARD, K. FORD (1981). Cis-diamminedichloroplatinum (II) in locally advanced and metastatic urothelial cancer. Cancer 47: 476

UICC (1978), Union Internationale Contre le Cancer: TNM-Classification Malignant tumors, Geneva

Uro-Oncology: Current Status
and Future Trends, pages 71–79
© 1990 Wiley-Liss, Inc.

FOLLOW UP OF PATIENTS RECEIVING TREATMENT FOR SUPERFICIAL
BLADDER CANCER WITH MITOMYCIN C AND BCG

Mark S. Soloway

Department of Urology, University of Tennessee,
Memphis, and Baptist Memorial Hospital, Memphis,
Tennessee. Address: 956 Court, Box 10,
Memphis, TN 38163

Bladder cancer represents a heterogeneous group of
neoplasms ranging from low grade, papillary, noninvasive
tumors to those which are high grade and deeply involve the
muscle wall of the bladder. The prognosis differs dramatically among these different types of tumors. The group of
tumors for which intravesical chemotherapy or immunotherapy
are indicated are those which are confined to the mucosa or
lamina propria and may be grade I-III. Tumors which are
high grade (grade III), flat, and confined to the mucosa
are termed carcinoma in situ. The initial task faced by
the clinician who has diagnosed a patient with superficial
bladder cancer is the eradication of all existing tumors in
the bladder and the prevention of subsequent neoplasms.

Following initial tumor resection, the likelihood that
a patient will develop a subsequent bladder tumor varies
from 30% to 80% and is dependent upon the number of initial
tumors, the grade, stage, and prior history of tumors.
Patients who have already developed several tumors are, of
course, more likely to continue to develop them unless an
attempt is made to alter the neoplastic diathesis occurring
in the urothelium. Patients with multifocal tumor, those
in whom mucosal biopsies from normal-appearing urothelium
contain severe dysplasia or carcinoma in situ, and those in
whom a cytology following the transurethral resection is
positive, are very likely to develop a subsequent tumor
despite adequate resection of the initial tumor(s).

Intravesical therapy is designed to either eradicate
tumor which persists in the bladder following biopsy or

transurethral resection (treatment) or prevent subsequent recurrence after all tumor has been resected (prophylaxis). The rationale for the use of intravesical therapy has been elaborated in other articles (Soloway, 1980; Soloway, 1987; Herr, 1987).

When intravesical therapy is used for treatment, the drug is usually instilled weekly for six to eight weeks. A marker will be present, either in the form of visible tumor or a positive cytology, and response can be determined after a course of therapy by repeat endoscopy and cytology.

On the other hand, if all endoscopically visible tumor has been resected and if a post resection cytology is devoid of tumor cells, intravesical therapy is used as prophylaxis. Such a schedule may consist of weekly therapy for four to six weeks and possibly followed by monthly instillations. A variety of schedules have been used, however, for prophylaxis. Effectiveness is based on failure to develop a subsequent neoplasm in a given period of time. An accurate idea of a drug's efficacy in this situation can only be obtained by comparing the patient's pre-intravesical therapy recurrence pattern to that after treatment, or in large trials, by comparing the time to recurrence interval between a treated and nontreated group, or by comparing two regimens. It is critical that the patients are stratified according to appropriate prognostic factors.

MITOMYCIN C

Mitomycin C (MMC) has been used for several years for the intravesical treatment and prophylaxis of superficial bladder tumors. The absorption of Mitomycin C following intravesical instillation is low, probably because its molecular weight is relatively high. Myelosuppression is sufficiently rare that there is no need to monitor the patients' blood counts during treatment.

I have used intravesical Mitomycin C for treatment of residual tumor in 80 patients. Mitomycin instillation was initiated 7-14 days following transurethral biopsy or incomplete resection of stages Ta, Tcis, or T1 bladder cancer. All patients had a history of bladder cancer and most had multiple recurrences. The majority had received

intravesical Thiotepa as treatment or prophylaxis and continued to develop tumor despite this agent. It was thus
felt that further transurethral resection as the only
treatment was ineffective and an alternative would be an
intensive course of intravesical chemotherapy in an attempt
to eliminate or reduce the frequent need for transurethral
resections. In patients at high risk for developing a muscle invasive tumor, MMC was offered as an alternative to
proceeding directly to cystectomy.

All patients started on MMC were requested to restrict
fluids for eight hours prior to intravesical instillation.
40 mg. MMC was diluted in 40 cc. of sterile water to produce a final concentration of 1 mg./ml. The instillation
time was two hours. Cystograms were not performed, as I
feel that vesicoureteral reflux is not a contraindication
to MMC instillation.

The criteria for a complete response in these patients
who received MMC as treatment included no tumor at the
three-month follow up cystopanendoscopy, negative biopsies
from selected or random sites, and no tumor cells identified from the bladder washing cytology specimen. Patients
who had any evidence of tumor, either a positive cytology,
biopsy, or visible neoplasm, were considered failures and
usually proceeded to alternative treatment which varied,
depending on the stage and grade of the tumor.

The average follow up for these 80 patients is 40
months. Fifty-four (67.5%) have been followed a minimum
of three years and 27 (34%) have been followed at least
five years with the longest eight years. The initial stage
was Ta in 41 patients (51%), TCis in 21 (26%), and T1 in 18
(23%).

Fifteen of the 41 patients (37%) who had an initial G
II - G III Ta lesion had a complete response. During the
subsequent period of follow up, only 15 (13%) of those who
had an initial complete response at three months eventually
had a cystectomy, and only one of the 15 (7%) subsequently
developed a tumor which invaded the muscle. None of these
complete responders have died from bladder cancer. On the
other hand, six of 26 (23%) of those who did have persistent tumor at the first response evaluation required a
cystectomy and four (15%) developed a tumor that invaded
the muscle. Three of these 26 failures (11%) eventually

died of bladder cancer.

It is of interest to note the pathology at the time of cystectomy for the eight patients with initial Ta tumors who required this procedure 6 to 39 months after the first dose of MMC. The stage in three of the eight was pT1 and two had pT2 tumors. Tumor in two patients was limited to the prostatic urethra or ducts and one patient had no tumor in the cystectomy specimen.

Multifocal carcinoma in situ was another indication for treatment with intravesical MMC. Twenty-one patients received eight weeks of MMC and at the first three-month evaluation, 33% had no tumor (CR). Only one (14%) subsequently had a cystectomy among the complete responders and this is the only patient who developed a tumor with muscle invasion. He eventually died of bladder cancer and was the only one of the complete responders to do so. On the other hand, 8 of the 14 (57%) nonresponders had a cystectomy, although only two (14%) developed a T2 tumor. Fortunately, none of these patients have died of bladder cancer.

Among the patients with CIS who eventually had a cystectomy from 3 to 63 months after MMC, only two of the nine had tumor limited to carcinoma in situ. Five had muscle invasive lesions and two had tumor limited to the prostatic ducts.

Eighteen patients with T1 lesions were given a treatment course of MMC and eight (44%) had a complete response. Only one (5%) of these complete responders subsequently had a cystectomy and none died of bladder cancer. There were 10 who had evidence of persistent tumor following the treatment course of MMC and three (30%) had a cystectomy and an equal number had muscle invasion and died of bladder cancer. Thus, although all of these patients would have been candidates for cystectomy in the hands of some who believe that patients with G II - G III, T1 bladder cancer is an indication for cystectomy, only four (22%) of the 18 who were given a treatment course of MMC had a cystectomy. The pathology at the time of cystectomy was pT2 in two patients, Cis in one, and no tumor in one.

Thus, in looking at the entire group of 80 patients who received MMC for treatment, 26% have had a cystectomy while 15% have subsequently developed a tumor which has been at least pT2. Seven of the 80 patients (9%) died of bladder cancer.

In summary, it appears that in this high-risk group of patients with superficial bladder cancer MMC may be effective in reducing the frequency of subsequent tumor, preventing some individuals from developing muscle invasive bladder cancer, and possibly reducing the number of patients who die of bladder cancer. Since this was not a prospective randomized trial comparing Mitomycin C to a TUR-only group, it is impossible to draw these conclusions from this analysis. One thing is apparent, however. The likelihood of retaining the bladder is much greater if a patient has a complete response than if they have evidence of tumor at the first three-month evaluation. Thus, it is my feeling that if there is persistent tumor at this interval, a change in treatment should be seriously considered.

BACILLUS CALMETTE-GUERIN (BCG)

BCG has been the only new intravesical agent introduced during the last five years. Although there are a number of strains of BCG that have been used, namely the Pasteur, Tice, Connaught, and the Dutch RIVM strain, there is no evidence that there is a difference in efficacy among these strains. Randomized trials have not been performed, however, to document this point. Repeated intravesical instillation of BCG produces an impressive inflammatory response and has been demonstrated to eradicate residual bladder cancer and, in patients in which BCG is used for prophylaxis, prevent the development of subsequent tumors (Morales, 1984; Lamm et al., 1980). To date, there have been only two large prospective randomized trials to compare the efficacy of BCG and chemotherapy and the results differ. The Southwest Oncology Group compared the use of BCG to Adriamycin, both for prophylaxis and treatment, and found BCG to be superior for both indications (Crawford et al., 1985). A large prophylaxis trial conducted in The Netherlands indicates no difference in treatment or toxicity between intravesical BCG, using the RIVM strain, and Mitomycin C (Debruyne et al., 1988). Many of the patients had low grade, Ta tumors and thus would not have had a recurrence without subsequent treatment. The entry of these patients may have diluted a difference between the agents. The trial is being repeated with both the Tice and RIVM strain.

I have used BCG in 55 patients with stages Ta, Tcis, and T1 bladder cancer. This is a relatively heterogeneous group, since prior to initiation of BCG, all patients did not have documentation whether residual tumor was present. Thus, they cannot be divided into treatment and prophylaxis.

The Tice strain of BCG was used and patients received one ampule dissolved in 60 ml. weekly for six consecutive weeks. Treatment was initiated approximately one week following biopsy or transurethral resection of the bladder tumor. No patient received dermal scarification. Reevaluation for response was six weeks following the last dose and the criteria for response was the same as had been utilized for Mitomycin C.

Twenty-two of the 55 patients (40%) developed tumor after receiving MMC and almost all of the remainder had received prior Thiotepa.

The average follow up is 20 months. Only nine (16%) have been followed more than three years and none have been followed more than five years.

Twenty-two patients had multifocal G II-III Ta bladder tumors prior to initiation of BCG. At the first three-month evaluation, 14 (64%) had a complete response and none of these subsequently required a cystectomy, developed an invasive bladder cancer, or died of bladder cancer. Eight (36%) had evidence of persistent tumor, either endoscopically visible, observed on biopsy, or had a positive cytology at the first three-month evaluation. One of these patients subsequently had a cystectomy and two developed an invasive bladder tumor. None died of bladder cancer.

There were 19 patients with multifocal carcinoma in situ and in this instance, none had eradication of all disease and all had a positive cytology prior to initiation of BCG. Eleven (58%) had a complete response at the first three-month evaluation and only one of these CRs (9%) have had a cystectomy, although three have developed muscle invasive disease. None died of bladder cancer. Of the eight who failed (42%), two of the eight have had a cystectomy and one developed a muscle-invasive bladder cancer. None of the patients died of bladder cancer.

Fourteen patients had tumor which invaded the lamina propria, T1, prior to initiation of BCG. Six (43%) had a complete response and in the follow up period, only one (17%) has had a cystectomy and this was for a tumor which invaded the muscle. None of the patients died of bladder cancer. Of the eight failures, 37% developed at least a T2 lesion. The only two deaths in the BCG-treated group had T1 tumors prior to initiation of BCG.

Thus, of the 55 patients who received BCG, 31 (60%) had a complete response and only two (6%) have had a cystectomy. This compares with 6 of the 24 (25%) failures. Seven of the failures (29%) have subsequently had a muscle invasive tumor and two (8%) died of bladder cancer.

It is of interest to compare the results of these 55 patients with the 104 patients who received BCG and were reported by Kavoussi et al. (1988). 37.5% were indicated to be tumor-free after six BCG instillations with 70% having no evidence of disease after 12 doses of BCG. Fourteen percent had a cystectomy and six percent died of metastatic disease.

SUMMARY

The approach that I have followed for patients with recurrent superficial transitional cell carcinoma of the urinary bladder has generally been to perform a thorough endoscopic evaluation of the bladder with appropriate evaluation of the prostatic urethra as well as the upper urinary tract, and if it is felt that the neoplasm is confined to the bladder (and possibly the mucosa of the prostatic urethra), then all obvious tumor should be resected and a three-month trial of intravesical therapy instituted. Based upon the results presented, the response at the first three-month evaluation has major prognostic importance. Those patients who had no evidence of tumor at this first three-month evaluation were less likely to have a subsequent cystectomy or die of bladder cancer than those who had evidence of persistent tumor. Among the 80 patients who received a treatment course of MMC, 13% of the complete responders compared to 34% of those who failed had a subsequent cystectomy, and among the 55 patients who received

BCG, 6% of the complete responders compared to 25% of the failures had a subsequent cystectomy during the follow up interval. Indeed, part of this difference can be explained by the gradual adherence to the philosophy that if there is persistent high grade tumor or a high grade tumor develops following an adequate treatment course of MMC or BCG, cystectomy is indicated in order to avoid the development of a tumor which invades into the muscle.

Nonetheless, it is evident from this report that in patients who fail Mitomycin C, yet have a tumor which is confined to the mucosa or lamina propria, a trial of BCG should be considered.

Many of the patients who developed a tumor following MMC instillations had a complete response with six weeks of BCG and a majority of those patients remain free of tumor.

The low death rates among the MMC patients, 9%, and the BCG patients, 4%, indicate that this approach is safe. This is true only if the urologist is absolutely certain he has accurately staged the patient. I always review the pathology material myself and I believe this is a practice all urologists should consider.

It must be emphasized that while monitoring patients who have had an excellent response to intravesical therapy, bladder washing cytology must be an integral part of the follow up. Transitional cell carcinoma of the prostatic urethra is not unusual in patients who have been successfully treated for urothelial malignancy of the bladder. We have yet to have a patient with a high grade tumor in the prostatic urethra which has not been detected by cytology. It is my feeling that if the tumor is confined to the mucosa of the prostatic urethra, one might consider transurethral resection and intravesical therapy; however, if there is any indication that tumor has spread into the prostatic ducts, cystoprostatectomy and urethrectomy is the treatment of choice.

REFERENCES

Crawford ED, Lamm DL, Montie JE, Scardino PT, Grossman B, Stanis IK, Smith JA, Sullivan JW (1985). Intravesical adriamycin for recurrent superficial bladder cancer:

a Southwest Oncology Group protocol. J Urol 133:213A.

Debruyne FMJ, Vandermeijden APM, Gebores ADH, Franssen MPH, Von Leeuwen MJW, Steerenberg PA, De Jong WH, Ruitenberg JJ (1988). BCG (RIVM) versus mitomycin intravesical therapy in superficial bladder cancer. Urology (supplement) 31:20-25.

Herr HW (1987). Intravesical therapy: a critical review. Urol Clin N Amer 14:399-404.

Kavoussi LR, Torrence RJ, Gillen DP, Hudson MA, Haaff EO, Dresner SM, Ratliff TL, Catalona WJ (1988). Results of six-weekly intravesical bacillus calmette-guerin instillations on the treatment of superficial bladder tumors. J Urol 139:935-940.

Lamm DL, Thor DE, Harris SC, Renya JA, Stogdill VD, Radwin HM (1980). Bacillus calmette-guerin immunotherapy of superficial bladder cancer. J Urol 124:38-42.

Morales A (1984). Long term results and complications of intracavitary bacillus calmette-guerin therapy for bladder cancer. J Urol 132:457-459.

Soloway MS (1987). Selecting initial therapy for bladder cancer. Cancer (supplement)60:502-513.

Soloway MS (1980). Rationale for intensive intravesical chemotherapy for superficial bladder cancer. J Urol 123:461-466.

Uro-Oncology: Current Status
and Future Trends, pages 81–86
© 1990 Wiley-Liss, Inc.

Percutaneous BCG perfusion of the upper urinary tract for
carcinoma in situ

U.E. Studer, G. Casanova, R. Kraft, E.J. Zingg

Department of Urology and Institute of Pathology, University of Bern, Inselspital, 3010 Bern,
Switzerland

INTRODUCTION

Intravesical administration of Bacillus Calmette-Guérin (BCG) is an effective therapy for flat carcinoma in
situ (Tis) of the bladder (Brosman, 1982; Herr et al.,
1983; Lamm, 1985; deKernion et al., 1985; Catalona et al.,
1987; Ackermann et al., 1986). While the importance of a
systemic host reaction to intravesical instillation is unknown and might either be a concomitant effect or a necessity for the therapeutic efficacy of BCG (Droller, 1986;
Ratliff and Gillen, 1986), the direct contact of BCG with
the diseased urothelium seems to be important: persistance
of ureteral or prostatic carcinoma in situ after successful
intravesical BCG therapy has been observed (Herr and Whitmore, 1987; Herr et al., 1986; Studer, 1987). This prompted
us to use BCG in the upper urinary tract for carcinoma in
situ.

PATIENTS AND METHODS

Between January 1986 and May 1987, 10 renoureteral
units of 8 patients were perfused with BCG. Their mean age
was 74 (66–86) years. All had a long history of urothelial
cancer, treated previously by repeated transurethral resections and intravesical instillations (n=7), and/or by radical cystectomy (n=3); one patient also underwent a nephroureterectomy on the contralateral side for invasive urothelial cancer of the renal pelvis, and two patients had ear-

lier had an organ-preserving open resection of a renal pelvis cancer in solitary kidneys.

All patients showed positive urine cytology during follow-up examinations. In the 5 non-cystectomized patients, the multiple random biopsies of the bladder mucosa and of the prostatic urethra were negative. In all patients the ureters were intubated with 7 Fr catheters and cytology of collected urine and/or washouts was positive. In 7 of 8 patients, the uretero-pyelogrammes showed no tumors.

Under ultrasound control, a percutaneous nephrostomy tube was placed under local anesthesia. An unobstructed flow from the renal pelvis to the ileal conduit or the bladder was checked under fluoroscopy. 360 mg of immune BCG Pasteur F were dissolved in 150 ml of 0.9 % saline. The flask was placed 20 cm above the kidney of the resting patient (figure 1). After filling the pyeloureteral system with 10-15 ml of the BCG solution, a continuous flow of approx. 1 ml per minute (= 15 to 20 drops per minute) was maintained. The perfusion was stopped after 2 hours. The patients received ampicilline prophylactically and were kept at the hospital for one night. This was repeated at weekly intervals for a total of 6 perfusions (= 1 treatment course). If 6 weeks later cytology remained positive, a further treatment course was started.1

FIGURE 1

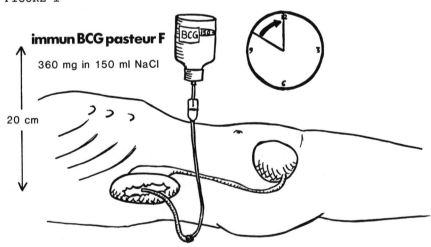

immun BCG pasteur F
360 mg in 150 ml NaCl

20 cm

RESULTS

5 patients had a single course of 6 BCG perfusions after which carcinoma in situ could no longer be found by cytology during an observation period of 12 to 24 months. In one of these, persisting papillary tumors were resected in the ureters (Table 1). 2 patients had bilateral perfusions and required several courses until cytology became negative and remained so for 12 and 15 months respectively. One of these showed a recurrent bladder cancer (T1 G3) one year later. In one patient the treatment was stopped after the first perfusion for severe septicemia.

TABLE 1.

4 patients	1 BCG course	cytology negative for 12-24 months
1 patient	1 BCG course	disappearance of Cis, persistence of papillary tumor
1 patient	2 BCG courses, left 2 BCG courses, right	cytology negative for 15 months, recurrence in bladder
1 patient	3 BCG courses, left 1 BCG course, right	cytology negative for 12 months
1 patient	premature stop after 1 BCG perfusion	severe septicemia

The side effects were comparable to those seen after BCG installation into the bladder: fever up to 38.6°C, fatigue and dysuria, pollakisuruia for 1 to 3 days. No significant change in serum creatinine, no systemic spread of BCG (miliaris), no major granulomatous renal masses and no urothelial cancer along the nephrostomy track have so far been observed.

DISCUSSION

A durable response of carcinoma in situ of the renal pelvis to topical BCG was probably first reported in 1985 by H. Herr (Herr, 1985): he performed renal autotransplantation with direct pyelovesical anastomosis followed by intravesical BCG.

BCG perfusion of the upper urinary tract must be considered as an experimental treatment. All the patients reported in this series had undergone previous surgery for urothelial cancer and were unwilling, unfit or unable to undergo further surgery. This is also reflected by this patient group's mean age of 74 years, and in half of the patients, a nephroureterectomy would have resulted in uremia, necessitating chronic hemodialysis. Interestingly, despite the poor patient selection, the percutaneous BCG perfusion did not result in major complications, except for the patient who developed septicemia. Repeated fluoroscopic monitoring of proper drainage of the pyeloureteral system towards the bladder or ileal conduit seems to be important, as well as a low perfusion pressure produced by only slightly elevating the flask containing the BCG solution (20 cm). Fever and chills during the first night are common, and the additional risk of septicemia may justify a stay at the hospital for the first night. It is unknown if a lower dosage of BCG would show less side effects. The dosage chosen by us (360 mg in 150 ml NaCl perfused during 2 hours) is arbitrary. It corresponds to the concentration of BCG usually used for treatment for carcinoma in situ in the bladder (120 mg BCG of the Pasteur strain dissolved in 50 ml NaCl).

Although never observed in our small series of patients, it is unknown if large granulomatous renal masses, which have occasionally been observed after intravesical BCG application, might occur more frequently when BCG is perfused through the renal pelvis (Schellhammer, 1987; Stanisic et al., 1986). The additional potential risk, that this form of treatment might spread urothelial cancer cells along the nephrostomy tube, has also never been observed.

Nevertheless, since multifocal carcinoma in situ is treated less frequently by radical cystectomy combined with resection of the distal ureters because of the successful use of intravesical BCG applications, it might be that carcinoma in situ of the upper urinary tract, mainly the distal ureters, may become an increasing problem in the future: According to H. Herr, ureteral carcinoma in situ after successful intravesical BCG therapy may occur in up to 29 %

of cases (Herr and Whitmore, 1987). This high incidence stresses the need to find new organ-preserving treatment possibilities. One of these could become the BCG perfusion of the upper urinary tract, provided our encouraging, preliminary results can be confirmed by others.

REFERENCES

Ackermann D, Schnyder M, Bandelier D, Studer UE (1986). Traitement des tumeurs superficielles de la vessie par le bacillus de Calmette-Guérin (BCG). J Urol (Paris) 92:33-38.

Brosman SA (1982). Experience with Bacillus Calmette-Guérin in patients with superficial bladder carcinoma. J Urol 128:27-30

Catalona WJ, Hudson MA, Gillen DP, Andriole GL, Ratliff TL (1987). Risks and benefits of repeated courses of intravesical Bacillus Calmette-Guérin therapy for superficial bladder cancer. J Urol 137:220-223.

Droller MJ (1986). Bacillus Calmette-Guérin in the management of bladder cancer (Editorial). J Urol 135:331-333.

Herr HW, Pinsky CM, Whitmore WF Jr, Oettgen HF, Melamed MR (1983). Effect of intravesical Bacillus Calmette-Guérin (BCG) on carcinoma in situ of the bladder. Cancer 51:1323-1326.

Herr HW (1985). Durable response of a carcinoma in situ of the renal pelvis to topical Bacillus Calmette-Guérin. J Urol 134:531-532.

Herr HW, Pinsky CM, Whitmore WF Jr, Sogani PC, Oettgen HF, Melamed MR (1986). Long-term effect of intravesical Bacillus Calmette-Guérin on flat carcinoma in situ of the bladder. J Urol 135:265-267.

Herr HW, Whitmore WF Jr (1987). Ureteral carcinoma in situ after successful intravesical therapy for superficial bladder tumors: incidence, possible pathogenesis and management. J Urol 138:292-294.

deKernion JB, Huang M-Y, Lindner A, Smith RB, Kaufman JJ (1985). The management of superficial bladder tumors and carcinoma in situ with intravesical Bacillus Calmette-Guérin. J Urol 133:598-601.

Lamm DL (1985). Bacillus Calmette-Guérin immunotherapy for bladder cancer. J Urol 134:40-47.

Ratliff TL, Gillen D (1986). Requirement for thymus-dependent immune response for the inhibition of intravesical mouse bladder tumor growth. J Urol 135:122A.

Schellhammer PF (1987). Letter to the Editor. Re: Intravesical Bacillus Calmette-Guérin therapy and associated
granulomatous renal masses. Stanisic et al. J Urol
137:315.

Stanisic TH, Brewer ML, Graham AR (1986). Intravesical Bacillus Calmette-Guérin therapy and associated granulomatous renal masses. J Urol 135:356-358.

Studer UE, Ackermann D, Schnyder v Wartensee M (1987). Im-
munotherapie bei oberflächlichen Harnblasentumoren. In
Sommerkamp H, Altwein JE, Klippel KF (eds): "Urologische
Onkologie I" München Bern Wien San Francisco: W. Zuck-
schwerdt Verlag, pp 129-135.

Uro-Oncology: Current Status
and Future Trends, pages 87–99
© 1990 Wiley-Liss, Inc.

OVERVIEW OF SYSTEMIC TREATMENT OF BLADDER CANCER AND RESULTS WITH M-VAC THERAPY

Alan Yagoda

Solid Tumor Service, Department of Medicine,
Memorial Sloan-Kettering Cancer Center, New
York, New York 10021

INTRODUCTION

Of the estimated 46,400 new urothelial tract tumors in the United States in 1988, approximately 65%-75% will present initially with local disease compared to 13% with regional and 20% with distant metastases (Silverberg et al., 1988). These malignancies account for 4.7% of all tumors, 6.8% in males and 2.5% in females, and for 0.2% or 10,400 deaths annually. Although the 5-year survival in white men has increased between 1960-63 and 1984 from 50% to 73%, respectively, this increase is due in part to earlier diagnosis of superficial non-muscle invading benign papilloma, and papillary and flat carcinoma-in-situ (CIS).

During the past 15 years there has been a systematic evaluation of single agents and multi-drug regimens for therapy of advanced disease; only recently have prospective randomized phase III trials been undertaken to define more precisely the efficacy of cytotoxic agents. It must be understood that enhanced antitumor activity attributed to many combination drug regimens, particularly those which contain effective agents when used singly, in limited non-randomized, so called extended phase II trials, can be misleading. However, when sufficient numbers of cases from multiple trials are culled from the literature, the 95% confidence intervals (95% CI) may be of value in determining those combinations which should be explored in prospective phase III trial.

With the recognition that transitional cell carcinoma

TABLE 1. Advanced Urothelial Tract Cancer: Stage Migration in Five Protocols in 13 Years

	ADM	ADM+ CTX	DDP	DDP+ CTX	M-VAC
No. Patients	31	20	30	23	121
Age (yrs)	63	57	63	58	62
Males (%)	74	70	76	82	88
KPS (%)	60	70	80	80	80
Prior Irradiation (%)	96	90	76	62	53
Prior Chemotherapy (%)	55	30	21	8	10
Ileo-Conduit (%)	50	55	27	39	30
Dx-Protocol (mos)	32	13	26	23	<10
Protocol-Death (mos)	4	8	6	7	13

of the renal pelvis, ureter, urinary bladder, urethra, and prostatic ducts are chemotherapeutically responsive tumors, patient selection and entry criteria for phase II trials have improved, so much so that some of the improvement in response rates and survival durations when compared to older studies, may simply reflect stage migration--the silent statistician (Feinstein et al., 1985). An example of this phenomenon with regard to patient selection for phase II trials is illustrated in Table 1. In five studies spanning 13 years at Memorial Hospital, the Karnofsky Performance Status (KPS) increased, the number of patients who had received prior radiation therapy and chemotherapy decreased, as did the time from diagnosis (DX) to protocol. Most investigators have found slightly better results in such good-risk compared to poor- risk (low KPS, extensive prior therapy, etc.) cases. Stage migration may also account for the difference in response found in a 1983 (Soloway et al.) and a 1986 (Hillcoat et al.) study of cisplatin (DDP) in advanced bladder cancer. The former cooperative group trial noted a 21% while the latter showed a 33% complete (CR) and partial (PR) remission rate.

LITERATURE REVIEW

Table 2 outlines results of 20 single agents in treatment of patients with advanced urothelial tract cancer (Yagoda, 1987). The most active drugs are DDP and methotrexate (MTX) with remission in 30% each (95% CI 25%-35%). It is still unclear if high-dose MTX is superior to the

standard low-dose of 40 mg/m2 administered weekly. In 57
patients given doses >100 mg/m2 with citrovorum factor, 45%
(95% CI 32%-58%) achieved CR + PR. The data for carboplatin, although not complete, are somewhat disappointing
except when the drug is given as a continuous infusion for
24 hours (Yagoda, 1987; Creekmore et al., 1986). Adriamycin (ADM) and vinblastine (VLB) induce response in 17% of
cases. A new investigational agent gallium nitrate has
demonstrated some antitumor activity, even in a limited
number of cases previously treated with DDP (Crawford et
al., 1983). However, bolus administration proved too toxic

TABLE 2. Single Agents for Advanced Urothelial Tract
Cancer

	Pts.	% CR + PR	(95% CI)
Cisplatin	320	30	(25-35)
Methotrexate	236	29	(23-35)
10-Deaza-aminopterin	15	20	(0-40)
Adriamycin	238	17	(12-22)
Gallium nitrate	41	17	(5-39)
bolus	26	27	(10-44)
infusion x 5 days	15	0	(0-20)
5-Flourouracil	141	17	(11-25)
Vinblastine	38	16	(4-28)
Vincristine	42	14	(3-27)
Mitomycin-C	42	13	(3-23)
Hexamethymelamine	24	13	(0-27)
Teniposide	212	12	(8-16)
Amsacrine	61	12	(4-20)
Carboplatin	80	11	(3-19)
bolus	61	8	(1-15)
infusion x 1 day	19	21	(3-40)
Etoposide	47	2	(0- 6)
Mitoxantrone	28	0	(0-10)
Cyclophosphamide	26	7	(0-17)
Dichloromethotrexate	20	0	(0-15)
Sparfosic acid	18	0	(0-16)
Diaziquine	16	0	(0-17)
Neocarcinostatin	16	0	(0-17)
Bisantrene	13	0	(0-20)

and few patients tolerated three doses: Utilizing a less
toxic schedule, a five-day continuous infusion, no activity

was found. (Sternberg et al., 1988a). Other agents which
have some antitumor activity include mitomycin-C, amsa-
crine, and possibly hexamethylmelamine and 5-fluorouracil.
Of importance, few patients (<5%) achieved CR status.

TABLE 3. Combination Regimens

	Pts.	%CR + PR
ADM	218	17
+ 5-Fluorouracil	103	39
+ Teniposide + Mitomycin-C	29	48
+ Teniposide	29	27
+ Bleomycin	7	0
+ Cyclophosphamide	56	23
+ 5-Fluorouracil (FAC)	58	19
+ Bleomycin	23	33
MTX	236	29
+ Vinblastine	47	40
+ Mitomycin-C	16	31
+ Vincristine + Bleomycin	22	32
+ Adriamycin + Cyclophosphamide	38	39
DDP	320	30
+ Adriamycin	142	51
+ Adriamycin + Cyclophosphamide	354	46
+ Cyclophosphamide	113	25
+ Dichloromethotrexate	49	47
+ Methotrexate	166	32
+ Methotrexate + Vinblastine (CMV)	62	42
+ Methotrexate + Vinblastine + Epirubicin (M-VEC)	53	72
+ Methotrexate + Vinblastine + Adriamycin (M-VAC)	121	72

As stated previously, most combinations (Table 3)
offer little more than that which can be obtained with the
single most active component of the multi-drug regimen
(Yagoda, 1987). Combinations that seem to be somewhat more
active, particularly in inducing CR, are DDP + ADM, DDP +
ADM + cyclophosphamide (the CISCA regimen), DDP + MTX, DDP
+ MTX + VLB (the CMV regimen), MTX + VLB + epirubicin + DDP
(the M-VEC regimen) (Reuther et al., 1987), and MTX + VLB +
ADM + DDP (the M-VAC regimen). At this time, it is difficult to determine if any one of these regimens is superior,

and only after prospective randomized phase III trials are
completed will a clear superiority become evident. Studies
comparing CISCA versus M-VAC (Logothetis et al., 1988), and
M-VAC to MTX or DDP, each used singly, have been initiated.
In a randomized trial comparing MTX versus MTX + DDP,
median survival was almost identical for both arms, 7.2 and
8.7 months, respectively, as was response, 45% for the
combination versus 33% for DDP alone, a non-statistically
significant difference (Hillcoat et al., 1986). Similarly,
while randomized studies of ADM + DDP and of CISCA have
consistently noted higher remission rates compared to
single agent therapy, with relatively small numbers of
cases entered into each arm of the study, statistical
significance was never found.

THE M-VAC REGIMEN

Since previous speakers have discussed results of DDP
+ MTX, CISCA, and CMV (Harker et al., 1985; Meyers et al.,
1988), this paper focuses on the 133 cases at Memorial
Sloan-Kettering Cancer Center who received M-VAC during the
first 3 years of protocol and had a minimum of 2.5 years
follow-up (Sternberg et al., 1988b; submitted). Protocol
criteria required patients to have metastatic (M+) and/or
advanced nodal (N3-4) urothelial tract tumors with bidimensionally measurable parameters for response. There were
217 evaluable disease sites: moreover, cystoscopy with
biopsy, urine cytology, and clinical (T) and surgical/
pathological (P) restaging procedures were performed in 43
of 60 adequately treated primary bladder cases not having
had cystectomy. Protocol eligibility included a KPS >30%,
white blood cell count (WBC) >3500 cells/mm3, platelets
(Plt) >150,000 cells/mm3, serum creatinine <1.7 mg%, blood
urea nitrogen <30 mg%, and/or a creatinine clearance of >50
ml/min. Following hospitalization, the patient was started
on intravenous hydration with D51/2NS and potassium supplement to insure a urinary output >100 ml/hour. MTX in a
dose of 30 mg/m2 was administered on day 1 and on day 2,
ADM 30 mg/m2, VLB 3 mg/m2, and DDP 70 mg/m2 were given with
antiemetics and 12.5 gm of mannitol. In patients having
had >20 Gy in five days to whole pelvis or irradiation to
>2 bone marrow-containing sites, ADM was reduced to 15
mg/m2. Identical doses of VLB + MTX were given together on
days 15 and 22 when the WBC was >2500 cells/mm3, Plt
>100,000 cells/mm3, and there was no evidence of mucositis.
DDP was withheld when the creatinine clearance was <40

ml/min. Although not part of the protocol, 14 (12%)
patients received their initial DDP dose in equally divided
doses on days 2 and 3. Patients having CR and significant
PR were urged to undergo surgical restaging after 3-4
cycles and when no tumor was found, chemotherapy was
stopped; in those having residual disease which could be
completely resected, two more cycles were given.

The median age was 62 years, KPS 80%, and the
male:female ratio was 4.1:1. Three patients had a
non-transitional cell histology, all of whom progressed
with M-VAC therapy. Twelve (10%) patients had had prior
systemic chemotherapy, most having had MTX, VLB, or DDP.
With 5 (4%) patients inadequately treated, there were 124
(93%) and 121 (91%) cases evaluable for survival and
response, respectively.

CR + PR occurred in 72% ± 8%. CR was achieved in 36%
± 9%, of whom 13/44 patients required surgical resection of
remaining residual disease. Median CR response duration
was 21 months, range 8->60, and with 23 (52%) still alive,
survivals at 1-, 2-, 3-, and 4 years were 91%, 68%, 54% and
49%, respectively. PR was noted in 36% ± 9%: median survival was 11 months. There were 6% ± 4% patients who had a
minor response with a median survival duration similar to
PR, 11 months; none lived two years. The median survival
of 27 (22% ± 7%) cases who progressed with M-VAC therapy
was 8 months with 19% alive at 1- and 4% at 2- years.
While there was no difference in response rate by sex or by
prior irradiation, N+ patients fared better than those with
more advanced disease, M+N0. CR was obtained in 33% of 100
M+ versus 52% of 21 N+M0 cases and of more importance,
median survival for the former was 12 months versus 33 for
the latter.

Clinical versus surgical restaging was performed in 32
cases who presented with metastatic and/or primary tumors.
There were 8/23 (35%) patients clinically staged as a PR
who, in fact, were pathologically proven to have CR status.
The staging error, therefore, was similar to that described
for cystectomy series. While objective tumor regression
occurred in all sites (54%-90%), the most responsive
lesions were intra-abdominal lymph nodes and pelvic masses,
subcutaneous nodules and lymph nodes, pulmonary lesions,
and bone (Table 4). Although hepatic metastases frequently

TABLE 4. M-VAC Response by Metastatic Site

	No.	% CR	% PR
Lung	37	24	57
Bone	31	26	32
Liver	15	15	54
Nodes/masses			
in CT scan	72	35	31
by physical	20	20	70

regressed (69%), most were for a short duration and not really of major clinical benefit since the median survival for patients who obtained CR or PR in liver was only 12 months (Table 5). A troublesome relapsing pattern was observed in 15% of responding cases, central nervous system metastasis, half of whom had not relapsed systemically. While the median onset of brain lesions occurred 6-22 months after starting protocol, therapy was ineffective and the median survival was only 2 months.

TABLE 5. M-VAC Responding Sites with Survival in Months

Metastasis	Response	Median
Bone CR	33	
	PROG	8
Lung CR	28	
	PROG	9
Liver	CR	13
	PROG	4
Nodes/masses:		
by CT scan	CR	30
	PROG	9
by Physical	CR	52
	PROG	4

Toxicity was significant with nausea and vomiting being universal despite antiemetic therapy; however, severe (3+) toxicity was distinctly uncommon. Renal dysfunction was noted in 38%, primarily being transient although cumulative persistent renal abnormalities did occur. Myelosuppression was moderately severe with 25% experiencing nadir sepsis and 3% a drug-related death.

There were 38% of cases who had a WBC <2000 cells/mm3 and
20% with a count <1000 cells/mm3. Platelet abnormalities
were less intense with 62% of cases having thrombocytopenia; 21% had 3+ toxicity. In a subsequent study using
granulocyte stimulating factor (G-CSF), doses of >3 ug/kg
given either daily or three times weekly almost totally
ameliorated the WBC nadir, the incidence of sepsis and
requirement for hospitalization and of note, the incidence
of mucositis decreased from 44% to 11% (Gabrilove et al.,
1988)

NEO-ADJUVANT M-VAC

These results in patients with advanced disease
stimulated the use of M-VAC neoadjuvantly in 71 patients
with bladder cancer and 11 with extravesical disease (Scher
et al., 1988a; 1988b; in press)

Criteria for patient entry required NOMO disease with
adequate hematologic, cardiac, and renal function.
Neoadjuvant response criteria for CR was strict and was
defined as no evidence of disease and a negative urine
cytology. When urine cytology was positive or a thickened
bladder wall was found by any non-invasive staging
procedure such as CT scan, physical examination and/or
ultrasonography, the patient was downstaged to a PR. Any
response less than a CR or PR was classified as incomplete
(IR). Clinical restaging was performed generally after 2
cycles and surgical staging after 2-4. While patients were
urged to undergo radical cystectomy, some refused which led
to laparotomy with lymph nodal dissection or sampling and a
partial cystectomy to document CR pathologically.

T3 and T4 disease were present in 60/71 (85%) cases
and 64 (90%) had transitional cell carcinoma. Mixed
histologies were more frequent with extravesical and
urethral tumors. Five cases received 1 cycle, 27 had 2, 8
had 3, 29 had 4, and 2 had >5 cycles. It seemed that the
greatest extent of tumor regression was observed after 3-4
cycles.

Of the 65 cases evaluable for response, clinical
downstaging to T0 occurred in 49% and to TIS in 13%. Urine
cytology converted from abnormal to normal in 54% of 48
evaluable patients; however, when all clinical T staging
parameters for response were evaluated, only 21% achieved

what would be considered total absence of disease (CR) and 39% were considered to have a PR; overall, the CR + PR rate was 60% with 95% CI of 49%-71%.

Of the 45 evaluable cases who underwent surgical restaging, 28 had a radical cystectomy, 12 a partial cystectomy, and 5 were found unresectable. Of note, no patient with an atypical histology achieved CR status. Of the transitional cell carcinoma cases, 11/45 (24% ± 11%) did achieve a pathologically proven CR, and 4 with total disappearance of muscle infiltrating disease still had remaining carcinoma-in-situ. Thirty-one patients had an IR. While there have been no relapses or deaths in the 15 responding cases, 14/30 (47%) with IR already have developed metastases within a median of 11 months (range 7-17), 10 of whom underwent complete resection of residual invasive disease.

TABLE 6. Neo-adjuvant M-VAC: Clinical versus Pathological Staging Accuracy

Clinical	No.	%CR	%PR	%IR
CR	9	78	22	0
PR	15	27	33	40
IR	21	0	0	100

The pre-operative clinical stage was compared with the post-operative pathological stage. Of the 15 T0 cases, 9 were indeed P0 and 1 had only PIS; but 1 was T1 and 4 were P3. Overall, clinical understaging was similar to that described for the advanced disease protocol, approximately 30%. Correlation of the clinical and pathological response was correct in 74% with 18% being understaged (Table 6). In those patients achieving PR status clinically, only 35% were correctly staged indicating a major difficulty in distinguishing fibrosis and/or post-operative changes from viable tumor by the non-invasive staging procedures undertaken. All IR patients were correctly staged.

There are 56% of neoadjuvantly treated patients alive disease-free and of note, 28% still have a functional bladder. The median followup for all 71 cases is 24 months

(range 2-42).   In the remaining patients, 23/33 have
developed M+ disease, 19 (27% of 71 cases) of whom have
died, 11 are alive with disease in the bladder (5), and in
node (N+) and viscera (M+) (3 each).

Results were similar for the extravesical group except
that mixed histologies were more frequent and more
difficulty was noted in determining the clinical stage by
the diagnostic techniques employed.   In fact, the accuracy
of clinical versus pathological staging in the small number
of cases with extravesical disease was inconclusive
suggesting, at this time, that surgery must follow any
neoadjuvant therapy for this group of tumors.

Conclusions from the neoadjuvant studies indicate that
M-VAC can effectively induce CR status in 27%, with an
additional 14% of cases being downstaged to carcinoma-in-
situ.   With 20/71 (28%) of patients still having a
functional bladder, and with 58% still free of disease,
neoadjuvant therapy may be beneficial and in selected cases
may permit bladder preservation.   Patients not responding
(IR) have a distinctly poor prognosis regardless of the
therapeutic maneuver after neoadjuvant therapy; in fact,
most will die suggesting that these non-responsive cases
represent a poor-risk group that will need a more
aggressive approach in the future.   It appears that M-VAC
is not effective against existing carcinoma or against the
prevention of new carcinoma-in-situ, or in forestalling the
development of new invasive disease.   Additionally,
although the numbers of cases are few, M-VAC is ineffective
against mixed and non-transitional cell histologies.
Reliance on clinical staging alone will underestimate the
extent of disease, particularly for extravesical lesions,
and while downstaging may be an important goal, the
ultimate end-point of neoadjuvant chemotherapy must be
survival.   Large prospective randomized trials have now
been undertaken to evaluate M-VAC + cystectomy versus
cystectomy alone, a CMV-like regimen versus no therapy
followed by either irradiation or surgery, and the concept
of bladder preservation using a multi-disciplinary approach
combining chemotherapy + irradiation.

SUMMARY

Cytotoxic chemotherapy is playing an increasingly
important role for advanced disease, and is being properly

evaluated in prospective trials as neoadjuvant therapy. There has been no major undertaking to examine adjuvant treatment, and hopefully randomized studies will be started in the future. There is sparse data concerning the effectiveness of immunological agents for treatment of this tumor, and phase II efficacy studies are needed. Future studies will need to define more accurately the poor-risk group in whom new agents or regimens using a more intensive schedule, perhaps with G-CSF, can be explored as initial therapy.

REFERENCES

Crawford ED, Saiers JH, Baker LH (1983). Treatment of metastatic bladder cancer with gallium nitrate. 13th International Congress of Chemotherapy (abstract)240: 12.1.7/A4, 84.

Creekmore SP, Waters WB, Vogelzang NJ, Micetich KC, Fisher RI (1986). Antitumor activity of 24-hour CBDCA infusions in metastatic transitional cell carcinoma. Proc Amer Soc Clin Oncol (abstract 393) 5:101.

Feinstein AR, Sossin DM, Wells CR (1985). The Will Rogers phenomenon: stage migration and new diagnostic techniques as a source of misleading statistics for survival and cancer. N Engl J Med 312:1604=1608.

Gabrilove JL, Jakubowski A, Fain A, Grous J, Scher HI, Sternberg CN, Yagoda A, Clarkson B, Morore MAS, Bonilla MA, Oettgen HF, Alton K, Bone T, Altrock B, Welte K, Sousa L (1988). A study of human recombinant granulocyte colony stimulating factor in patients with transitional cell carcinoma. N Engl J Med 318:1414-1422.

Harker WG, Meyers FJ, Frehia FS, Palmer JM, Shortliffw LD, Hannigan JF, McWhirter KM, Torti F (1985). Cisplatin, methotrexate and vinblastine (CMV): an effective chemotherapy regimen for metastatic transitional cell carcinoma of the urinary tract: a Northern California Oncology Group study. J Clin Oncol 3:1463-1470.

Hillcoat BL, Raghavan D (1986). A randomized comparison of cisplatin (C) versus cisplatinum and methotrexate (C+M)in advanced bladder cancer. Proc Amer Soc Clin Oncol (abstract 426) 5:110.

Logothetis C, Chong C, Dexeus F, Sella A, Finn L (1988). Preliminary results of a prospective randomized trial comparing CISCA to M-VAC chemotherapy for patients (pts) with advanced transitional cell carcinoma (TCC) of the urothelium. Proc Amer Soc Clin Oncol (abstract

517) 7:134.

Meyers FJ, Palmer JM, Hannigan JF (1988). Chemotherapy of disseminated transitional cell carcinoma. In: Williams RD (ed), Advances in Urologic Oncology (Vol I): General Perspectives. New York: Macmillan Publ. Co; 183-192.

Reuther U, Bauerle K, Rassweiler J, Tripp T, Eisenberger F (1987). Chemotherapy with MVFC in advanced carcinoma of the bladder and upper urinary tract. Proc 4th Europ Conf Clin Oncol and Cancer Nursing (Madrid, November 17, 1987), (abstract 235)4:65.

Scher HI, Yagoda A, Herr H, Sternberg CN, Bosl G, Morse MI, Sogani PC, Watson RC, Dershaw DD, Reuter V, Geller N, Hollander PS, Vaughn ED, Whitmore WF, Fair WR (1988a). Neoadjuvant M-VAC (methotrexate, vinblastine, adriamycin and cisplatin) effect on the primary bladder lesion. J Urol 139:470-474.

Scher HI, Yagoda A, Herr H, Sternberg CN, Morse MJ, Sogani PC, Watson RC, Reuter V, Whitmore WF, Fair WR (1988b). Neoadjuvant M-VAC (methotrexate, vinblastine, adriamycin, and cisplatin) for extravesical urinary tract tumors. J Urol 139:475-477.

Scher HI, Herr H, Sternberg C, Bosl G, Morse M, Sogani P, Watson R, Dershaw DD, Reuter V, Curley T, Darracott V Jr, Whitmore W, Fair W, Yagoda A (in press). Neo-adjuvant chemotherapy for invasive bladder cancer: experience with the M-VAC regimen. Brit J Urol.

Silverberg E, Lubera JA (1988). Cancer statistics. CA 38:5-22.

Soloway MS, Einstein A, Corder MP, Bonne W, Prout GR, Coombs J (1983). A comparison of cisplatin and the combination of cisplatin and cyclophosphamide in advanced urothelial cancer. Cancer 52:767-772.

Sternberg CN, Yagoda A, Scher HI, Bosl GJ, Rosado L (1988a). Phase II trial of gallium nitrate in patients with metastatic transitional cell carcinoma. Proc Amer Soc Clin Oncol (abstract 488) 7:126.

Sternberg CN, Yagoda A, Scher HI, Watson RC, Herr HW, Morse MJ, Sogani PC, Vaughan ED, Bander N, Weiselberg L, Geller N, Hollander PS, Lipperman R, Fair WR, Whitmore WF Jr (1988b). M-VAC (methotrexate, vinblastine, adriamycin and cisplatin) for advanced transitional cell carcinoma of the urothelium. J Urol 139:461-469.

Sternberg CN, Yagoda A, Scher HI, Watson RC, Geller N, Herr HW, Morse MJ, Sogani PC, Vaughan ED, Bander N, Weiselberg L,Rosado K, Smart T, Lin SY, Penenberg D,

Fair WR, Whitmore WF Jr (submitted). M-VAC for advanced transitional cell carcinoma of the urothelium: efficacy and patterns of response and relapse.
Yagoda A (1987). Chemotherapy of urothelial tract tumors. Cancer 60:574-585.

Uro-Oncology: Current Status
and Future Trends, pages 101–106
© 1990 Wiley-Liss, Inc.

INTRAARTERIAL CHEMOTHERAPY FOR BLADDER CANCER

Stephen C. Jacobs, MD and David S. Menashe, MD

Department of Urology

Medical College of Wisconsin
Milwaukee, Wisconsin, USA

INTRODUCTION

Cisplatin(CDDP) has emerged as the single most
active drug in the treatmentof bladder cancer. In this
regard, increasing the therapeutic index ofcisplatin
might lead directly to increasing tumor response rates.
Two techniques recently explored to increase
thetherapeutic index of various drugs include 1) the
continuous infusion of a drug rather than bolus therapy
and 2) the intra-arterial(IA) rather than IV route of
administration. It has been demonstrated that the IA
response rate to CDDP increases from 2-10 fold over the
IV route of the drug for the same disease (1). The
continuous infusion of CDDP has also been shown to
result in an increased tumor cell exposure to the
active drug and to decrease systemic toxicity (2,3).
In the present study a 48 hour continuous IA CDDP
infusion was used as a primary or adjuvant therapy in 30
patients with invasive bladder cancer.

PATIENT SELECTION AND TREATMENT

Thirty patients with T3 or T4 bladder cancer
limited to the pelvis were staged preoperatively with
cystoscopy, deep transurethral biopsy, bimanual
examination, CT scan abdomen and pelvis, bone scan, and
chest x-ray. Bilateral IA infusion catheters were

placed via a percutaneous femoral artery route in 28 patients. Two patients had their catheters placed at the time of laparotomy. The catheter tips were located, whenever possible, just beyond the origin of the superior gluteal artery from the hypogastric artery or in the main trunk of the hypogastric artery. Three patients had unilateral catheter placement on the side of their bladder masses, while 27 patients had bilateral hypogastric artery infusions.

CDDP 75-150 mg/m^2 was administered as a constant IA infusion over 48 hours. Patients were kept at bedrest, hydrated with 150 cc/h NS, and given antiemetics as required. Four patients received 2 courses of CDDP 6-8 weeks apart. If a curative resection was planned, laparotomy with possible tumor resection was performed at 4 weeks.

COMPLICATIONS

Treatment complications were relatively minor. Two hospital acquired lower urinary tract infections were treated with antimicrobials. Nausea occurred in all but 1 patient; vomitting occurred in 18 of the 30 patients and was treated with metoclopramide. Leukopenia (wbc <3000) occurred in 5 patients, but only 1 patient developed wbc <1000. Two patients developed thrombocytopenia with a platelet count <50,000. Three patients suffered creatinine elevations. Peripheral neuropathy in all 4 extremities occurred in 1 patient. Gluteal pain and an ecchymotic discoloration of the buttocks occurred in 1 patient.

The most disabling complications were in 3 patients who suffered lower extremitiy neuropathies consistent with selective S2-4 nerve injury. These required 2-3 months before remission.

EFFECT ON THE BLADDER MASS

Twenty patients could be evaluated for a change in the size of their local bladder mass. This was done by either examination of the resected tumor specimen or by followup cystoscopy and/or CT scan. In 19 of the 20 bladders examined significant tumor necrosis and mass

shrinkage was seen, with 8 bladders being rendered free
of cancer by the IA CDDP. Six of the PO bladders were
in patients with negative lymph nodes, but in 2 cases
the bladders became PO while the lymph nodes were
positive. It appears that the IA CDDP is a reasonable
palliative treatment for pelvic pain, a bulky mass, or
hematuria. Only 1 of the 30 patients died from bladder
hemorrhage and that patient died 10 months following
treatment.

EFFECT ON SURVIVAL

The effects on survival were not as great as would
be desired. Apparently the treatment does not affect N+
disease. There were 15 patients with N+ disease: four
of these patient underwent cystectomy. Three of these 4
died (average survival 13 months) and the only 1 alive
is at only 3 months. Eleven N+ patients did not undergo
cystectomy, but were treated with chemotherapy (usually
MVAC) or radiation therapy. Only 3 of these 11 are
alive: 7 died of their cancers and 1 died of
chemotherapy complications.

In the T3-4 N+ group then, 11 patients died at 14 $\pm$
2 SEM months and only 4 are alive, but they are only 10$^-$
$\pm$ 6 SEM months out.

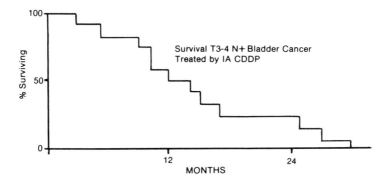

Figure 1.

The T3 N0 patients fared better. Of the 15 T3 N0
M0 patients, 3 were treated without cystectomy (2
palliatively, 1 refused). Two of these 3 died at 2 and
7 months of untreated sepsis and 1 patient remains alive
and well with a functioning bladder. Twelve patients
then underwent an attempt at curative cystectomy. Four
of these patients have died of causes other than bladder
cancer, though 1 died 3 months postop of pulmonary
insufficiency, having never left the hospital. The
other 8 cystectomy patients are all alive with NED at 28
± 8 SEM months.

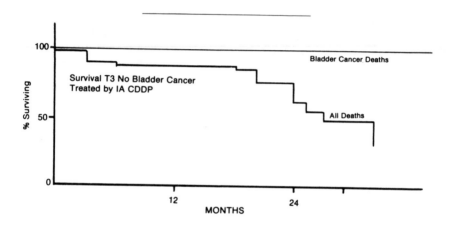

Figure 2.

DISCUSSION

Direct comparison of this series with other series
of IA CDDP treated bladder cancer patients is difficult.
To date none of the series have used similar CDDP
schedules. Maatman et al (4) achieved a 77% CR + PR
rate, but gave a smaller dose (40-75 mg/^{m}2) of IA CDDP

along with cytoxan and adriamycin over only 30 minutes. Wallace et al (5) achieved a 60% CR + PR rate by giving 80-120 mg/^{m}2 over 24 hours. Stewart et al (6) achieved a 67-86% CR + PR rate by giving 25-120 mg/m2 over 2 hours. While the patients are very difficult to directly compare, a clear trend is present showing that IA CDDP has a high response rate in transitional cell carcinoma, but it is probably not high enough for IA CDDP to be uniformly used alone as treatment.

Maatman's series also included cystectomy and the PO rate in the bladder was 23% (4). Our PO rate in cystectomy specimens was equivalent at 40%, showing that in some select patients IA CDDP alone might be sufficient treatment. However, identification of the patients pre-cystectomy is not yet possible.

The N+ patients in the present series have been followed long enough to conclude that while this therapy may provide helpful palliation, it cannot handle N+ disease. Our initial followup of the T3N0 group is very encouraging in that no patient currently has bladder cancer or has died from bladder cancer, though these patients average only 28 months followup and some later deaths are to be anticipated.

In summary, IA CDDP appears to provide good palliation from bleeding and mass effects in bulky bladder cancer patients. This therapy can be delivered with a defined set of side effects that are acceptable. However, even if the bladder is completely freed of malignancy,the patients will die if lymph nodes are positive. For T3N0 patients, pre-cystectomy IA CDDP affords an excellent adjuvant which may prove difficult to improve upon.

REFERENCES

1. Lehane, DE (1984): Intra-arterial cis-platinum in advanced solid tumors. Intra-arterial and Intracavitary Cancer Chemotherapy, SB Howell,ed. Boston, Martinus Nijhoff, pp 111-124.
2. Belliveau,JF, Posner,MR, Ferrari,L (1986) Cisplatin administered as a continuous 5-day infusion: plasma platinum levels and urine platinum excretion. Cancer Treat. Rep. 70:1215-1217.

3. Posner, MR, Ferrari,L, Belliveau, JF, Cummings, FJ, Wiemann, MC, O'Rourke,
   A, Weitberg, AB, Calibers,P (1987) A Phase I trial of continuous infusion cisplatin. Cancer 59:15-18.
4. Maatman, TJ, Montie, JE, Bukowski, RM, Risius, B, Geisinger, M (1986) Intra-arterial chemotherapy as an adjuvant to surgery in transitional cell carcinoma of the bladder. J. Urol. 135:256-260.
5. Wallace, SS, Chuang, VP, Samuels, M, Johnson, D (1982) Transcatheter intra-arterial infusion of chemotherapy in advanced bladder cancer. Cancer 49:640-645.
6. Stewart, DJ, Eapan, L, Hirte, WE, Futter, MG, Moors, DE, Murphy, PG, Irvine, AH, Genest, P, McKay, DE, Evans, WK, Rasuli, P. Peterson, RA, Maroun, JA (1987) Intra-arterial cisplatin for bladder cancer. J. Urol.138: 302-305.

Uro-Oncology: Current Status
and Future Trends, pages 107–114
© 1990 Wiley-Liss, Inc.

THE IMPACT OF CHEMOTHERAPY ON THE SURVIVAL OF PATIENTS WITH
METASTATIC UROTHELIAL TUMORS

Christopher J. Logothetis, Francisco H. Dexeus,
Clayton Chong, Avishay Sella and Sheryl Ogden

Department of Medical Oncology, Section of Genito-
urinary Oncology, The University of Texas M. D.
Anderson Cancer Center, 1515 Holcombe Boulevard,
Box 13, Houston, Texas   77030, U. S. A.

INTRODUCTION

CISCA chemotherapy has been used at M. D. Anderson
Cancer Center for the treatment of metastatic urothelial
tumors. Throughout that time, large numbers of patients
have been treated. Despite the high response rate reported
for adriamycin- and cisplatin-based therapy, its effect on
survival has been disputed by various investigators. The
goal of this brief manuscript is to assess the impact of
CISCA chemotherapy on long-term disease-free survival and
cure rates among patients with metastatic, local-regional,
and resected urothelial tumors at high risk for relapse.

INITIAL CISCA TRIAL

Before the development of cisplatin-based chemotherapy, the
prognosis for patients with metastatic urothelial tumors was
very poor. A clinical trial at M. D. Anderson Cancer Center
assessing the value of VM-26 revealed that patients with
metastatic urothelial tumors had a median 17-month survival.

The dosages of CISCA used are shown on Table 1.

TABLE 1. CISCA

Cyclophosphamide	650 mg/m^2 B.S.A. Day 1
Adriamycin	50 mg/m^2 B.S.A. Day 1
Cisplatin	70 mg/m^2 B.S.A. Day 2

Throughout the study, the full dosage of chemotherapy was maintained and not compromised. Therefore, we can assess the impact on survival of full-dose CISCA chemotherapy as delivered at our institution. At M. D. Anderson Cancer Center, a total of 97 previously untreated patients were treated with the combination of cisplatin, cyclophosphamide, and adriamycin (CISCA) for metastatic urothelial tumors (Logothetis et al., in press 1988).

Tissue from each study patient was available for histologic review, and radiographic studies were available to assess the extent of tumor dissemination. Patients were divided into three groups according to histologic subtype: pure transitional cell carcinoma, mixed cell types, and squamous cell carcinoma (Table 2). The extent of disease spread was divided into local-nodal and visceral.

TABLE 2. CISCA Disseminated Bladder Cancer
Patient Characteristics

Histologic type	Total Patients
TCC	74
Mixed	20
SCC	3
Disease spread	
Local nodal	62
Visceral	35

The response rate of patients with disseminated bladder cancer was highest for those with pure transitional cell carcinoma and those with nodal spread only. Patients with mixed tumors who had visceral involvement had a very low response rate.

TABLE 3.   CISCA
                      Response Rate

Histologic type	Response	
	CR	PR
TCC	39%	31%
Mixed	20%	25%
+SCC	-	33%
Disease spread		
Local nodal	45%	19%
Visceral	20%	12%

+Total 3 patients only

Thirty-five patients achieved a complete remission. For 17 of the 35, the duration of the complete remission was less than 100 weeks. For the 18 patients who maintained a complete remission for longer greater than 100 weeks, the probability of their dying of a second primary tumor, however, was equal to the probality of their dying of recurrent urothelial tumors. Seventy-two percent of the patients in complete remission for longer than 100 weeks have continued to maintain their complete remission. Many patients have now been monitored in excess of five years.

We conclude from this experience with select patients that complete remissions occur frequently with adriamycin- and cisplatin-based chemotherapy delivered at full dosage, and that almost half of the complete remissions are maintained for longer than 100 weeks. In the presence of a complete remission longer than 100 weeks, the likelihood of a patient's remaining disease-free for five years and potentially cured is 72%. The most important predictor for the long-term disease-free survival of these patients was their ability to respond to CISCA chemotherapy.

The results of this trial cannot be compared to the experience of other investigators. This, because of the select nature of the patients treated and the intensity of the therapy. In addition, a relatively high portion of patients with unresectable local-regional disease was included in this trial. These patients had the highest complete-remission rate, suggesting that earlier delivery of therapy may increase the likelihood of achieving a complete remission.

ADJUVANT CISCA TRIAL

Following the preliminary results of this experience, a prospective trial of adjuvant postoperative CISCA chemotherapy was conducted for patients with invasive urothelial tumors. Five courses were delivered at full dose. The selection of five courses was based on our clinical experience in patients with metastatic disease, in which long-term disease-free survival (≥ 100 weeks disease free) was not attained by any patient who had received less than five full courses of CISCA chemotherapy.

All patients in whom a cystectomy was performed at M. D. Anderson Cancer Center throughout the study period were evaluated (Logothetis et al., in press 1988). These patients were divided into three groups: Group I consisted of patients at low risk for relapse (no adverse pathologic findings suggesting a high likelihood of relapse; low risk controls); Group II included patients who were at high risk for tumor recurrence but did not receive adjuvant chemotherapy, because of either patient refusal or medical contraindications for therapy (high risk controls); and Group III consisted of the 71 patients at high risk for recurrence who received adjuvant chemotherapy. The indications for adjuvant chemotherapy included: vascular invasion in the primary tumor, nodal metastases that had been resected, tumor invasion of the prostate or vagina, or extravesicular extension of the tumor. Each of these pathologic findings is associated with an adverse outcome, in both our experience and the experience of other investigators.

TABLE 4. Comparison of disease free survival

		NED/TOTAL %		
I.	Low risk control (Favorable Pathology)	157/206	76%	
	High risk control (Unfavorable Pathology)	23/62	37%	p < .00001
II.	Low risk control (Favorable Pathology)	157/206	76%	
	Adjuvant (Unfavorable Pathology)	50/71	70%	p = .33
III.	High risk control (Unfavorable Pathology)	23/62	37%	
	Adjuvant (Favorable Pathology)	50/71	70%	p = .00012

A comparison of these three populations (Table 4) reveals that the low-risk control group and the high-risk control group had very different long-term disease-free survival rates. This difference in survival confirms the significance of the pathologic findings as predictions of a poor outcome. A comparison between the low-risk controls and those patients with very adverse pathologic findings who received CISCA chemotherapy reveals no statistically significant difference in long-term disease-free survival rates (76% and 70%, P=.33). This, we believe, is the strongest evidence of the effect of adjuvant CISCA chemotherapy. The fact that the similar disease-free survival rates are similar for patients with nodal metastases, urothelial tumor invasion into the extravesicular spaces, and direct invasion of adjuvant organs and for a population with high-grade diffuse superficial disease or minimal muscular invasion can only be explained by a positive effect from the chemotherapy. Futhermore, when the patients at high risk for relapse who did not receive adjuvant chemotherapy were compared to those who received adjuvant chemotherapy, a significant difference in survival rate became evident (70% vs 37%, $\underline{P}$=.00012). This significant difference also supports a positive impact for adjuvant chemotherapy.

All patients in this study population have been monitored for a minimum of two years. Therefore they are beyond the major risk for tumor recurrence. Although tumor may still recur, we believe that this data are now mature and that adequate numbers of patients have been treated to suggest strongly that adjuvant chemotherapy has a positive effect on the outcome of patients with metastatic urothelial tumors.

Unless new and more effective chemotherapy regimens are developed, the most profound impact on disease-free survival is likely to come from the appropriate integration of primary chemotherapy with local therapy (surgery or radiation). The comparison of the relative effectiveness between neoadjuvant (preoperative) chemotherapy and adjuvant chemotherapy needs to be made prospectively. The clinical staging error for patients with bladder carcinoma is notoriously high. Because of this clinical staging error, meticulously controlled trials are required to compare pre- vs postoperative chemotherapy. To address the issue of how best to integrate primary chemotherapy with surgery, a prospective randomized trial is currently underway at our institution comparing preoperative chemotherapy with methotrexate, vinblastine, adriamycin, and cisplatin (MVAC) to a cystectomy followed by postoperative (MVAC) chemotherapy. The results of this trial remain preliminary.

The selection of chemotherapeutic agents for patients with metastatic urothelial tumors remains in question. Recent encouraging reports for methotrexate- and cisplatin-based chemotherapy and cisplatin, methotrexate, and vincristine (MVAC [CMV]) imply that such combinations may have a higher response rate than the one we report for CISCA chemotherapy (Yagoda A., 1986). Because of changes that may have occurred in the natural history of bladder carcinoma and referral patterns of physicians, attributed to the recent enthusiasm for treating this disease, we believe that a prospective trial comparing the MVAC and CISCA regimens is required. To evaluate their relative effectiveness and to confirm the prognostic significance of tumor dissemination and histologic types, we are currently conducting a prospective randomized trial comparing CISCA and MVAC chemotherapy in patients with metastatic unresectable urothelial tumors. The preliminary data reveal no significant difference in response rates and confirm both that patients with nodal disease have the highest complete-remission rate and that histologic type does influence the response to chemotherapy.

TABLE 5. CISCA vs MVAC
Preliminary results of randomized trial

	Partial Response (PR)		Complete Response (CR)	
	CISCA %	MVAC %	CISCA %	MVAC %
Nodal metastasis	2/12 (16)	6/15 (40)	6/12 (50)	6/15 (40)
Visceral metastasis	4/15 (26)	5/16 (31)	0/15 (0)	4/16 (25)
TCC	5/21 (24)	9/24 (37)	4/21 (19)	7/24 (29)
TCC + mixed	1/06 (16)	2/07 (28)	2/06 (33)	3/07 (43)

CONCLUSION

We believe that this retrospective review of the M. D. Anderson Cancer Center experience with CISCA chemotherapy demonstrates a definite survival advantage for patients with metastatic disease who receive CISCA chemotherapy. In addition, we believe that the survival advantage for patients is highest when the therapy is delivered early and is integrated with local therapy. Further major therapeutic advantages and prolongation of survival are likely to be achieved with appropriate integration of systemic and local therapy. The best chemotherapy regimen for patients with metastatic urothelial tumors has yet to be identified, and the most appropriate manner to integrate systemic and local therapy (preoperative vs postoperative) remains unclear.

REFERENCES

Logothetis CJ, Dexeus FH, Chong C, Sella A, Pilat S and
    Ogden S (1988).   CISCA chemotherapy for unresectable
    urothelial tumors: The M. D. Anderson experience.   In
    press to The Journal of Urology.
Logothetis CJ, Johnson DE, Chong C, Dexeus FH, Sella A,
    Ogden S, Terry Smith, Swanson DA, Babaian RJ, Wishnow KI
    and von Eschenbach A (1988).   Adjuvant CISCA chemotherapy
    for bladder cancer: an update.   In press to Journal of
    Clinical Oncology.
Yagoda A (1986).   Chemotherapy for advanced bladder cancer.
    Adv Cancer Ther 87-106.

Uro-Oncology: Current Status
and Future Trends, pages 115–127
© 1990 Wiley-Liss, Inc.

THE EVOLUTION OF ACTIVE CHEMOTHERAPY IN METASTATIC AND
LOCALLY ADVANCED BLADDER CANCER

D.W.W. NEWLING for the E.O.R.T.C. G.U. Group

Consultant Urologist

Princess Royal Hospital, Saltshouse Road
Hull, U.K. HU8 9HE

INTRODUCTION

Over the last 10 years the EORTC GU Group has
investigated a number of agents singly and in combination
in an effort to find the best and safest chemotherapy for
advanced bladder cancer. All the completed studies have
been Phase II but now the scene seems to be set for the
first large scale Phase III study in T3 and T4
non-metastatic disease. In the development of the Group's
strategy cognisance has been taken of other Phase II/III
studies carried out elsewhere in the world and those
apposite to the development of our protocols will be
described in this paper along with the EORTC studies
themselves.

In the early 1970's the majority of urologists were
dissatisfied with the results of surgery or radiotherapy in
advanced bladder cancer which yielded five year survival
rates at best of 42–45% (Clark 1978, Edsmyr et al 1978).

The majority of patients died from metastatic disease
and in approximately half of these there was no evidence of
local disease recurrence. It seemed, therefore, likely
that they had micro metastases present at the time of
curative treatment of the primary and that if some method
could be devised of eliminating these early on in the
management of the cancer then the patient's outlook would,
clearly, be greatly improved.

TABLE 1. Cumulated results of cystectomy with and without preoperative radiotherapy for invasive bladder cancer

	Operative mortality	5 year survival
Partial cystectomy	4%	30%
Simple cystectomy	3% - 10%	35%
Radical cystectomy	4% - 12%	38%
Preoperative radiotherapy and cystectomy	4% - 9%	42%
Preoperative radiotherapy and radical cystectomy	3% - 13%	43%

TABLE 2. Results obtained with radical radiotherapy at the Karolinksa Institute

Survival	Category			Grade	
	T2	T3	T4	G2	G3
		%			%
5 years	31	20	10	26	18
10 years	22	14	4	19	13

Coffey and Isaacs (1979) had demonstrated quite clearly that systemic chemotherapy would be most effective on small groups of cancer cells, such as micro metastases, and it therefore seemed sensible that the ultimate aim of the Group should be to define suitable chemotherapy which would be safe and practical to use in an adjuvant situation along with standard methods of control of the locally advanced disease. It seemed only sensible to the members of the Group that the development of this strategy should take place in three stages. Firstly, there should be a search for effective agents which would eliminate tumor masses. Secondly, these agents had to be acceptable alongside standard local therapy in the patient population in which they were going to be used and thirdly, suitable tests should be undertaken to define the optimal scheduling for these drugs.

The search for active agents commenced in 1976 to a background of a successful Phase II study carried out by the Yorkshire Urological Cancer Research Group which showed that two of the agents identified by Carter and Wasserman (1975) as effective when used singly in bladder cancer viz Adriamycin and 5 Fluorouracil, had shown a response rate of 35% when used in combination (Cross et al 1976). The initial pilot study then carried out by the EORTC Group B looked at this combination of 5 Fluorouracil in a dose of 500 mg/m^2 and Adriamycin 50 mg/m^2 administered at three-weekly intervals for a minimum of four courses in patients with metastatic transitional cell carcinoma. The study in 52 patients showed an overall response rate of 40% but there were only 10% complete responders and the duration of complete response was only three months (EORTC GU Group 1977). The same year that this study was carried out it was decided to embark, with some ambition, on a Phase III study comparing the same dose of Adriamycin plus Cyclophosphamide 400 mg/m^2 with Adriamycin and 5 Fluorouracil in the same concentration as had been employed in the initial pilot study. This study, co-ordinated by Robinson, was not successful. Only 58 patients were entered over a two year period and the study was aborted due to unsatisfactory accrual. Both regimes had proved to be toxic and neither yielded complete response rates of more than 10% (Robinson 1979).

In 1977 Yagoda described eight partial responses in 23 patients with advanced bladder cancer treated with Cisplatinum alone (Yagoda et al 1978). Other workers, Peters and O'Neill (1980) and Soloway et al (1981) confirmed that this was an effective single agent and apparently more effective than any of the previously employed ones. It was suggested by the latter worker that a combination of Cisplatinum and Cyclophosphamide would probably be more effective than Cisplatinum alone. From a study of cell cycle kinetics it seemed likely that the micro metastases could be completely destroyed if that combination was further augmented by Adriamycin as all three agents apparently worked at different stages of the cell cycle and should, therefore, be capable of killing the majority of cells actively dividing. In 1977 the EORTC started its second Phase II study, No.30771 — (Co-ordinator, Mulder JR), looking at this combination in a dose of Cyclophosphamide, 400 mg/m^2, Adriamycin 40 mg/m^2, Cisplatinum 40 mg/m^2 given every three weeks over a period of six months. Forty two evaluable patients were recruited. The complete response rate was 12%, the partial response rate was 28%, the duration of response was five to seven months. The response rate, therefore, with this combination was really no greater than that of Cisplatinum alone (Mulder et al 1982).

At this stage it has to be said that the response criteria in the early Phase II studies carried out by the EORTC were different from those employed subsequently. Evaluable lesions as well as those strictly measurable were accepted and, therefore, the complete response and certainly the partial response rates were probably too optimistic.

Still searching for the most single effective agent in advanced bladder cancer, the next Phase II study (No.30797) was carried out employing the vinca alkaloid, Vincristine. Thirty six evaluable patients were included in this study and there was only one complete response and three partial responses. The toxicity of Vincristine appeared to be greater than with any of the other vinca alkaloids. Bone marrow toxicity led to dose modification in 40% and there was a 30% incidence of neurotoxicity. With these poor responses and this high incidence of toxicity Richards concluded that Vincristine was not an active or suitable agent in this group of patients (Richards et al 1983).

In 1979 a Phase III randomised study of Adriamycin plus 5 FU vs control in patients with T3 N0 N1 M0 bladder tumors after flash radiotherapy and radical cystectomy was embarked upon (No.30784 - Co-ordinator, Martinez Pinero). This complex protocol did not recruit a satisfactory number of patients and was abandoned after two years (Prout et al 1979).

In the next Phase II study the criteria for inclusion and criteria of response were clearly laid down and subsequently these criteria have been used for all the Phase II protocols the Group has carried out since that time (Appendix). In the next study (No.30802) the combination of Cisplatinum and VM26 was investigated. This study which was co-ordinated by Stoter recruited 41 evaluable patients. There was a complete response rate in four, again only 10%, with partial response in another 17 (41%). Once more, the combination of Cisplatinum with another derivative which should, apparently, have been synergistic, had proved negative and the overall response rate was no better than with Cisplatinum used as a single agent (Stoter et al 1984).

In 1980-1982 a Phase III study of Radiotherapy with or without chemotherapy in T3 patients was carried out in Yorkshire investigating the combination of Adriamycin and 5-Fluorouracil with radiotherapy and radiotherapy alone. In this study, a total of 110 evaluable patients were investigated and the results are well known. There was no difference in the two arms of the study. Both groups of patients seemed to fare equally badly and in terms of survival or times to progression (Table 3) no difference was found from the addition of chemotherapy (Richards et al 1983).

At the same time as this study was being carried out and the EORTC was still looking for the most effective single or combination therapy in very advanced disease, Socquet in Belgium (1981) published a study of adjuvant methotrexate given after radical local therapy to the primary tumor in patients presenting with T3 bladder tumors. His initial and subsequent results were unbelievable but sufficiently inspirational for a group in the North East of England under the direction of Hall to carry out a similar study. This study employed methotrexate in an initial dose of 2 g monthly reducing to 1 g monthly after the first dose following radical transurethral resection or partial cystectomy of the primary T3 tumor. At three years, the survival figure of 60% is as good as that obtained by any other modality of treatment. At five years the figure still stands up against either cystectomy or radical radiotherapy or even cystectomy following pre-operative irradiation therapy (Hall et al 1984).

At this stage then it seemed that in Cisplatinum and Methotrexate, the two most active chemotherapeutic agents in advanced bladder cancer had been identified. It also seemed that the overall survival figures were little altered by the local therapy, be it radical TUR, partial cystectomy, total cystectomy or radiotherapy. Nevertheless, the rate of complete response to chemotherapeutic agents was not high enough to be certain that the most active agents had been found or, indeed, to improve the overall survival in these patients presenting with locally advanced disease as much as had been hoped.

TABLE 3. Comparison of survival of patients with T3 carcinoma of bladder following various treatments (%)

	1 year	3 years	5 years
Institute of Urology 1982:			
Radiotherapy	54	44	33
YUCRG:			
Radiotherapy	70	54	37
Institute of Urology:			
Radiotherapy and cystectomy	63	50	45
Socquet:			
Partial cystectomy/methotrexate	98	85	85
North Eastern Study:			
TUR and Methotrexate	81	60	52

By 1982 work in the United States had confirmed that there was a synergistic effect with Cisplatinum and Methotrexate and that the combination of the two was probably more beneficial than Cisplatinum on its own (Yagoda 1982). In 1982 the EORTC embarked upon a study of Cisplatinum and Methotrexate and the scheduling was Cisplatinum 70 mg/m^2 on Day 1 with Methotrexate 40 mg/m^2 on Days 8 and 15 of a 21 day cycle. For the first time in this study the Group saw an improvement in CR and PR over and above Cisplatinum alone and with an overall response rate of some 46% in patients with metastatic disease, 23% of which were complete responders with a median survival of over 18 months. The Group was greatly encouraged and it seemed that the most effective combination thus far had been confirmed (Stoter et al 1986). While encouraged with these complete and partial response rates, it was felt that possibly they could be improved further with less toxicity with a different scheduling of the drugs. Of great concern to the study co-ordinator in this first combination study of Cisplatinum and Methotrexate was the high incidence of marrow toxicity which occurred in 35%. In addition, nephrotoxicity was a problem in 8% of cases. Kaye showed in a series of pharmokinetic studies that Cisplatinum and Methotrexate could be given together on the first day of the cycle with a lessening of bone marrow toxicity and no increase in nephrotoxicity (Kaye et al 1984). It was, therefore, decided that following the success of the initial protocol a second protocol should be carried out using the same combination of drugs giving Methotrexate on Day 1 plus Day 15 of the cycle. This study, protocol 30842, recruited 47 patients and the response was extremely disappointing. From an overall response rate (CR + PR) in the first study of some 46%, the response rate in the second study dropped to 25%. Toxicity was less with higher white cell and platelet nadirs but with a deterioration in the overall response rate, clearly this different scheduling was not the best (Stoter 1987). A careful analysis has been made comparing the two studies by Sylvester and the conclusion is that since patient characteristics and tumor characteristics were identical in the two studies, it can only be the scheduling which has led to a diminution in the response rate (Sylvester 1987). It seems that Methotrexate does not have an opportunity to work when it is given at the same time as the diuresis following Cisplatinum therapy. It seems likely that Methotrexate is washed out of the circulation before it can have a chance to have an effect on the malignant cells.

In the North East of England Hall has continued to look at the combination of Cisplatinum and Methotrexate with local surgery, radical TUR or partial cystectomy and the overall response appears slightly better than the initial study with partial cystectomy and Methotrexate alone (Hall et al 1986). Meanwhile in the EORTC two further Phase II studies have been carried out investigating Mitoxanthrone and TGU as single agents. With Mitoxanthrone there were no responders amongst 28 patients (Van Oosterom 1985) and with TGU the drug was found to be too toxic and without any effect in the first five patients and, therefore was withdrawn by the pharmaceutical company. To bring the situation right up to date the most recently closed Phase II study investigated 4 Epirubicin, 90 mg/m^2 weekly in patients with metastatic disease, when it was found to bring about only a 15% partial response rate with no complete responders but minimal toxicity (Fossa 1988). It was concluded that possibly in a higher dose the drug may be more effective. The ongoing study at present is a randomized study of Cisplatinum and Methotrexate against Cisplatinum, Methotrexate and Vinblastine in patients with metastatic urothelial tumors and this study has already recruited some 70 patients. The results will, hopefully, answer the question as to whether the addition of Vinblastine is of sufficient benefit in this group of patients to warrant the risk of further toxicity.

Meanwhile the EORTC has decided to investigate further the concept of neoadjuvant therapy and a study started in

1985 has looked at first line chemotherapy with a combination of Cisplatinum and Methotrexate in the same schedule as employed in 30821 with Methotrexate being given on Days 8 and 15 of a three week cycle. The patients are assessed after two courses, complete and partial responders go on to receive a further two courses and then whatever local therapy the clinician wishes. In the neoadjuvant setting it is clearly important that this study is continued until a sufficient number of patients have been evaluated after total cystectomy to see if the combination improves overall survival.

As Stoter has recently pointed out (1987), the toxicity of this regime is only acceptable if the response rate is maintained and further evaluation of the first Cisplatinum and Methotrexate study has shown that median response rates for complete responders was 81 weeks, for partial responders 37 weeks and 35 weeks for those where no change was detected in the measurable lesion. Clearly, these are a great improvement on previous studies and the neoadjuvant study at present ongoing will, hopefully, confirm these figures.

The studies from the Memorial Sloan Kettering and other American groups have shown that at the present time probably the most effective combination is Cisplatinum and Methotrexate plus Vinblastine and Adriamycin. It is, however, an extremely toxic combination and in the first study in metastatic disease there was a 7% mortality from drug toxicity. This has improved in later studies. The response rates both in metastatic and locally advanced disease appear at this stage to be slightly better than for the combination of Cisplatinum and Methotrexate together (Sternberg et al 1988). Workers at Stanford (Meyers et al 1985) have achieved similar response rates with the CMV combination of Cisplatinum, Methotrexate and Vinblastine and it is this combination which is being evaluated by the Medical Research Council as a neoadjuvant treatment in a study recently embarked upon in the United Kingdom. Elsewhere in the United Kingdom, in Newcastle, Epic-M, a combination of Methotrexate, Cisplatinum and Epirubicin is being evaluated as neoadjuvant therapy in patients with locally advanced disease and the results, so far, appear to stand up against the M–VAC and CMV combinations.

CONCLUSIONS

Cisplatinum/Methotrexate combination chemotherapy appears to be the most effective available at the present time. For the management of patients with very advanced bladder cancer response rates of 30-40% are being consistently produced in metastatic and locally advanced disease. Phase II studies of chemotherapy plus surgery or radiotherapy are showing improved response rates in patients with advanced disease over any single modality alone. There are, at present, a number of Phase III studies in locally advanced disease, the results of which are eagerly awaited, comparing standard therapy plus combination chemotherapy with standard therapy alone and also studies where the previously acceptable standard therapy of radical or total cystectomy has been reduced to a more local therapy with bladder preservation. At a recent meeting the EORTC and a group of its friends decided to embark on a Phase III study of neoadjuvant chemotherapy, probably using Cisplatinum and Methotrexate with or without Vinblastine followed by whatever local treatment the clinician wishes to use with an evaluation of duration of survival and time to progression after surgery or radiotherapy. In an attempt to recruit a large number of patients, the Protocol is to be kept simple and its most likely form is shown in Figure 1.

FIGURE 1. Study Design

T2 G3	R	3 courses of CMV followed by definitive
	A	local therapy as per
T3	N	policy for that centre
	D	
T4 MO	O	
	M	
	I	
	S	
	E	definitive local therapy

From all the studies reported here and elsewhere it is clear that we have not yet found the perfect chemotherapeutic regime but we have found effective regimes with acceptable toxicity for use in patients with advanced bladder cancer. For proof of an improvement in overall survival we need to await the results of the first

prospective studies using chemotherapy plus standard
therapy against standard therapy alone. In the meantime
the EORTC still feels it important to look in a
standardized Phase II format at new compounds which may be
more effective than those at present employed.

REFERENCES

Carter SK, Wasserman TH (1975) The chemotherapy of
    urological cancer. Cancer 36: 729-747
Clark PB (1978) Radical cystectomy for carcinoma of the
    bladder. Br J Urol 50: 492-495
Coffey DS, Isaacs JT (1979) Experimental concepts in the
    design of new treatments for human prostatic cancer. In:
    Coffey, Isaacs (eds) Prostatic Cancer. UICC, Basel, p
    233 (Technical Reports Series, vol 48): 233
Cross RJ, Glashan RW, Humphrey CS, Robinson MRG, Smith PH,
    Williams RE (1976) The treatment of advanced bladder
    cancer with adriamycin and 5-fluorouracil. Br J Urol 48:
    609-610
Edsmyr F, Esposti P-L, Andersson L (1978) Radiotherapy in
    the management of bladder cancer. In: Pavone Macaluso M,
    Smith PH, Edsmyr F (eds) Bladder tumors and other topics
    in urological oncology. New York, Academic Press, p 279
EORTC GU Group (1977) The treatment of advanced carcinoma
    of the bladder with a combination of adriamycin and
    5-fluorouracil. Eur J Urol 3: 276-279
Fossa S (1988) Personal Communication
Hall RR, Bloom HJG, Freeman JE, Nawrock A, Wallace DM
    (1974) Methotrexate treatment for advanced bladder
    cancer. Br J Urol 46: 431-438
Hall RR, Newling DWW, Ramsden PD, Richards B, Robinson MRG,
    Phillips PA (1984) Treatment of invasive bladder cancer
    by local resection and high dose Methotrexate. Br J Urol
    56: 668-672
Hall RR, Powell PH, Ramsden PD, Newling DWW, Richards B,
    Robinson MRG, Smith PH (1986) TUR and systemic chemo-
    therapy as primary treatment for T3 bladder cancer - read
    at 7th Congress of E.A.U., Budapest 1986
Kaye SB, McWhinnie D, Hart A, Deane RF, Billaert P, Welsh
    J, Milsted RV, Stuart JFB, Kalman KC (1984) The treat-
    ment of advanced bladder cancer with methotrexate and
    cisplatinum - a pharmacokinetic study. Eur J Cancer Clin
    Oncol 20: 249-252
Mulder et al. Mulder JH (1982) Cyclophosphamide, adria-

mycin and cisplatinum – combination chemotherapy in advanced bladder cancer. An EORTC phase II study. Eur J Cancer Clin Oncol 18: 111-112

Myers FJ, Palmer JM, Freyha FS, Harker EG, Shortliffe LD, Hannigan J, McWhirter K and Torti FM (1985) The Fate of the Bladder in Patients with Metastatic Bladder Cancer treated with C.M.V. J Urol 134: 1118

Peters PC, O'Neill MR (1980) Cisplatinum as a therapeutic agent in metastatic transitional cell carcinoma. J Urol 123: 375-377

Prout GR, Griffin PP, Shipley WU (1979) Bladder cancer as a systemic disease. J Cancer 43: 2532

Richards B, Newling D, Fossa S, Bastable JRG, Denis L, Jones WB, De Pauw M (1983) Vincristine in advanced bladder cancer – an EORTC phase II study. Cancer Treat Rep 67: 575-577

Richards B, Bastable JRG, Glashan RW, Harris G, Newling DWW, Robinson MRG, Smith PH, YUCRG (1983) Adjuvant therapy with adriamycin and 5-fluorouracil in T3NXMO carcinoma of the bladder treated with radiotherapy. Br J Urol 55: 386-391

Smith PH, Childs JA, Mulder JH, Van Oosterom A, Martinez Pinero JA, Richards B, Stoter G, Dalesio O, De Pauw M, Sylvester R (1983) Co-operative studies of systemic chemotherapy. Clin Chemother Pharmacol II (Suppl): 25-31

Socquet Y (1981) Combined surgery and adjuvant chemotherapy with high-dose methotrexate and folinic acid rescue for infiltrating tumours of the bladder. Br J Urol 53: 439-443

Soloway MS, Kard M, Ford K (1981) Cisplatinum in local advanced and metastatic bladder cancer. Cancer 47: 467-480

Sternberg CN, Yagoda A, Scher HI, Watson RC, Herr HW, Morse MJ, Sogani PC, Vaughn ED, Bander JN, Weiselberg LR, Geller N, Hollander PS, Lipperman R, Fair WR, Whitmore JR Jnr (1988) M-VAC for advanced transitional cell carcinoma of the urothelium. J Urol 139: 461

Stoter G, Van Oosterom A, Mulder J, De Pauw M, Fossa S (1984) Combination chemotherapy – cisplatinum, VM26 in patients with advanced transitional cell carcinoma of the bladder. Eur J Cancer Clin Oncol 20: 315-317

Stoter G, Child JA, Fossa SD, Denis L, Splinter TAW, Van Oosterom AT, De Pauw M, Sylvester R for the EORTC GU Group (1986) Combination chemotherapy with cisplatinum and methotrexate in advanced transitional cell cancer of the bladder. J Urol (in press)

Stoter G (1987) Systemic chemotherapy in advanced trans-
    itional cell cancer of the bladder - read at Int.Workshop
    in Urology, Cannes. Oct 1987
Sylvester R (1987) Personal communication
Van Oosterom A, Fossa SD, Mulder JH, Calciati A, De Pauw M,
    Sylvester R (1985) Mitoxanthrone in advanced bladder
    carcinoma - a phase II of the EORTC GU Co-operative Group
    Eur J Cancer Clin Oncol 21: 1013-1014
Yagoda A, Watson RC, Kemenyn Barzell WE, Grabstald H,
    Whitmore WF (1978) Cisplatinum and cyclophosphamide in
    the treatment of advanced urothelial cancer. Cancer 41:
    2121-2136
Yagoda A (1982) Chemotherapy of advanced bladder cancer.
    In: Denis L, Smith PH, Pavone Macaluso M (eds) Clinical
    Bladder Cancer.

APPENDIX

Master   Protocol   for   Phase   II   studies   of   new
chemotherapeutic agents in advanced bladder cancer.

Conditions for patient eligibility

1. Histologically proven transitional cell cancer of the
   urinary tract, including bladder, ureter and renal
   pelvis.
2. Measurable distant metastases (M1, stage IV):
   a) Skin and subcutaneous metastases.
   b) Superficial lymph nodes.
   c) Lymph nodes in the mediastinum and in the retro-
      peritoneal region if they can be measured by CT-scan.
      The initial diameters must be > than 3 cm to allow
      reliable measurements during follow up.
   d) Liver metastases if they can be measured by CT-scan
      or echography. The initial diameters must be > than
      3 cm to allow reliable measurements during follow up.
   e) Lung metastases.
3. Unresectable primary bladder cancer and pelvic recurrences only if the tumor can be measured by CT-scan.

Criteria of Response

Complete Response will be defined as the complete
disappearance of all detectable tumor, determined by two
observations, not less than 4 weeks apart, with no new

lesions having developed.

Partial Response will be defined as at least a 50% reduction in the sum of the products of the two largest perpendicular diameters of all measurable lesions, determined by two observations not less than 4 weeks apart, with no new lesions having developed.

Stable Disease will be defined as a change of less than 50% reduction or less than 25% increase in the sum of the products of the largest perpendicular diameters of all measurable lesions.

Progressive Disease will be defined as an increase greater than 25% in the sum of the products of the two largest perpendicular diameters of all measurable lesions, or the appearance of new lesions.

Uro-Oncology: Current Status
and Future Trends, pages 129–140
© 1990 Wiley-Liss, Inc.

OVERVIEW OF HORMONAL THERAPY FOR PROSTATE CANCER

H. Ballentine Carter and John T. Isaacs

Department of Urology, The Johns Hopkins
University School of Medicine
Baltimore, Maryland 21205, USA

Prostate cancer is now the second most commonly diagnosed cancer in males and the second most common cause of male cancer deaths (Silverberg and Lubera, 1988). The trends in prostate cancer incidence and mortality would indicate that minimal therapeutic impact has been made on this disease. Controversies regarding the timing and extent of hormonal therapy for prostate cancer continue, despite evidence that tumor cell heterogeneity manifested by androgen independent cells is responsible for therapeutic failure after androgen ablation. The relationship between these failures and increasing tumor volume would suggest that earlier therapy of low stage disease should be considered for the high risk patient instead of emphasis on early therapy of metastatic disease. In addition, new therapeutic alternatives need to be developed to target androgen independent cells for treatment of patients with advanced disease.

THE PROBLEM

Prostate cancer accounts for 10% of the total annual incidence of all forms of cancer in the U.S. and in 1988 will total 99,000 new cases (Silverberg and Lubera, 1988). Of these cases approximately 20% occur under the age of 65 (NCI, 1987). This means that in 1988 there will be 19,800 cases of prostate cancer in men under the age of 65 which will account for more cancer cases than all renal cancers and leukemias in males of all ages, and more than all brain and CNS cancers in males and females of all ages (Silverberg and Lubera, 1988). The age adjusted incidence

of prostate cancer (new cases per 100,000 males per year)
has been increasing over the 13 year period from 1973 to
1985 at the rate of 2.2% per year for all races combined
(NCI, 1987). Because the incidence of prostate cancer
increases with age faster than any other human cancer, the
aging of the U.S. population will lead to further increases
in the number of cases seen in the next decade. In
addition, the age adjusted mortality (deaths per 100,000
males per year) for prostate cancer has increased at 0.8%
per year for all races over the same time period (NCI,
1987) and in 1988 will account for 28,000 deaths
(Silverberg and Lubera, 1988). Another way of looking at
the magnitude of the problem is to assess the risk of
developing or dying of prostate cancer (Seidman et al.
1985). The probability of developing prostate cancer has
risen since 1975 and now is equivalent to the chance of
developing lung cancer or approximately 1 in 10 to 12
depending upon the race (higher chance in blacks). The
lifetime risk of a black male dying of prostate cancer (1
in 23) has risen 65% since 1975 and the risk for a white
male (1 in 38) has risen 30% over the same time period.
The stage or extent of the disease at the time of diagnosis
has prognostic importance, and it is generally agreed that
patients with disease outside the prostate have little
chance for cure with surgery alone. Approximately 50-60%
of patients diagnosed with prostate cancer yearly are felt
to have disease confined to the prostate by current
clinical staging modalities. However, at the time of
surgery 40% of these patients are upstaged to non organ
confined disease (Carter and Coffey, 1986). Therefore,
around 60% of patients diagnosed yearly with prostate
cancer have the disease outside the organ of origin and
have a much poorer prognosis than patients whose disease is
confined to the prostate gland. It is these patients at
high risk for progression who would benefit from new
approaches to therapy. The trends in incidence and
mortality described above are a sobering reminder that even
though the earlier diagnosis of prostate cancer has led to
an increase in the 5 year relative survival (lead time
bias), new approaches to therapy will be required to have
an impact on this disease.

COMPLETE VS PARTIAL ANDROGEN ABLATION

Controversies surrounding the extent of androgen
withdrawal continue despite a lack of objective evidence to

support total androgen ablation in the treatment of advanced disease. Objective human data have shown no advantage for additional attempts at androgen withdrawal (adrenalectomy, hypophysectomy and antiandrogens) after relapse with standard testicular androgen ablation (Schulze et al., 1987). In addition, early non randomized trials suggested a survival advantage for total androgen ablation (LHRH analogue plus antiandrogen) compared to testicular androgen ablation alone (Labrie et al., 1985; Labrie et al., 1987) but these results have not been supported by prospective randomized trials (Trachtenberg, 1987; Crawford et al., 1988). Animal models of prostate cancer have shown no advantage for total androgen ablation when compared to testicular androgen ablation in terms of tumor growth rate or survival (Ellis and Isaacs, 1985). In the Dunning G and H rat prostatic tumors (androgen responsive tumors) growing subcutaneously in rats, castration plus an antiandrogen (cyproterone acetate) fails to increase survival or decrease tumor growth rate over castration alone. If adrenal androgens are not responsible for the failure of standard hormone withdrawal in the treatment of prostatic cancer, what is the explanation for this phenomenon? The well differentiated Dunning H tumor growing in rats initially responds to castration with a decrease in tumor volume, followed by relapse and tumor progression as is seen in the treatment of advanced human prostate cancer. It has been shown that relapse is due to the presence of androgen independent cells within the H tumor prior to androgen ablation and not their development as a result of androgen withdrawal (Isaacs and Coffey, 1981). These androgen independent cells then become the predominant cell population as the androgen dependent cells die which results in a hormone independent tumor that kills the host. This preexisting heterogeneity (androgen dependent and independent cell populations) precludes the chance of curing a tumor with androgen withdrawal alone and explains the lack of response seen with total androgen ablation. As shown in Figure 1, the origin of this tumor cell heterogeneity is genetic change that occurs in cells within a tumor as the tumor grows (Nowell, 1982; Nowell, 1986). This eventually results in a range of morphological and functional diversity over time. The presence of androgen independent cells is one of the many functional manifestations of tumor cell heterogeneity which is present early in the life of a prostatic tumor (Smolev et al., 1977). It follows then that early therapy of tumors at a time when heterogeneity is minimized is more likely to be curative.

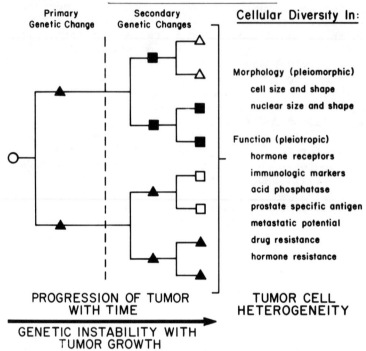

Figure 1. Diagrammatic representation of genetic changes leading to tumor cell heterogeneity. (O, normal cell; ■, ▲, □, Δ, cancer cells)

EARLY TREATMENT OF ADVANCED DISEASE VS TREATMENT OF EARLIER STAGE DISEASE

The timing of androgen ablation for advanced prostate cancer is of relatively little consequence in terms of overall survival. When a tumor is at an advanced stage there is a wide range of heterogeneity present which determines the outcome of the patient. Therefore, whether androgen ablation is initiated early or late for advanced stage disease has no effect on survival, since androgen independent cells present in the advanced tumor will result in relapse and progression. This was shown in the VACURG study which demonstrated no advantage for early hormonal therapy of advanced prostate cancer (Blackard, 1971). On the other hand, the concept of aggressive treatment of earlier stage disease is supported by animal tumor models of prostate cancer. As discussed previously, an animal bearing the Dunning H tumor responds initially to androgen withdrawal and then relapses because of overgrowth of androgen independent cells. Despite early androgen ablation no animal has ever been cured by this therapy alone because of preexisting androgen independent cells (heterogeneity) (Isaacs, 1984). However, the early combined treatment of these animals bearing H tumors with androgen ablation and chemotherapy results in increased host survival compared to either treatment alone when given early. This demonstrates that early multimodal therapy confers maximal benefit in this animal model. The benefit of early therapy has also be shown in an androgen independent metastatic tumor model combining surgery and chemotherapy (Henry and Isaacs, 1988). The Dunning MAT-Lu tumor when growing in the hind legs of rats will result in 100% of animals with lung metastases at a 1cc primary tumor volume. At a primary tumor volume of 0.5-0.8cc 50% of animals will develop lung metastases and at this tumor volume 100% of animals can be cured with chemotherapy and surgery. In comparison only 50% of animals can be cured by surgery alone (hind leg removal) at this tumor volume. When the primary tumor volume reaches 1-2cc and 100% of animals have lung metastases, neither chemotherapy or surgery alone is curative. However, when both treatments are combined at this tumor volume 90% of animals can be cured. Despite a combination of surgery and chemotherapy no animals can be cured with greater than 1-2cc tumor volumes. Prospective, randomized data on combined therapy for patients with early stage prostate cancer at high risk for progression (approximately 40% of patients undergoing radical prostatectomy) is limited (Huben and Murphy, 1988). There are retrospective studies which suggest a survival advantage when combined androgen withdrawal and surgery are used to treat patients with locally advanced disease (stage C) or small volume metastases (D1) (Myers et al., 1983; Zincke et al., 1986; Zincke et al., 1987). Based on animal models for prostate cancer it would seem that trials of multimodal therapy for these patients are warranted. Failure to demonstrate a survival advantage when chemotherapy is used to treat far advanced disease does not preclude a benefit when used at an earlier stage. The studies presented above suggest an important relationship between tumor volume and progression in solid tumors.

RELATIONSHIP BETWEEN TUMOR VOLUME AND PROGRESSION

The previous discussion of tumor cell heterogeneity emphasized the genetic instability occurring within a tumor as it grows. This process leads to genetic changes which result in cells with a growth advantage that eventually overgrow other cell populations without a growth advantage. As this process continues further genetic changes occur resulting in a tumor with phenotypic diversity (metastatic ability, chemotherapy resistance, androgen independence). Therefore, it can be seen that tumor volume is directly related to the heterogeneity within a tumor. In prostate cancer this relationship was first shown by the morphometric study of Cantrell, which documented that in stage A (incidentally discovered cancer) the percentage of gland involved with tumor was important with regard to outcome (Cantrell et al., 1981). Since then tumor volume in stage B disease (nodule confined to gland) has been shown to be an adverse prognostic indicator (McNeal et al., 1986; Partin et al., 1988). This relationship would be expected from what is known about the origin of tumor heterogeneity and lends support to the argument for multimodal therapy at an earlier stage. Although the role of early adjuvant therapy is supported by studies in other solid tumors (Bonadonna et al., 1986; Clark et al., 1987) and in animal models of prostate cancer, there is as yet no evidence that this approach would be curative in prostatic cancer. The low proliferation rate of prostatic cancer cells and their low death rate present significant problems for therapy directed at proliferating cells.

CONCLUSIONS

Currently there are many approaches to eliminating the androgen-dependent cells within a prostatic tumor including surgical ablation of testicular androgens and medical ablation of both testicular and adrenal androgens. Because genetic instability and resulting tumor heterogeneity leads to the presence of androgen-independent cells, it is unlikely that therapy directed only at androgen-dependent cells will be curative regardless of the extent of androgen ablation. The search, therefore, for effective agents targeted at the androgen-independent human prostatic cancer cells must continue. Most of the presently available chemotherapeutic agents are targeted at proliferating cancer cells, therefore, it is not surprising that there is a good correlation in a large variety of cancers between the effectiveness of these agents and the respective cancer's rate of cell proliferation (Shackney et al., 1987). These previous studies have demonstrated that in cancers with high cell proliferation rates, chemotherapy can achieve high initial fractional cell kills per course of therapy, producing complete clinical responses. In contrast, in cancers with a low cell proliferation rate, it has been found that the fractional cell kills are small, producing partial responses and shallow complete responses at best. The strong correlation between a high cell proliferation rate and chemotherapeutic sensitivity in human cancer is demonstrated from the studies of Tubiana and Malaise (1976). These data affirm that slow growing cancers have very low rates of cell proliferation and respond with small fractional cell kills per course of therapy.

These data also suggest that in order for chemotherapy to be effective, not only the rate of cell proliferation, but also the rate of cell death, must be high. The importance of this statement is emphasized by the following two examples using the data of Tubiana and Malaise (1976). In an average embryonal cancer, approximately 44% of the cells are proliferating per day and 41% of the cells are dying per day. If this embryonal cancer is treated with a chemotherapeutic agent which produces a decrease in the cell proliferation rate of as little as 10% (i.e., changes it from 44% to 40% per day) with no effect on the daily cell death rate, then the cancer will actually involute since the rate of cell death (i.e., 41% per day) is now greater than the rate of cell proliferation (i.e., 40% per day). In contrast, in a typical adenocarcinoma, approximately 2.9% of the cells are proliferating per day and 2.0% are dying per day. If this adenocarcinoma is treated with a chemotherapeutic agent which reduces the daily cell proliferation rate by 10% (i.e., changes it from 2.9% to 2.6% per day) with no effect on the daily cell death rate, then the cancer will still continue to grow since the rate of cell proliferation (i.e., 2.6% per day) is still greater than the rate of cell death (i.e., 2.0% per day). In fact, it can be calculated from cell kinetic equations (Steel, 1977) that this response will only change the tumor doubling time of the adenocarcinoma from 83 to 116 days, a response having little effect upon host survival. These examples demonstrate that, if the daily cell death rate in a cancer is high enough, then anti-proliferative chemotherapy which induces even a small (e.g., 10%) reduction in the daily cell proliferation rate can produce tumor regression, resulting in a high rate of complete durable response (e.g., a fast growing cancer). In contrast, if the daily cell death rate is too low (i.e., in slow growing cancers), then anti-proliferative chemotherapy must induce a much larger reduction in the daily cell proliferation rate (i.e., a large fractional cell kill) to produce a similar response. Unfortunately, the fractional cell kills achievable at maximum tolerated therapeutic intensity in slow growing cancers are not high enough to produce high complete response rates or durable complete responses (Shackney et al., 1978). These examples demonstrate that a high death rate is critically important in allowing even small decreases in the cell proliferation rates, induced by chemotherapy, to be clinically useful.

While the exact magnitude of the daily cell proliferation rate has been determined for only a small number of human prostatic cancer patients (Meyer et al., 1982; Sufrin and Coffey, 1975), the published results demonstrate that prostatic cancers are typical of most other solid adenocarcinomas in their low rate of cell proliferation. The daily rate of cell death has not been precisely determined for any human prostatic cancers, but from preliminary analysis, it would appear to be in the same low range as for other slow growing solid cancers. This would suggest that the successful treatment of slow growing prostatic cancers will require simultaneous androgen ablation for the removal of the androgen responsive clones of tumor cells, coupled with chemotherapy targeted at the androgen-independent clones of cells. The chemotherapy, itself, may have to include two different types of agents; one agent having anti-proliferating activity affecting the small number of dividing androgen-independent cells, and the other agent targeted at increasing the low rate of cell death among the majority of non-proliferating androgen-independent prostatic cancer cells present. Since there appears to be a large variety of adequate anti-proliferative chemotherapeutic agents presently available, it would appear most appropriate for the future to attempt to develop new agents of the latter type specifically targeted at increasing the rate of cell death of non-dividing cancer cells. Along these lines, recent studies have demonstrated that the involution of the normal prostate following androgen withdrawal is due to activation of a series (i.e., cascade) of discrete biochemical steps induced by androgen withdrawal leading to the "programmed death" of the androgen-dependent cell within the prostate (Kyprianou and Isaacs, 1988). This programmed cell death is an active process and involves a calcium activated endonuclease activity. Studies are presently being performed to determine if androgen-independent prostatic cancer cells can be made to undergo this same programmed cell death by nonhormonal agents which activate the cascade distal to the point normally blocked by androgens.

REFERENCES

Blackard CE (1971). Treatment of advanced carcinoma of the prostate. Surg Gynecol Obstet 133:97-98.

Bonadonna G, Valagussa P, Tancini G, Rossi A, Brambilla C, Zambetti M, Bignami P, Di Gronzo G, Silvestrini R (1986). Current status of Milan adjuvant chemotherapy trials for node-positive and node-negative breast cancer. NCI Monogr 1:45-49.

Cantrell BB, DeKlerk DP, Eggleston JC, Boitnott JK, Walsh PC (1981). Pathological factors that influence prognosis in stage A prostatic cancer: The influence of extent versus grade. J Urol 125:516-520.

Carter HB, Coffey DS (1986). Prostate cancer: The magnitude of the problem in the United States. Proceedings of meeting held in Prouts Neck, Maine, In press.

Clark JR, Fallon BG, Frei E III (1987). Induction chemotherapy as initial treatment for advanced head and neck cancer: A model for the multidisciplinary treatment of solid tumors. In DeVita JT, Hellman S, Rosenberg SA (eds): Important Advances in Oncology, Philadelphia, JB Lippincott, pp 175-195.

Crawford ED, McLeod D, Donn A, Spaulding J, Benson R, Eisenberger M, Blumenstein B. Treatment of newly diagnosed stage D2 prostate cancer with Leuprolide alone, Phase III, intergroup study 0036. Presented at the 1988 American Urological Meeting, Boston, MA (Abstract #3706).

Ellis WJ, Isaacs JT (1985). Effectiveness of complete versus partial androgen withdrawal therapy for the treatment of prostatic cancer as studied in the Dunning R-3327 system of rat prostatic adenocarcinoma. Cancer Res 45:6041-6050.

Henry JM, Isaacs JT (1988). Relationship between tumor size and the curability of metastatic prostatic cancer by surgery alone or in combination with adjuvant chemotherapy. J Urol 139:1119-1123.

Huben RP, Murphy GP (1988). Management of advanced cancer of the prostate. In Skinner DG, Liewkovsky G (eds): Genitourinary Cancer. Philadelphia, WB Saunders Co, pp. 473-482.

Isaacs JT (1984). The timing of androgen ablation therapy and/or chemotherapy in the treatment of prostatic cancer. Prostate 5:1-17.

Isaacs JT, Coffey DS (1981). Adaptation versus selection as the mechanism responsible for the relapse of prostatic cancer to androgen ablation therapy as studied in the Dunning R-3327-H adenocarcinoma. Cancer Res 41:5707-5075.

Kyprianou N, Isaacs JT (1988). Activation of programmed cell death in the rat ventral prostate after castration. Endocrinology 122:552-562.

Labrie F, Dupont A, Belanger A et al. (1985). Antiandrogens and LHRH agonists in the treatment of prostatic cancer. Medicine/Science 1:435.

Labrie F, Dupont A, Giguere M, Borsanyi JP, Lacourciere Y, Belanger A, Lachance R, Emond J, Monfette G (1987). Combination therapy with flutamide and castration (orchiectomy or LHRH agonist): The minimal endocrine therapy in both untreated and previously treated patients. J Steroid Biochem 27:525-532.

McNeal JE, Kindrachuk RA, Freiha FS, Bostwick DG, Redwine EA, Stamey TA (1986). Patterns of progression in prostate cancer. Lancet 1:60-63.

Meyer JS, Sufrin G, Martin SA (1982). Proliferative activity of benign human prostate, prostatic adenocarcinoma and seminal vesicle evaluated by thymidine labeling. J Urol 128:1353-1356.

Myers RP, Zincke H, Fleming TR, Farrow GM, Furlow WL, Utz DC (1983). Hormonal treatment at time of radical retropubic prostatectomy for stage D1 prostate cancer. J Urol 130:99-101.

National Cancer Institute: Division of Cancer Prevention and Control. Annual Cancer Statistics Review. NIH Publication No. 88-2789: III.13, IV.9, V. 14. (1987).

Nowell PC (1982). Genetic instability in cancer cells: Relationship to tumor cell heterogeneity. In Owens AH Jr, Coffey DS, Baylin SD (eds): Tumor Cell Heterogeneity: Origins and Implications. New York, Academic Press, pp 351-364.

Nowell PC (1986). Mechanisms of tumor progression. Cancer Res 46:2203-2207.

Partin AW, Epstein JI, Cho KR, Gittelsohn AM, Walsh PC (1988). Morphometric measurement of tumor volume and percent of gland involvement as predictors of pathologic stage in clinical stage B prostate cancer. J Urol (In press).

Schulze H, Isaacs JT, Coffey DS (1987). A critical review of the concept of total androgen ablation in the treatment of prostate cancer. In Murphy GP, Khoury S, Kuss R, Chatelain C, Denis L (eds): Progress in Clinical and Biological Research. New York, Alan R Liss, Vol 243A, pp 3-5.

Seidman H, Mushinski MH, Gelb SK, Silverberg E (1985). Probabilities of eventually developing or dying of cancer: United States, 1985. CA 35:36-56.

Shackney SE, McCormack GW, Cuchural GJ (1978). Growth rate patterns of solid tumors and their relation to responsiveness to therapy. Ann Intern Med 89:107.

Silverberg E, Lubera JA (1988). Cancer Statistics. CA 38(1):14-15.

Smolev JK, Heston WDW, Scott WW, Coffey DS (1977). Characterization of the Dunning R3327H prostatic adenocarcinoma: An appropriate animal model for prostatic cancer. Cancer Trtm Rep 61:273-287.

Steel GG (1977). Growth Kinetics of Tumors. Oxford, Clarendon Press, p 71.

Sufrin G, Coffey DS (1975). Differences in the mechanism of action of medrogestone and cyproterone acetate. Invest Urol 13:1-9.

Trachtenberg J (1987). Hormonal management of stage D carcinoma of the prostate. Urol Clin North Amer 14(4):685-692.

Tubiana M, Malaise EP (1976). Growth rate and cell kinetics in human tumors: Some prognostic and therapeutic implications. In Symington T, Carter RL (eds): Scientific Foundations of Oncology, Year Book Medical Publs Inc, p 126.

Zincke H , Utz DC, Taylor WF (1986).   Bilateral pelvic
    lymphadenectomy and radical prostatectomy for clinical
    stage C prostatic cancer: Role of adjuvant treatment
    for residual cancer and in disease progression J Urol
    135:1199-1205.
Zincke H, Utz DC, Thule PM, Taylor WF (1987).   Treatment
    options for patients with stage D1 adenocarcinoma of
    prostate.   Urology 30:307-315.

Uro-Oncology: Current Status
and Future Trends, pages 141–148
© 1990 Wiley-Liss, Inc.

THE IMPORTANCE OF PRETREATMENT TESTOSTERONE AND OTHER PROG-
NOSTIC VARIABLES IN THE RESPONSE TO ANDROGEN DEPRIVATION
THERAPY

Mark S. Soloway

Department of Urology, University of Tennessee,
Memphis, Veterans Administration Hospital,
Memphis, and Baptist Memorial Hospital, Memphis,
Tennessee. Address: 956 Court, Box 10,
Memphis, TN 38163

Although androgen deprivation will provide a symptomatic and often objective clinical tumor regression in a
high percentage of men with advanced prostate cancer, most
will relapse in approximately 18 to 24 months. Chemotherapy may be offered to patients who initially do not respond
to androgen deprivation and may be considered for those
patients who eventually relapse following initial successful androgen deprivation therapy. Unfortunately, an effective single or combination chemotherapy regimen has not
been reproducibly demonstrated to have significant activity
in advanced prostate cancer. Among the possible reasons
for the lack of successful chemotherapy is the advanced
nature of the tumor when chemotherapy is initiated. It
might be possible to select patients who will not have a
response to androgen deprivation, thus initiating chemotherapy earlier. Thus, the bone marrow reserve might be
greater and the patient's performance status at a higher
level, allowing appropriate doses of chemotherapy to be
used.

Another reason to identify prognostic factors in regard to androgen deprivation therapy is to select important
stratification variables for trials which are performed to
determine the efficacy of alternative forms of androgen
deprivation. The primary methods for reducing the male
hormone level in the past have been bilateral orchiectomy
and exogenous estrogens. More recently, luteinizing
hormone-releasing hormone (LH-RH) analogues have been developed and have been demonstrated in comparative trials to
be equally efficacious to both orchiectomy and estrogens

(Koutsilieris et al., 1986; Leuprolide Study Group, 1984). Evaluation of new treatment modalities for prostate cancer does require prospective randomized trials to compare them with traditional therapy. Unfortunately, most patients with prostate cancer do not have bidimensionally measurable disease, e.g., pulmonary or soft tissue metastasis, and thus the bone scan is the study most commonly utilized to evaluate response. Bone is the only site of metastasis in 65% of patients who present with metastatic prostate cancer. Other criteria used to evaluate response are the performance status, serum acid phosphatase, prostate specific antigen (PSA), analgesic requirement, and the size of the prostate. Although the PSA level may be incorporated into the response criteria of future trials, the change in the bone scan over time remains the most important method for evaluation of response.

The designation of the most important prognostic indicators, particularly with their relationship to the patient's progression-free survival, are important for stratification on entry into phase II or III clinical trials. When effective chemotherapy becomes available for prostate cancer, those patients who are unlikely to respond to androgen deprivation might be the first considered for early intervention with such a regimen.

PRETREATMENT TESTOSTERONE

Approximately 20% of patients with advanced prostate cancer never respond to androgen deprivation therapy and virtually all patients will eventually progress. Two theories have been offered to explain the resistance to androgen deprivation (Isaacs, 1984). One suggests that all prostatic tumor cells are initially hormone sensitive, but following androgen deprivation, a proportion of these cells become androgen independent and eventually predominate. The second hypothesis suggests that prostatic cancer initially consists of a heterogeneous group of cells, some of which are androgen independent, and presumably in those patients who do not respond to androgen deprivation therapy, this androgen independent population of cells predominate and grow despite the reduction in androgen.

The eventual progression in virtually all patients with advanced prostate cancer might be explained by the adaptation of the prostate tumor cells to a low androgen environment with subsequent proliferation. If the population of patients who had predominantly androgen independent cells could be identified before commencement of androgen deprivation therapy, then chemotherapy alone or combined with hormone therapy might be started immediately when the number of tumor cells was lower.

A series of studies over the last several years suggests that patients whose pretreatment serum testosterone is below normal are less likely to favorably respond to androgen deprivation therapy. Adlercreutz et al (1981) noted that the mean serum testosterone level was significantly higher in patients who had a good response, compared to those with a poor response. Harper and associates (1984) studied 222 patients and reported that those patients who died within one year of androgen deprivation therapy had significantly lower pretreatment serum testosterone levels than those who survived for longer than one year. Young and Kent (1968) also noted a direct correlation between pretreatment serum testosterone and survival. Wilson et al (1985) reported that patients with serum testosterone levels greater than 400 ng/dl had a better prognosis.

Hickey et al (1988) reviewed the pretreatment serum testosterone levels and correlated this with response in 53 patients treated at the University of Tennessee. All patients had stage D2 adenocarcinoma of the prostate and a positive bone scan. A variety of forms of androgen deprivation were used, but were all thought to be equivalent. Before commencement of treatment, all patients had their serum testosterone determined from blood drawn at 8:00 a.m. Evaluation of the best response revealed that there were 6% complete and 32% partial responders while 41% remained stable and 21% had progression. The pretreatment serum testosterone levels ranged from 150 to 879 ng/dl. Of interest was the fact that the mean serum testosterone level for those patients who had a complete response was 524 ± 18 ng/dl, whereas the mean pretreatment testosterone for those patients whose tumor progressed despite endocrine manipulation was 279 ± 110 ng/dl. Fifteen patients had a pretreatment serum testosterone of more than 500 ng/dl and only one (7%) progressed, while none of the patients whose pretreatment testosterone was less than 200 ng/dl had objective tumor regression. These results were consistent with prior studies indicating patients with a higher pretreatment testosterone were more likely to have an objective response following androgen deprivation therapy.

In a recent prospective randomized trial performed in the United States comparing the depot LH–RH analogue Zoladex to surgical castration for patients with metastatic prostate cancer, it was observed that the pretreatment serum testosterone level correlated with the time to treatment failure (Soloway, 1988). The two most important factors influencing time to treatment failure were the patient's performance status using the Eastern Cooperative Oncology Group (ECOG) scoring system from 0-4 and the pretreatment testosterone level. Patients with a pretreatment serum testosterone > 200 ng/dl had a significantly longer time to treatment failure than those with a value of less than 200. Likewise, patients with an ECOG performance of 0-1 had a statistically significant longer time to treatment failure than those with a performance status of 2-4. When this was analyzed by the likelihood of a patient achieving a tumor response, either complete, partial, or stabilization of disease (nonprogression), once again, those patients with a higher serum testosterone and better performance status were more likely to achieve a clinical response than those patients who had low performance status and low serum testosterone.

Eighty-nine percent of 113 patients with an initial serum testosterone greater than 200 ng/dl had nonprogression compared to 65% of 26 patients whose serum testosterone was less than 200.

MULTIVARIATE ANALYSIS OF SELECTED PROGNOSTIC FACTORS

Recently, Soloway et al (1988) proposed a new semi-quantitative grading system based upon the extent of disease observed on the bone scan. A scale of 1-4 was devised and it was found that those patients with less than six metastatic deposits on the pretreatment bone scan had a significantly better two-year survival than those with more extensive metastasis. Patients who had a superscan or its equivalent, that is, more than 75% of the ribs, vertebrae, and pelvic bones with areas of increased uptake consistent with metastatic disease had a significantly poorer two-year survival than those with less sites of disease.

110 patients with metastatic prostate cancer were then
analyzed with particular attention to selected pretreatment
prognostic factors in order to determine which were most
important as an indicator of progression-free survival.
All of these patients had histologically proven prostate
adenocarcinoma and a positive bone scan and no patient had
received endocrine therapy prior to detection of bone
metastasis. The forms of androgen deprivation varied.
Forty-six patients received an LH-RH analogue, 33 received
3 mg. daily of diethylstilbestrol, 22 underwent bilateral
orchiectomy, seven received megestrol acetate, and three
were placed on estramustine phosphate. Current data would
suggest that all of these forms of androgen deprivation
have equivalent activity. The patients' ages ranged from
47 to 92 years with a mean of 67.7. Forty-seven men were
white and 63 black. Forty-eight patients had an ECOG performance status (PS) of 0, 51 had a PS of 1, and 11 had a
PS of 2. The median follow up was 21 months with a range
of 4-89 months.

Because the pretreatment serum acid phosphatase was
determined by an enzymatic assay in 19 patients and by
radioimmunoassay in 91 patients, an index was used to compare the values among the patients. The correlation coef-
ficient of the enzymatic assay and the RIA is approximately
1.0.

The pretreatment testosterone level was determined in
79 patients. The normal range is 300-800 ng/dl.

The time to progression of disease was calculated from
the time of initiation of androgen deprivation therapy to
documented disease progression. The criteria for response
was that of the National Prostatic Cancer Program (Slack et
al., 1980). For practical purposes, a new area of uptake
on the bone scan was the criteria for progression in almost
all of the patients.

Time to progression was analyzed for possible association with a number of covariates. These covariates were
age, race, performance status, pretreatment serum testosterone, extent of disease on the bone scan, and the prostatic acid phosphatase level. The univariate analysis of a
single covariate consisted of estimating the progression-
free survival by means of the Kaplan-Meier product limit
method for each level of the covariate. The time at which

progression was detected was the end point in this application of a standard survival analysis method. The survival
curves for each level of a single covariate were compared
by means of the Lee-Desu statistic. For this univariate
analysis, age was coded into the categories as less than
64, 65-74, and greater or equal to 75; PAP was coded 1,
2-15, 16-40, and greater than 40; testosterone was coded
less than 300 or greater and equal to 300.

Cox's proportional hazards model was used to examine
all covariates simultaneously in a multivariate model.

The univariate survival analysis of time to progression resulted in three significant associations. Pretreatment testosterone (P = 0.0004), extent of bone metastases
(P = 0.0024), and performance status (P = 0.0418) were all
significant indicators. The remaining covariates which
were examined, namely, age, race, and pretreatment prostatic acid phosphatase were not significantly associated with
time to progression (P > 0.05).

Patients with pretreatment testosterone levels less
than 300 ng/dl had shorter progression-free intervals than
patients with pretreatment testosterone levels greater than
300. The median progression-free intervals were 14 months
and 31 months, respectively. Proportions of patients without progression at 24 months were 26% and 57%, respectively.

In agreement with our earlier report on the extent of
disease on the bone scan, those patients with an EOD I,
that is, with less than six bony metastases, had the longest progression-free interval. The median progression-free
interval was greater than 89 months for those with EOD I
bone scans but 17, 16, and 15 months, respectively, for
bone scan levels II, III, and IV. At two years, 76% were
progression-free for bone scan EOD I but only 34%, 28%, and
34% for those with EOD II, III, and IV, respectively.

When analyzed according to performance status, those
patients with the best performance status had the longest
median progression-free interval, 39 months, and 59% were
still progression-free at 24 months. Patients with a poorer performance status (1 and 2) had median progression-free
intervals of 16 and 22 months, respectively, and 38% and
35% were free of progression at 24 months.

Cox's proportional hazards model identified pretreatment testosterone level and the extent of disease on the bone scan as the only two covariates significantly associated with time until progression. Bone metastases EOD II-IV were combined for the multivariate analysis. When this was performed, a relative risk of progression could be determined. Patients with the bone scans EOD II-IV have approximately 2.7 times the risk of progression as patients with a bone scan EOD I. A patient with a pretreatment serum testosterone less than 300 ng/dl has approximately 2.2 times the risk of progression as a man with a level greater than 300.

Based upon these analyses, it seems reasonable that prospective randomized studies comparing treatments for patients with newly diagnosed metastatic prostate cancer should consider using the pretreatment serum testosterone level and the extent of disease on the bone scan for stratification. If our population of patients and treatment philosophy is similar to other centers, it appears that patients with metastatic prostate cancer begin therapy before there is a decline in performance status and thus this does not serve as an important prognostic variable. Most patients had a good performance status when therapy was initiated.

It might be time to reconsider our strategy for patients less likely to have a satisfactory response to androgen deprivation. Patients with a pretreatment serum testosterone which is less than 300 are less likely to achieve a satisfactory response to further lowering the testosterone level. A combination of chemotherapy plus androgen deprivation might produce an improved progression-free interval. Only a properly designed randomized trial, of course, can answer this question.

Supported by the Lillian and Morrie Moss Urologic Research Fund and a grant from Dr. Armand Hammer.

REFERENCES

Adlercreutz H, Ranikko S, Karento AL, Karonen SL (1981). Hormonal pattern in prostate cancer. II. Correlation with primary response to endocrine treatment. ACTA Endocr 98:634-640.

Harper ME, Pierrepoint CG, Griffiths K (1984). Carcinoma
  of the prostate: relationship of pretreatment hormone
  levels to survival. Eur J Cancer Clin Oncol 20:477-482.
Hickey D, Todd B, Soloway MS (1988). Pretreatment testosterone levels: significance in androgen deprivation
  therapy. J Urol 136:1038-1040.
Isaacs JT (1984). The timing of androgen ablation therapy
  and/or chemotherapy in the treatment of prostatic cancer. Prostate 5:1.
Koutsilieris M, Faure N, Tolis G, Laroche B, Robert G,
  Ackman, CFD (1986). Objective response in disease outcome in 59 patients with stage D2 prostatic cancer treated with either buserelin or orchiectomy. Urology
  27:221-228.
Leuprolide Study Group (1984). Leuprolide versus diethylstilbestrol for metastatic prostate cancer. N Engl J Med
  311:1281-1286.
Slack NH, Karr JP, Chu TM, Murphy GP (1980). An assessment
  of bone scans for monitoring osseous metastases in
  patients being treated for prostate carcinoma. Prostate
  1:259-270, 1980.
Soloway MS, Hardeman SW, Hickey D, Raymond J, Todd B,
  Soloway S, Moinuddin M (1988). Stratification of
  patients with metastatic prostate cancer based on extent
  of disease on initial bone scan. Cancer 61:195-202.
Soloway MS (1988). A phase III, multicenter comparison of
  depot zoladex and orchiectomy in patients with
  previously-untreated, stage D$_2$ prostate cancer. Oral
  communication at International Symposium on GnRH Analogues in Cancer and Human Reproduction, Geneva,
  Switzerland, February 18.
Wilson DW, Harper ME, Jensen HM, Ikeda RM, Richards G,
  Peeling WP, Pierrepoint CG, Griffiths K (1985). A prognostic index for the clinical management of patients with
  advanced prostatic cancer: a British Prostate Study
  Group investigation. The Prostate 7:131-141.
Young HH II, Kent JR (1968). Plasma testosterone levels in
  patients with prostatic carcinoma before and after treatment. J Urol 99:788-792.

Uro-Oncology: Current Status
and Future Trends, pages 149–157
© 1990 Wiley-Liss, Inc.

IS THERE A ROLE FOR PURE ANTIANDROGENS IN THE TREATMENT OF ADVANCED PROSTATIC CANCER?

M. Pavone-Macaluso, V. Serretta, G Daricello, C. Pavone, M. Cacciatore, C. Romano, N. Cavallo

Institute of Urology and Interdepartment Center for Research in Clinical Oncology,

University Polyclinic Hospital, 90127 Palermo, Italy

INTRODUCTION

New modalities of treatment have been introduced in recent years and some views and concepts have been re-evaluated. A greater emphasis has been put on the quality of life. The modalities of treatment for the localised disease remain the same as they were 5 years ago: radical surgery, external irradiation, interstitial irradiation and even no treatment, i.e. the wait and see policy, adopted by many urologists in England and Denmark. The initial success of interstitial radiation was mainly due to the possibility of preservation of sexual function, which represents an important aspect of the quality of life, at least for some patients, irrespective of their age. The same holds true for the increasing popularity of nerve- sparing radical surgery and of postoperative treatment of impotence, especially by the intracavernous injection of papaverine. The effort to preserve sexual function and to improve the quality of life has been criticized because it may lead to a less radical surgery according to the traditional rules of oncological surgery. Strangely enough, this same aspect has not been generally taken in consideration, with regard to the treatment of metastatic disease. In fact, some people have defined as unethical any new treatment which offers our patients the chance of maintaining their sexual potency. This is a rather peculiar attitude, especially since it is almost invariably assumed that our current modalities of treatment cannot be proved as being capable of improving the survival rate of the patient, but they only have a palliative effect, or, in other words, can merely improve the quality of life. It has been stated that the use of pure antiandrogens in patients with prostatic cancer must be banned because it produces an extremely high rise in plasma testosterone level in intact rats. Few people are aware of the fact that in elderly patients, such modifications are inconstant and, even when they occur, are of minor magnitude, never exceed the upper normal values and tend to disappear within 12 months.

PURE ANTIANDROGENS

Two "pure antiandrogens" have been submitted to clinical evaluation in recent years. A third one, which does not produce a rise in circulating androgens, is presently under evaluation (1). Obviously, cyproterone acetate, which is a steroid and produces a blockade of LH and a fall of plasma testosterone is not included in the category of pure antiandrogens.

a) Flutamide (Eulexin)

Flutamide is a well known antiandrogen, which acts by a peripheral blockade of intranuclear androgen receptors. It has been recently advised as a necessary supplement to orchidectomy (or to chemical castration by the LHRH analogues) in order to achieve a "complete androgen blockade". However, this "combination therapy" may have some influence on survival, but usually induces sexual impotence.

One of the unique features of flutamide is that is does not necessarily abolish libido and potency in sexually active patients. Results from phase III studies showed that flutamide, administered alone, is at least as effective as DES in the treatment of advanced prostate cancer (2). In a Danish randomized study, flutamide 750 mg daily was compared with DES 3 mg. At 12 months either an objective response or a stabilization was seen in 13 of 20 patients treated with flutamide as compared to 8 of 20 patients treated with DES (3). The difference was not statistically significant, but DES caused more frequent and more severe side effects than flutamide. Gynecomastia was prevented by irradiating the breasts before treatment. No significant alteration of libido or potency was observed in patients treated with flutamide, while all those treated with DES became impotent. In the flutamide group, rise in plasma testosterone was moderate and inconstant, with a very large standard deviation. After 12 months, plasma testosterone concentrations had reverted to normal levels.

Clinical results have been very encouraging in previously untreated patients (4). In a randomized study comparing flutamide (750 or 1500 mg daily) with DES (1 mg daily) there were no apparent differences in response between patients on flutamide and those receiving DES (5). In Italy, a large cooperative group has treated with flutamide patients with either stage C or stage D prostate cancer (6). Other patients were treated with a combination of flutamide and the LHRH superagonist, Zoladex. Not only was it impossible to detect any difference in response rate, but there was even a trend in favour of flutamide. This was not a randomized trial and thus the results must be taken with caution.

In our experience (7), response rate, time to progression and survival were not different, stage by stage, to those reported in historical series, in which "classical" drugs, such as DES 3 mg, CPA, or estramustine were employed. A direct comparison is impossible but the indication can be drawn that some patients benefit from flutamide and remain potent, if they wish so.

As mentioned before, the use of pure antiandrogens in prostate cancer has been criticized on the ground that they produce a marked rise in plasma testosterone levels in the intact experimental animals. On the other hand, it is uncertain to what an extent flutamide is capable of producing a total blockade of the androgen receptors in the nuclei of the androgen-sensitive cells. It is feared therefore that a rise in circulating (and, possibly, intracellular) androgens, not associated with a complete inhibition of their intracellular activity, may result in excessive androgenic stimulation. A rise in plasma testosterone is very marked in rats but its extent does not seem to be identical in other animal species and in particular, in men. In young adults flutamide brings about a rise in circulating LH, testosterone and oestradiol, but this effect is of much lower magnitude than in rats (8). In older subjects, namely in patients with prostate cancer treated with flutamide, the rise in plasma testosterone has been inconstant and quite moderate (9).

No correlation between testosterone fluctuations and clinical response has been observed so far. No data have been reported on intracellular levels of DHT and no Leydig cell hyperplasia has been observed in patients treated with flutamide. It is our feeling that, unless the data reported by ourselves and by other authors can be disproved, the theoretical objections are of insufficient value. It is hoped that randomized clinical trials comparing flutamide alone with flutamide and castration (or LHRH analogues) will be performed in the near future. The only randomized study reported so far compared flutamide with estramustine phosphate (10). The preliminary results seem to indicate that these two drugs produce a similar initial response, but that its duration is more prolonged in the estramustine treated group. However, the numbers are small and these results await confirmation. Meanwhile, it can be concluded that flutamide is a legitimate therapeutic option in informed patients with a strong motivation to maintain their sexual activity.

It is relatively well tolerated, but it must be administered with caution in patients with borderline liver insufficiency because its side effects may occasionally be rather severe (11). Subjective and objective responses may also occur in patients progressing after initial response to castration (12, 13).

b) Nilutamide (Anandron[R])

Nilutamide is given usually in association with LH-RH agonists (14, 15) or as a complement to orchidectomy (16, 17). Its use in monotherapy is still preliminary, and no results have been published so far, although an Italian study (18) showed results that were not inferior to those obtainable with conventional hormonal therapy of untreated patients. Of 37 patients (36 with metastases) evaluable for response at 3 months from start of therapy, 23 were previously untreated. There were 39 % partial responses and 61 % of the patients remained with stable disease. Pain decreased in 62 % of patients including those in relapse after previous treatments and completely disappeared in 52 % of all cases. A marked decrease in serum prostatic acid phosphatase reaching almost normal values was observed also in some patients with stabilization and progression. Increase in plasma testosterone was moderate and never rose above normal values. It is unknown whether nilutamide - treated patients maintain potency if sexually active. The side effects were moderate, although emeralopia was a disturbing phenomenon in 23.1 % of cases. Other side effects were: hot flushes (54 %), nausea or vomiting (48 %), gynecomastia (39 %), gastralgia (9 %), diarrhoea (9 %), antabuse effect (8 %), skin rash (6 %). The advantages over flutamide consists of more favourable pharmacokinetics enabling a lower daily dose, usually 300 mg. The experience is still limited and further data are needed.

c) ICI 176, 334 (Casodex[R]) This drug is presently under evaluation.

PERSONAL EXPERIENCE

Our personal experience with flutamide was reported earlier (7).

Since October 1982, 22 patients, 60 - 84 years old, entered the study. 17 patients had a stage C (15 T3N0M0 and 2 T4N0M0) and 5 a stage D2 (M1) prostatic carcinoma. Only 4 patients had previously received an endocrine therapy. Every patient at entry into the study should have an histological confirmation of the disease, a good performance status (WHO 0, 1, 2), a life expectancy over 3 months and no severe anemia.

Every patient received a daily oral dose of 750 mg of flutamide, in 3 administrations. Response was evaluated according to the EORTC criteria. The first evaluation of the objective response was at 3 months: patients showing stabilizations or objective response remained on treatment until progression. The average follow-up duration was 18 months (6 - 35). At the 6 months follow-up, 18 patients (82 %) showed a partial or complete local response, 2 patients (9 %) were stable and other 2 (9 %) had a local progression. Of 5 patients having bony metastases at the start of the treatment, 1 had a partial response, 3 were stable and 1 showed progression.

At the end of follow-up, (average duration: 18 months) only 1 patient (4.5 %) showed a complete objective response, 7 (31.8 %) had a partial response, 4 (18.1 %) were stable and 10 patients (45.4) showed an objective progression.

Regarding subjective response, the performance status improved in 18 patients (81.8 %), was stable in 2 (9 %) and worsened in 2 (9 %). The voiding abnormalities suffered by 6 patients, improved in 5 (83.3 %) and remained stable in 1 (16.7 %). The bony pain, present in 3 patients, improved in 2 and remained stable in 1.

Plasma testosterone levels were evaluated before and during flutamide treatment by standard radioimmunological assays. An increased level was detected only in 3 patients (13.6 %), while it was decreased in 3 (13.6 %) and stable in 16 (72.7 %). Practically, all patients whose sexual life was normal before the treatment with flutamide remained potent thereafter, except one. Another patient who had lost his sexual potency during a previous treatment with cyproterone acetate, recovered it. The side effects, muscular cramps, diarrhoea, dryness of mouth, increased transaminase levels and gynecomastia, were relatively mild. In only 2 cases (9%) it was necessary to stop the administration of flutamide: one patient who suffered from liver insufficiency showed an increased level of serum transaminase and another one had severe diarrhoea. These side effects regressed after therapy suspension.

Gynecomastia was seen in 20 patients, but was reported as painful only in 8 (36.3 %). In one patient gynecomastia was prevented by pre-treatment irradiation (400 rads x 3) of the mammary glands.

CONCLUSION

In conclusion, our experience is in agreement with previous reports indicating that flutamide is a safe and effective form of hormonal treatment of advanced prostate cancer in previously untreated patients. Unless these results can be disproved, flutamide or its analogues still represent a valid therapeutic modality for sexually active patients with prostatic cancer who wish to remain potent. Under this regard, flutamide in monotherapy appears to be a more interesting and innovative modality of treatment than "complete androgenic blockade", whose merits still remain to be confirmed, insofar as the preliminary results of the on- going randomized trials have failed to confirm the original results from Canada (14) that the addition of flutamide to orchidectomy produce a dramatic improvement of survival rate and other parameters as compared to orchidectomy alone.

A careful monitoring of plasma testosterone is suggested and the treatment may be modified if plasma testosterone exceeds normal levels. The patient should be left free to express their option.

Further investigations are needed. No data regarding intracellular DHT concentrations in patients treated with pure antiandrogens are available so far. It is desirable that further clinical studies take this parameter into account in patients treated with flutamide or nilutamide.

Furthermore, on-going controlled clinical trials only compare surgical or medical castration versus castration plus antiandrogens. There is a need for a study comparing antiandrogens alone versus antiandrogens plus castration. Such a study has been recently implemented in Italy, under the form of a randomized multicentric trial. Pure antiandrogens can also be useful in patients relapsing after an initial response to hormonal treatment. It may represent a good alternative to weekly epirubicin or other forms of secondary treatment.

SUMMARY

Our preliminary experience shows that flutamide is an effective treatment in patients with stage C and D prostate cancer. Local and distant response rates appear to be comparable with those obtained by "classic" hormone therapy. Libido and sexual potency are generally not affected. Palliation of symptoms is frequent and is usually accompanied by improvement of performance status and quality of life. The side effects are slight or moderate, but an elevation of transaminases in patients with borderline liver insufficiency is possible.

REFERENCES

1) Furr B.J.A. (1988): ICI 176, 334: a novel non-steroidal, peripherally selective antiandrogen. In: Smith P.H., Pavone-Macaluso M.: Management of advanced cancer of the prostate and bladder. Alan R. Liss, New York, p. 13 - 26.

2) Neri R (1987) Clinical utility of flutamide. J. Drug Dev 1, suppl 1: 5-9

3) Lund F and Rasmussen F (1988) Flutamide versus stilboestrol in the treatment of advanced prostatic cancer: a randomized prospective study. Brit. J. Urol. 61: 140-142

4) Sogani PC, Whitmore WF (1979) Experience with flutamide in previously untreated patients with advanced prostatic cancer. J Urol 122: 640-643

5) Jacobo E, Schmidt JD, Weinstein SH, Flocks RH (1976) Comparison of flutamide (SCH-13521) and diethylstilbestrol in untreated advanced prostatic cancer. Urology 8: 231-234

6) Consoli C, Corrado F, Di Silverio F, Fontana D, Lotti T, Micali F, Pavone-Macaluso M, Piccinno A, Pisani F, Usai E, Recchia M, Granata P, Pintus C (1987) Risultati preliminari di uno studio multicentrico sul trattamento del carcinoma della prostata con flutamide. Proc. 60th Congress Italian Urological Society (Abstract) Acta Urol Ital 1:231

7) Daricello G, Serretta V, Pavone-Macaluso M (1987) Flutamide in the treatment of advanced prostate cancer J Drug Dev 1, suppl. 1: 17-22

8) Knuth UA, Hano R, Nieschlag E (1984) Effect of flutamide or cyproterone acetate on pituitary and testicular hormones in normal men. J Clin Endocr Metab 59: 963-969

9) Prout GR, Irwin RJ, Kliman B, Daly JJ, MacLaughlin RA, Griffin PP (1975) Prostatic cancer and SCH-13521. II: Histological alterations and the pituitary gonadal axis. J Urol 113:834

10) Johansson JE, Andersson SO, Beckman KW, Lindgardh G, Zador G (1987) Clinical evaluation of flutamide and estramustine as initial treatment of metastatic carcinoma of prostate. Urology 29: 55-59

11) MacFarlane JR, Tolley DA (1985) Flutamide therapy for advanced prostatic cancer: a phase II study. Brit. J. Urol. 57: 172-174

12) Kaisary AV, Fellows GJ, Smith JC (1987) Antiandrogen (flutamide) therapy in management of relapsing metastatic prostatic carcinoma. J Urol 137, (4, part 2), 256A, abstr. 612

13) Di Silverio F, Tenaglia R, Bizzarri M, Biggio A, Saragnano R (1987) Experience with flutamide in advanced prostatic cancer patients refractory to previous endocrine therapy. J Drug Dev. 1: Suppl. 1, 10 - 16

14) Labrie F, Dupont A, Belanger A, Lacourcière Y, Raynaud JP, Husson JM, Gareau J, Fazekas ATA, Sandow J, Monfette G, Girard JG, Emond J, Houle JG (1983) New approach in the treatment of prostate cancer: complete instead of partial withdrawal of androgens. Prostate 4: 579-594

15) Navratil H (1987) Double blind study of anandron versus placebo in stage D2 prostate cancer patients receiving Buserelin. In: Murphy GP, Khoury S, Küss R, Chatelain C, Denis L (eds) Prostate Cancer. Part A: Research, endocrine treatment and histopathology, Alan R Liss, New York, p. 401-410

16) Beland G, Elhilali M, Fradet Y, Laroch B, Ramsey EW, Benner PM, Tewar HD (1987) Total androgen blockade vs orchiectomy in stage D2 prostate cancer. In: Murphy GP, Khoury S, Küss R, Chatelain C, Denis L (eds): Prostate Cancer. Part A: Research, endocrine treatment and histopathology. Alan R Liss, New York, p 391-400

17) Brisset JM, Boccon-Gibod L, Botto H, Camey M, Criou G, Duclos JM, Duval F, Gonties D, Jorest R, Lamy L, Le Duc A, Mouton A, Petit M, Prawerman A, Richard F, Savatovsky I, Vallancien G (1987) Anandron (RU 23908) associated to surgical castration in previously untreated stage D prostate cancer: A multicenter comparative study of two doses of the drug and of a placebo. In: In: Murphy GP, Khoury S, Küss R, Chatelain C, Denis L (eds): Prostate Cancer. Part A: Research endocrine treatment and histopathology, Alan R Liss, New York, p 401-410

18) Boccardo F, Decensi AU, Guarneri D, Martorana G, Fioretto P, Mini E, Pavone-Macaluso M, Giuliani L, Santi L, Periti P and other participants in the Italian Prostatic Cancer Project (P.O.N.CA.P.) (1989): Anandron (RU 23908) as sole chemotherapy in metastatic prostate cancer: preliminary results of a multicentric Italian study. In: Murphy GP and Khoury S (eds): Therapeutic progress in urological cancer. Alan R Liss, New York, p 831-832

Uro-Oncology: Current Status
and Future Trends, pages 159–170
© 1990 Wiley-Liss, Inc.

CHEMOTHERAPY OF ADVANCED CANCER OF THE PROSTATE

M. P. Wirth

Department of Urology, School of Medicine, University of Würzburg, Josef-Schneider-Str. 2, 8700 Würzburg, FRG

Prostatic cancer is the second most common malignant tumor in men in the Federal Republic of Germany and in the United States of America (1,3,26). At the time of diagnosis 42 % of patients have stage C or D lesions (22). Of the prostate cancers, 20-30 % are hormone resistant and 50 % of patients with symptomatic metastatic disease will relapse within 3 years after initiation of hormonal therapy (25). Median survival after relapse during hormonal treatment is less than 40 weeks (8).

These data indicate clearly that additional forms of treatment in locally incurable prostate cancer are needed.

As yet, however, the results of chemotherapeutic treatment of prostate cancer have been disappointing. Several reasons are conceivable for this low response rate. In almost all patients with cancer of the prostate treated by chemotherapy, prior local and/or systemic therapy had already failed. The high tumor volume present in these patients is another limiting factor for chemotherapy. The tumor itself is the other problem. The low growth fraction of less than 5 % could be responsible for failure of chemotherapy since only dividing cells can be destroyed by most drugs administered. The tumor cell heterogeneity of prostate cancer, possibly with chemotherapy-resistant tumor cell clones, may also be a cause of the low response rates. On the other hand, the chemotherapeutic agents available today may not be sufficiently effective.

One problem in discussing the literature about chemotherapy in prostate cancer is the various definitions of response rates used. The EORTC-criteria (Table 1) require a measurable lesion to prove response, whereas the National Prostatic Cancer Project of the United States includes a stable disease for 12 weeks as a response criteria. This classification obviously leads to different results.

Table 1 EORTC - response-criteria in prostate cancer

Complete response:

(all criteria have to be fulfilled)

- Decrease of prostatic volume of 30 % or more, if measured by ultrasound

- Disappearance of all preexisting bone lesions

- Return of elevated acid phosphatase to normal

Partial response

(all criteria have to be fulfilled)

- No increase of primary tumor which is sufficient to state objective progression

- Decrease of measurable lesions by 50 % at least on two observations with a time interval of 4 weeks

- Decrease of elevated acid phosphatase of at least 50 %

- No deterioration in performance status or pain

- No new lesions appear

"No change" or "stable disease" is observed when the patient is not classified as having progression or a complete or partial response.

RESULTS OF PHASE II TRIALS IN HORMONE REFRACTORY PROSTATE CANCER

Single Agent Chemotherapy

In Table 2 the average overall response rates of single-agent chemotherapy in prostate cancer are given. The wide range of response rates is explained by the different dosages, treatment intervals and response criteria used in these trials. The overall response rates given in these studies usually refer due to stable disease during chemotherapy. Complete or partial response rates are also listed in Table 2, if given. These objective response rates are low and only cisplatin, epirubicin, and mitomycin C showed complete or partial response rates of more than 20 %.

Table 2   Single agent chemotherapy in hormone refractory prostate cancer (Phase II trials)

Drug	No. of patients evaluable	Response rates (%)		CR + PR only (%) (if given)	References
		Mean	Range		
Cisplatin	117	27	0 - 44	24	6
Cyclophosphamide	57	14	-	-	2
Doxorubicin	139	31	14 - 84	9	6
Epirubicin	60	36	27 - 47	23	2, 15 a)
Etoposide	43	7	3 - 40	5	6, 38
Estracyt	421	30	20 - 74	17	6, 16
Mitomycin C	35	26	0 - 29	29	6, 12
5-Fluorouracil	24	50	14 -100	-	

a) Medroxyprogesterone acetate was also given.

Combination chemotherapy

The average overall response rates for combination chemotherapy in phase II studies reported in the literature are higher than those for single agent treatment (Tables 2,3). However, if only the complete and partial response rates found in the small group of patients treated with cyclophosphamide, doxorubicin or cisplatin are considered, acceptable results have been achieved.

Table 3   Combination chemotherapy in hormone refractory prostate cancer (phase II trials)

Treatment	No. of patients	Response rates (%)		CR + PR only (%) (if given)	References
		Mean	Range		
CYC, DOX	93	41	18 - 57	13	10, 17, 19, 31, 37
DOX, 5-FU, MMC	92	50	44 - 64	3	9, 14, 18
MPL, MTX, 5-FU, VCR, PREDN.	84	61		4	24
CYC, DOX, DDP	17	71		41	11

CYC, cyclophosphamide; DOX, doxorubicin; 5-FU, 5-flourouracil; MMC, mitomycin C; MTX, methotrexate; VCR, vincristine; Predn., prednisone; DDP, cisplatin

Table 4   Combination chemotherapy versus monotherapy
           in hormone refractory prostate cancer

randomized studies

Combination chemotherapy	Response rate	Monotherapy	Reference
CYC + 5-FU + DOX b)	=	CYC	4
CYC + 5-FU + MTX b)	=	CYC	23
CYC + 5-FU + DOX b)	>	5-FU	30
MMC + 5-FU + DOX b)	=	CYC	14
CYC + DOX b)	-	Hydroxyurea	34
DOX + DDP a)	=	DOX	36
EST + VCR a)	=	EST	32
	=	VCR	
EST + DDP a)	>	EST	33
	>	DDP	

CYC, cyclophosphamide; 5-FU, 5-fluorouracil; DOX, doxorubicin; MTX, methotrexate, MMC, mitomycin C, DDP, cisplatin; EST, estracyt, VCR, vincristine

a)   Dosage and time intervals the same in monotherapy and combination therapy.

b)   Dosage and/or time intervals different in monotherapy and combination therapy.

Prospective Randomized Trials

In prospective randomized trials combination chemotherapy showed no superiority over a single agent treatment (Table 4). In five of the eight studies in the monotherapy arm summarized in Table 4, different drugs, dosages and/or time intervals were used in comparison to the combination therapy. This makes interpretations almost impossible because the alterations obviously influence the results. Stephens and coworkers (34) reported combination therapy to be superior. However, hydroxyurea, which was used in the monotherapy arm is regarded as an ineffective drug in prostate cancer. Torti and coworkers (36) tested cisplatinum plus doxorubicin versus doxorubicin alone using the same dosage and time intervals in both arms. Significantly higher toxicity was observed with the combination chemotherapy than with monotherapy with doxorubicin. Renal dysfunction was only seen when cisplatin was also used. Torti et al. thus did not show that combination chemotherapy with doxorubicin and cisplatin was better than doxorubicin alone.

In the study reported by Soloway et al.(32) an advantage of estracyt plus vincristine over estracyt or vincristine alone was also not found. A synergistic effect of combining estracyt with cisplatin has however been reported by Soloway and coworkers (33).

Weekly Chemotherapeutic Regimen

Weekly treatment regimens have also been used in prostate cancer. Instead of giving a 3- to 4-week cycle, a lower dose of cytostatic drugs is administered weekly. The reason for this kind of treatment is that almost all cytostatic drugs kill only dividing cells and after the growing cells are destroyed cells are recruited from the G 0 phase into the growth fraction. The cells recruited from the G 0 phase can be destroyed by cytotoxic therapy. In tumors like prostate cancer with a low growth fraction (less than 5 %), treatment at shorter intervals seems to be of advantage. Torti et al. (35) found good reponse rates using doxorubicin 20 mg/m^2 weekly (Table 5). However, with a total dose of only 20 mg doxorubicin per week, Fossa et al.(7) found only a minor response. The different results may due to the reduced dosage administered by Fossa et al. (Table 5). Epirubicin was also effective in a weekly treatment schedule used in an outpatient setting by Burk et al.(2). The toxicicty of this treatment modality was acceptable. Merrin et al.(20) reported a partial response of 43 % using weekly cisplatin 1 mg/kg for 6 weeks, and thereafter the same dose at 3-week-intervals. Moore et al.(21) used almost the same regimen and observed only a partial response in 10% of their patients. An explanation for these discrepancies is again the different response criteria used in the two studies.

Table 5   Weekly chemotherapeutic regimen
            in hormone refractory prostate cancer

Drug	No. of patients	Response rate (%)	PR only (%)	Reference
Doxorubicin	25	84	16	35
	22	27	0	7
Epirubicin	30	51	20	2
Cisplatin	21	43	43	20
	33	10	10	21

Primary Chemotherapy

The reasons for primary chemotherapy in prostate cancer are the following:

1.   Prostate cancer is heterogeneous with hormone-resistant cell clones

2.   Chemotherapy is probably more effective in low tumor volumes.

Protocol 500 of the National Prostatic Cancer Project (28) did not find any advantage of primary chemotherapy with cyclophosphamide and estracyt versus orchiectomy and diethylstilbestrol. Rübben and Altwein (27) reported primary chemotherapy to be superior in metastasized prostate cancer. In their non randomized study, tumor progression occured after 6 months in 41 % of the patients when orchiectomy had been performed. When chemotherapy consisting of 5-fluorouracil, doxorubicin and mitomycin C was given in addition to orchiectomy, only 17 % of the patients were in progress after 6 months.

Servadio et al.(29) described primary chemotherapy of stage C and D 2 prostate cancer consisting of cyclophosphamide and 5-fluorouracil after orchiectomy and additional estrogen therapy. They administered the drugs during the first 2 years at weekly intervals and thereafter at 3- and 4-week intervals. They reported a 5 year survival rate of 63.5 % in stage D2 disease and of 87.6% in stage C. These results, however, need to be corroborated by larger series.

LITERATUR

1. Altwein, J.E., Jacobi, G.H. (1980) Hormontherapie des Prostata-Carcinoms. Urologe A, 19: 350 - 357

2. Burk, K., Schultze-Seemann, W., de Riese, W., Hanke, P., Weber, W., (1986) Die ambulante cytostatische Therapie des hormon-refraktären Prostata-Carcinoms mit 4-Epirubicin (ab stract) Deutscher Kongreß für Urologie. 150

3. Carter S.K., Wassermann T.H. (1975) The chemotherapy of urologic cancer. Cancer 36: 729 - 747

4. Chlebowski, R.T., Hestorff, R. Sardoff, L. Weiner, J., Bateman, J.R. (1978) Cyclophosphamide (NSC 26271) versus the combination of adriamycin (NSC 123127), 5-fluorouracil (NSC 19893), and cyclophosphamide in the treatment of metastastic prostate cancer. Cancer 42: 2546 - 2552

5. Cutler, S.J., Young, J.L. (1975) Third national cancer survey: incidence data. Natl. Cancer. Inst. Monogr. 41

6. Eisenberger, M.A., Bezerdjian, L. Kalash, S. (1987) A critical assessment of the role of chemotherapy for endocrine-resistant prostatic carcinoma. Urol. Clin. North Am. 14: 695 - 706

7. Fossa, S.D., Urnes, T., Kaalhus, O. (1987) Weekly low-dose adriamycin in hormone-resistant metastatic cancer of the prostate. Scand. J. Urol. Nephrol. 21: 13 - 16

8. Gibbons, R.P. (1987) Prostate cancer chemotherapy. Cancer 60: 586 - 587

9. HSU, D.S., Babaian, R.J. (1983) 5-fluorouracil, adriamycin, mitomycin-C (FAM) in the treatment of hormonal resistant stage D adenocarcinoma of the prostate (abstract). Proc. Am. Soc. Clin. Oncol. 133

10. Ihde, D.C., Bunn, P.A., Cohen, M.H., Dunnick, N.R., Eddy, J.C., Minna, J.D. (1980) Effective treatment of hormonally unresponsive metastatic carcinoma of the prostate with adriamycin and cyclophosphamide: methods of documenting tumor response and progression. Cancer 45: 1300 - 1310

11. Ihde, D.C., Bunn, P.A., Cohen, M.H. (1981) Combination chemotherapy as initial treatment for stage D 2 prostatic cancer (abstract). Proc. Am. Assoc. Cancer Res: 648

12. Jones, W.G., Fossa, S.D., Bono, A.V., Croles, J.J., Stoter, G., de Pauw, M., Sylvester, R., members of the EORTC Genito-Urinary Tract Cooperative Group. (1986) Mitomycin-C in the treatment of metastatic prostate cancer: report on an EORTC phase II study. World J. Urol. 4: 182 - 185

13. Kasimis, B.S., Miller, B.J., Kaneshiro, C.A., Forbes, K.A., Moran, E.M., Metter, G.E. (1985) Cyclophosphamide versus 5-fluorouracil, doxorubicin, and mitomycin-C (FAM) in the treatment of hormone-resistant metastatic carcinoma of the prostate. A preliminary report of a randomized trial. J. Clin. Oncol. 3: 385 - 392

14. Kasimis, B.S., Moran, E.M., Miller, J.B. (1983) Treatment of hormone-resistant metastatic cancer of the prostate with 5-FU, doxorubicin and mitomycin-C (FAM): preliminary report. Cancer Treat. Rep. 67: 937 - 939

15. Kontturi, M., Sotarauta, M., Tammela, T., Lukkarinen, O., Romppainen, W. (1988) Sequentially alternating hormone chemotherapy with high-dose medroxy-progesterone acetate and low-dose epirubicin for the treatment of hormone-resistant metastatic prostate cancer. Eur. Urol. 15: 43 - 47

16. Leistenschneider, W., Nagel, R. (1980) Estracyt therapy of advanced prostatic cancer with special reference to control of therapy with cytology and DNA cytophotometry. Eur. Urol. 6: 111 - 115

17. Lloyd, R.E., Jones, S.E., Salmon, S.E., Durie, B.G.M., McMahon, C.J. (1976) Combination chemotherapy with adriamycin (NSC-123127) and cyclophosphamide (NSC-26271) for solid tumors: phase II trial. Cancer Treat. Rep. 60: 77 - 83

18. Logothetis, C.J., Samuels, M.L., von Eschenbach, A.C., Trindale, A., Ogden, S., Grant, C., Johnson, D.E. (1983) Doxorubicin, mitomycin-C and 5-fluorouracil (DMF) in the treatment of metastatic hormonal refractory adenocarcinoma of the prostate, with a note on the staging of metastatic prostate cancer. J. Clin. Oncol. 1: 368 - 378

19. Merrin, C., Etra, W., Wajsman, Z., Baumgartner, G., Murphy, G.P. (1976) Chemotherapy of advanced carcinoma of the prostate with 5-fluorouracil, cyclophosphamide, and adriamycin. J. Urol. 115: 86 - 88

20. Merrin, C. (1978) Treatment of advanced carcinoma of the prostate (stage D) with infusion of cis-diaminedichloroplatinum (II NSC 119875): a pilot study. J. Urol. 119: 522 - 524

21. Moore, M.R., Troner, M.B., DeSimone, P., Birch, R. Irwin, L. (1986): Phase II evaluation of weekly cisplatin in metastatic hormone-resistant prostate cancer: a Southeastern Cancer Study Group Trial. Cancer Treat. Rep. 70: 541 - 542

22. Murphy, G.P. Natarajan, N., Pontes, J.E., Schmitz, R.C., Smart, C.R., Schmidt, J.P., Mettlin, C. (1982) The national

    survey of prostate cancer in the United States by the American College of Surgeons. J. Urol. 127: 928 - 234

23. Muss, H.B., Howard, V., Richards, F., White, D.R., v. Jackson, D., Cooper, R.M., Stuart, J.J., Resnick, M.I., Brodkin, R., Spurr, C.L. (1981) cyclophosphamide versus cyclophosphamide, methotrexate, and 5-fluorouracil in advanced prostatic cancer. Cancer 47: 1949 - 1953

24. Paulson, D.F., Berry, W.R., Cox, E.B., Walker, A. Laszlo, J.(1979) Treatment of metastastic endocrine unresponsive carcinoma of the prostate gland with multiagent chemotherapy: Indicators of response of therapy. J. Natl. Cancer Inst. 63: 615 - 622

25. Reiner, W.G., Scott, W.W., Eggleston, J.C., Walsh, P.C. (1979) Long-term survival after hormonal therapy for stage D prostate cancer. J. Urol. 122: 183 - 184

26. Ross, R.K., Paganini-Hill, A, Henderson, B. (1983) The etiology of prostate cancer: what does epidemiology suggest? Prostate, 4: 333 - 344

27. Rübben, H., Altwein, J.E. (1987) Das fortgeschrittene Prostata-Carcinom - Ein therapeutisches Dilemma? Urologe A 26: 7 - 14

28. Schmidt, J.D. (1983) Combination of chemotherapy and hormones in prostatic cancer. In: Pavone Macaluso M., Smith P.H. (eds): Cancer of the prostate and kidney. Plenum, New York, P., 397

29. Servadio, C., Mukamel, E., Kahan, E. (1984) Carcinoma of the prostate in Israel: Some epidemiological and therapeutic considerations. Prostate 5: 375

30. Smalley, R.V., Bartolucci, A.A., Hemstreet, G., Hester, M. (1981) A phase II evaluation of a 3-drug combination of cyclophosphamide, doxorubicin and 5-fluorouracil and of 5-fluorouracil in patients with advanced bladder carcinoma or stage D prostatic carcinoma. J. Urol. 125: 191 - 195

31. Soloway, M.S., Shippel, R.M., Ikard, M. (1979) Cyclophosphamide, doxorubicin-hydrochloride and 5-fluorouracil in advanced carcinoma of the prostate. J. Urol. 122: 637 - 639

32. Soloway, M.S., DeKernion, J.B., Gibbons, R.P., Johnson, D.E., Loening, S.A., Pontes, J.E. Prout, G.R. Jr., Schmidt, J.D., Scott, W.W., Chu, T.M. Gaeta, J.F., Slack, N.H., Murphy, G.P. (1981) Comparison of estramustine phosphate and vincristine alone or in combination for patients with advanced hormone refractory, previously irradiated carcinoma of the prostate. J. Urol. 125: 664 - 667

33. Soloway, M.S., Beckley, S., Brady, M.F., Chu, T.M., DeKernion, J.B. Dhabuwala, C., Gaeta, J.F., Gibbons, R.P., Leoning, S.A., McKiel, C.F., Mc Leod, D.G., Pontes, J. E., Prout, G.R., Scardino, P.T., Schlegel, J.U., Schmidt, J.D., Scott, W.W., Slack, N.H., Murphy, G.P. (1983) A comparison of estramustine phosphate versus cisplatin alone versus estramustine phosphate plus cisplatin in patients with advanced hormone refractory prostate cancer who had had extensive irradiation to the pelvis or lumbosacral area. J. Urol. 129: 56 - 61

34. Stephens, R.L., Vaughn, C., Lane, M., Costanzi, J., O'Bryan, R., Balcerzak, S.P., Levin, H., Frank, J., Coltman, C.A. (1983) Adriamycin and cyclophosphamide versus hydroxyurea in advanced prostatic cancer. Cancer 53: 406 - 410

35. Torti, F.M., Aston, D., Lum, B.L., Kohler, M., Williams, R., Spaulding, J.T., Shortliffe, L., Freiha, F.S. (1983) Weekly doxorubicin in endocrine-refractory carcinoma of the prostate. J. Clin. Oncol. 1: 477 - 482

36. Torti, F.M., Shortliffe, L.D., Carter, S.K., Hannigan, J.F., Aston, D., Lum, B.L., Williams, R.D., Spaulding, J.T., Freiha, F.S. (1985) A randomized study of doxorubicin versus doxorubicin plus cisplatin in endocrine-unresponsive metastatic prostatic carcinoma. Cancer 56: 2580 - 2586

37. Uzbicki, R.M., Amer, R.H., Al-Sarraf, M. (1979) Combination of adriamycin and cyclophosphamide in the treatment of metastatic prostatic carcinoma. Cancer Treat. Rep. 63: 999 - 1001

38. Walther, P.J., Williams, St. D., Troner, M., Greco, A.F., Birch, R., Einhorn, L.H., and the Southeastern Cancer Study Group (1986) Phase II study of etoposide for carcinoma of the prostate. Cancer Treat. Rep. 70: 771 - 772

Uro-Oncology: Current Status
and Future Trends, pages 171–185
© 1990 Wiley-Liss, Inc.

STANFORD EXPERIENCE WITH CHEMOTHERAPY FOR METASTATIC
PROSTATE CANCER

Frank M. Torti, Jeffery Reese and Fuad Freiha

Divisions of Oncology and Urology, Stanford
University Medical Center, Stanford Ca. 94305
and Veterans Administration Medical Center,
Palo Alto, Ca. 94304

DEFINITION OF PROBLEM

More than ten percent of all cancer deaths in the
United States are attributable to cancer of the prostate.
In 1988, it was estimated that there were 99,000 new cases
of prostate cancer, and 28,000 deaths due to the disease.
In spite of attempts at early diagnosis and surveillance,
the majority of men have regional or distant metastatic
disease at diagnosis. Even among the small subset who
have disease completely confined to the prostate, nearly
half of these patients will recur after radical surgery or
irradiation, suggesting that even among this most
favorable group, tumor cells had spread beyond the
prostate prior to treatment. Unfortunately, then, most
patients with prostate cancer face therapy of a systemic
disease.

Death from prostate cancer seldom occurs before the
age of 50; mortality from the disease increases
dramatically with age (Blair and Fraumeni 1978; Franks
1973). Death rates from prostatic carcinoma show
considerable international geographical variation. The
age-adjusted mortality rate in 1974-1975 ranged from 0.1
per 100,000 population in Honduras, to 1 to 2 per 100,000
in Asian countries, and peaked at 22 per 100,000 in Sweden
(Silverberg 1980). Whether this difference is due to
genetic or environmental factors is speculative, although
studies of Polish and Japanese immigrants to the United
States suggest that environmental factors play an
important role (Staszewski and Haenszel 1965; Haenszel
and Kurihara 1968; Dunn 1975). In all countries, however,

roughly equivalent distributions of stage of disease at diagnosis prevail. Thus advanced stage at diagnosis is a common biologic manifestation of a wide range of ethnic, geographical and environmental variables which may contribute to the disease.

This manuscript will review the actual trials undertaken at Stanford and in the Northern California Oncology Group in recent years, and then review some of the generic issues of response measurement, as addressed by our group as well as other investigators.

PROSTATE CANCER CHEMOTHERAPY TRIALS

The first Stanford/NCOG trial randomized 37 patients with hormonally-refractory prostatic carcinoma between doxorubicin and doxorubicin plus cisplatin (Torti, 1985).

TABLE 1. Comparison of Sites of Disease at Study Entry
Weekly versus Three-weekly Doxorubicin Trials

	Doxorubicin		Doxorubicin + cisplatin		Weekly Doxorubicin	
	No.	%	No.	%	No.	%
Prostate: measurable						
tumor	5/20	25	7/17	41	8/25	32
Bone	20/20	100	13/17	76	24/25	96
Lymph nodes						
Peripheral	1/18	6	2/17	12	2/25	8
Pelvic or						
para-aortic	2/17	12	2/14	14	4/17	24
Pulmonary						
Lung nodules	3/20	15	0/16	0	1/25	4
Mediastinal mass	1/20	5	1/16	6	2/25	8
Pleural effusion	3/20	15	1/16	6	3/25	12
Liver	2/20	10	1/15	7	1/25	4
IVP/ureteral						
obstruction	5/18	28	6/15	40	1/17	6
Soft tissue	2/17	12	1/15	7	1/25	4

The header "No. of patients positive/ Total no. evaluated" spans the three data groups.

All patients had failed prior hormonal treatment, and the majority had failed two prior hormonal treatments. Mean Karnofsky performance status (76% doxorubicin versus 75% combination), percent of patients with prior palliative irradiation (40% doxorubicin versus 35% combination), and hemoglobin levels of <12 g/dl (30% doxorubicin versus 24% combination) were roughly equivalent in the two treatment groups. More patients treated with doxorubicin than the combination treatment had an elevated acid phosphatase level at study entry (90% versus 65%). Measurable bidimensional tumors were present in 13 patients in 16 sites in the doxorubicin arm and in 10 patients in 11 sites in the combination arm. Partial responses were seen in 1 of 13 patients in the doxorubicin arm and 2 (20%) of 10 patients in the combination arm. Improvement in Karnofsky performance status of 20% or greater was rarely observed with either treatment (7% doxorubicin versus 8% combination). Acid phosphatase levels normalized or improved by 50% in 39% of patients who received doxorubicin and 27% of patients who received the combination. The overall response rate by National Prostatic Cancer Project Criteria was 53% for doxorubicin and 59% for doxorubicin plus cisplatin. Bone marrow and gastrointestinal toxicity were severe, particularly in the combination arm, and required discontinuation of treatment in some patients who responded to treatment. Moderate renal dysfunction (creatinine value 2.0 - 3.0 mg/dl) occurred only in the combination arm at an incidence of 23%. Time to progression and survival were similar for the two treatment groups. In this small group of 37 patients, the combination of cisplatin and doxorubicin showed no improvement over doxorubicin alone in response, response duration, or survival, and was difficult to administer in this patient population. It is important to recognize that such a trial does not reflect on the single agent activity of cisplatin, which was not addressed in this trial.

We next investigated weekly doxorubicin as a single agent, which results which contrasted those reported above (Torti, 1983 a). Twenty-five patients with endocrine-refractory prostatic carcinoma were treated with doxorubicin, 20 mg/m^2 given weekly. All patients had prior hormonal therapy (68% had two or more prior hormonal maneuvers), and 21 (84%) had prior therapeutic or palliative irradiation. Median Karnofsky performance status at the time of entry was 70. Hemoglobin was less than 12.0 g/dl in 15 patients (See Table 1). Bidimensional tumors were present in 12 patients in 19 disease sites; four of the 12 patients (33%) responded in eight of the 19 sites (42%); and three of eight patients had a 75% decrease in prostatic nodule size. Ten of 20 evaluable patients had an improvement of 20% or greater in Karnofsky performance status and 67% (14 of 21) had marked improvement in pain. A greater than 50% reduction or normalization of acid phosphatase occurred in 19% and of alkaline phosphatase in 53%. Using the National Prostatic Cancer Project criteria, overall response rate was 84%.

TABLE 2. Effects of Treatment on Functional Sites and Phosphatase Levels Weekly versus Three-weekly Doxorubicin Trials

	No. responding/no. evaluable at entry*					
	Doxorubicin + cisplatin		Doxorubicin		Weekly Doxorubicin	
	No.	%	No.	%	No.	%
>-20% increase in Karnofsky Performance Status	1/15	7	1/13	8	10/20	50
Acid phosphatase Reduced by 50% or normalized (NCOG criteria)	7/18	39	3/11	27	3/16	19
Normalized	1/18	6	2/11	18	2/17	12
Alkaline phosphatase Reduced by 50% or normalized (NCOG criteria)	2/13	15	8/11	72	10/19	53
Normalized	1/13	8	5/11	45	4/22	18
>-20% decrease in bone pain	3/11	27	4/10	40	14/21	67

Gastrointestinal toxicity and alopecia were minimal and myelosupression was not life threatening in any patient. However, administration of adequate drug dosage required careful attention to the dose attenuation scheme (Table 3, below).

TABLE 3. Dose Reduction for Weekly Doxorubicin

Leukocytes (cells/uL)	>-150,000	149,999 100,000	(cells/uL) 99,999 75,000	<75,000
>-3,500	100	100*	50	0
3,000-3,499	100	75	50	0
2,500-2,999	50	0	0	0
<2,500	0	0	0	0

*Values represent percentage of calculated dose.

Our conclusion from this trial of weekly doxorubicin was that the therapeutic index was improved with weekly treatment over either of the three weekly regimens discussed above issues such as pain status of patients was carefully assessed (Table 4). Could we build on the reproducible responses and acceptable toxicity of the weekly doxorubicin, particularly to improve the response duration while maintaining acceptable toxicity? Recently completed trials, which are still undergoing final analysis, include investigations of the use of weekly doxorubicin plus methotrexate, as well as weekly doxorubicin plus difluoromethyl ornithine (DFMO) in the treatment of advanced endocrine-refractory disease.

One aspect of the toxicity of doxorubicin warrants further mention, that of cardiotoxicity. Cardiotoxicity is the chonic dose limiting toxicity of doxorubicin, and is the main reason for drug discontinuation in responding patients. Thus, simultaneously with these therapeutic trials of doxorubicin, we undertook to investigate the cardiotoxicity of the weekly and three weekly drug

TABLE 4. Stanford/NCOG Pain Status Scale

Status (%)	Definition
100	Normal, without pain
90	Able to carry on normal activity, minor pain, no special care
80	Normal activities with effort, some pain, no special care
70	Cares for self, unable to carry on normal activity or do active work due to pain
60	Requires occasional assistance in self-care but can accomplish most of own needs, pain is reason for assistance
50	Requires considerable assistance with personal needs and frequent medical care due to pain
40	Disabled, requires special medical care and assistance due to pain
30	Severely disable, hospitalization is indicated for pain
20	Hospitalization necessary; active supportive therapy needed for pain control; intravenous narcotics not completely effective
10	Intractable, constant, and completely debilitating pain

administration schedules. The endpoint of our analyses was the degree of myocardial damage observed in tissue obtained by endomyocardial biopsy and evaluated by electron microscopy; independent of other patient and tumor characteristics, the weekly regimen of doxorubicin was less cardiotoxic than the three weekly schedule. Almost two additional months of treatment could be administered on a weekly schedule to reach the same degree of myocardial damage as observed with a three weekly schedule (Torti, 1983 b).

RESPONSE CRITERIA IN PROSTATIC CARCINOMA

In most solid tumors, response to chemotherapy is easily quantitated by measuring changes in tumor diameter clinically or radiographically. In prostate cancer, measurable disease in the lung, lymph nodes, and soft tissue is uncommon; bone remains the most common clinically apparent site of metastatic spread and the predominant site of symptomatic disease. The skeletal distribution of metastases makes accurate measurement of response difficult. This creates variability in response criteria and patient eligibility requirements for clinical trials. Further, prostatic carcinoma patients with bone metastasis are frequently excluded form drug-oriented phase II trials because bone is a "non-measurable" disease site.

Quantitation of the Prostatic Tumor Nodule

Sequential digital examination of the prostate gland by the same observer may be a useful measure of disease activity and appears to parallel other measures of response. Occasionally, local response may occur during progression of bone disease (Slack et al. 1980). The response of local disease may occur later than response in other disease sites; patients responding to hormonal therapy as evidenced by decreasing acid phosphatase level and bone pain may show little local tumor change at three months, but demonstrate continued improvement in nodule size between three and six months. Anatomical grids displaying the prostate gland in at least two axes are essential for quantitation of local response.

In our Stanford/NCOG trials, the criteria for local disease response have been defined more rigorously than conventional response criteria. This is done specifically to avoid the well-known problems of assessing prostatic cancer dimensions by digital rectal examination. Thus, the response criterion for partial response in the prostate (Table 5) demands a 75% reduction in the area of the involved prostatic nodule.

TABLE 5. Stanford\Northern Oncology Group Definitions of Response for Prostatic Cancer

Category	Definition
Complete response	Complete disappearance of tumor; all sites initially involved must be reevaluated (including bone scan) prior to scoring an overall CR

Partial response	1. Bidimensional tumor
	  a. Prostate nodule: 75% decrease in the product of the two largest perpendicular diameters by sequential rectal exam or rectal
	  b. Other than prostate nodule: 50% decrease in the product of the two largest perpendicular diameters of soft tissue mass, palpable lymph nodes, liver mass or retroperitoneal mass on computerized tomographic scan, pulmonary nodes, etc; no evidence of progression on bone scan or bone roentgenograms and no deterioration in pain or Karnofsky performance status (as defined under progression)
	2. Evaluable disease, not bidimensional
	  a. Ureteral obstruction on intravenous pyelogram or ultrasound: complete resolution
	  b. Pleural effusion: complete resolution
	  c. Diffuse interstitial (lymphangitic) disease: complete resolution
	3. Acid phosphatase (evaluable if greater than 2 times normal): 50% reduction

Ancillary response	1. Pain: 20% improvement on pain status scale* not attributable to analgesic therapy

(TABLE 5 continued on page 179.)

(Continued from page 178.)

	2. Alkaline phosphatase (evaluable if greater than 2 times normal): 50% reduction or normalization
	3. Karnofsky performance status (evaluable if <80): 20% improvement
Progression	1. Bone scan: >three new lesions at 6 months; >three new leasions at any time of symptomatic progression
	2. Bidimensional disease
	a. Prostate nodule: 50% increase in the product of the two largest perpendicular diameters of any measurable lesion; appearance of any lesion
	3. Evaluable disease, not bidimensional
	a. Ureteral obstruction: occurrence of partial or complete ureteral obstruction while on therapy
	b. Pleural effusion: occurrence of cytologically positive effusion while on therapy
	4. Acid phosphatase: 50% increase over baseline maintained for at least 1 week apart
	5. Symptomatic measures
	a. Pain: 20% or greater increase in pain on pain status scale that persists over 3 weeks
	b. Karnofsky performance status: 20% decrease that persists for at least 3 weeks and is attributable to tumor
	c. Use of radiation therapy for pain control during therapy

Further, a nodule must be readily measurable before treatment in order to qualify as a "measurable" site. Areas of induration are excluded, although they likely represent cancer tissue, because their margins are too indiscreet to qualify for sequential measurement.

We have been moderately encouraged by the use of the rectal ultrasound for measuring changes in the local tumor in response to treatment. This technique can accurately measure prostate volume and assess state (periprostatic invasion and/or seminal vesicle involvement). Response to hormonal therapy has been monitored with ultrasonography with good results. However, the utility of this method in determining chemotherapeutic response or progression has been questioned (Resnick 1981). Recent advances at Stanford and at other institutions in quantifying prostatic size, as well as measuring the extent of localized prostatic cancers prior to radical prostatectomy, make it likely that such techniques will be applied more effectively in the future to measuring hormonal and chemotherapeutic responses.

Acid Phosphatase

The acid phosphatases are lysosomal enzymes found in glandular epithelium and are present in many body fluids and tissues, including serum, red blood cells, spleen, liver, kidney, and bone, especially in osteoclasts. These enzymes hydrolyze orthophosphoric acid esters in acid environments. Per unit weight, prostatic tissue has 1,000 times the concentration of this enzyme than any other tissue, and malignant prostatic tissue has been demonstrated to have less measurable enzyme activity than normal prostate tissue (Yam 1974). The primary role of prostatic acid phosphatases appears to be extracellular; they supply phosphate and catalyze phosphate group activity in spermatozoa (Bodandsky 1972). No major metabolic role in prostate cells has been recognized. Prostatic acid phosphatase (PAP) is heterogeneous, with at least two molecular variants (isoenzymes) (Smith and Lolutby 1968). Most acid phosphatase-containing tissues have two or more isoenzymes (Yam 1974; Bodansky 1972; Foti et al. 1977; Lam et al. 1973). Acid phosphatase level in the serum of healthy volunteers is primarily from enzyme contributed from red blood cells and platelets. Various substrates and enzyme inhibitors have been used to identify and quantitate enzyme activity attributable to the prostate, but prostatic acid phosphatase has not been shown to be more useful than serum acid phosphatase. Although serum acid phosphatase levels may be elevated by hemolysis of red cells and release of platelets during clotting and as a result of a number of malignant and nonmalignant diseases, Murphy et al. (Murphy et al. 1969) found conventional serum acid phosphatase to be as useful as the more specific enzyme assay.

The degree of initial elevation of acid phosphatase has prognostic significance in most series. A comparison of patients with or without metastases, who present with elevated serum acid phosphatase at diagnosis, and patients with normal levels, shows that patients with normal serum acid phosphatase levels live longer (Murphy et al. 1969; Nesbit et al. 1951). One exception to this was a study by Ishibe et al. (Ishibe et al. 1974), in which degree of initial elevation of serum acid phosphatase did not correlate with survival following hormonal therapy.

Serum acid phosphatases, when elevated, parallels other measures of response, although imperfectly. Johnson et al. (Johnson et al. 1976) demonstrated normalization of serum acid phosphatase correlated with pain relief and decreased tumor size; in this series, 17 of 91 patients achieved a 50 percent or greater reduction of tumor mass with chemotherapy. Of these 17 responders, 59 percent normalized their serum acid phosphatase levels. As a single-response parameter, the reduction or normalization of serum acid phosphatase level correlates with improved outcome in most series (Ishibe et al. 1974; Byar 1972; Citrin et al. 1983).

The radioimmunoassay (RIA) method for serum acid phosphatase determinations appears to be a more sensitive tool than enzymatic assays, although its lack of specificity has been questioned (The clinical utility of the RIA method for measuring response to treatment has been studied in a limited number of patients with encouraging results (Vihko et al. 1981; Moon et al. 1983).

Prostatic Specific Antigen (PSA)

Recent work at Stanford (Stamy, 1987), as well as other institutions, has shown a higher degree of correlation between volume of prostatic tissue and PSA than acid phosphatase, as well as a more complete disappearance of PSA than acid phosphatase after radical prostatectomy. Whether the improved diagnostic accuracy of the PSA over acid phosphatase in localized disease also holds for metastatic disease is currently being investigated in prospective trials at Stanford.

REFERENCES

Armenian HK, Lilienfeld AB, Diamond EL, et al. (1974). Relation between benign prostatic hyperplasia and cancer of the prostate. Lancet ii:115.

Blair A, Fraumeni JF (1978). Georgraphic patterns of prostate cancer in the United States, J Natl Cancer Inst 61:1379.

Bodansky O (1972). Acid phosphatase. Adv Clin Chem 15:43.

Bruce AW, Mahan DE (1982). The role of prostatic acid phosphatase in the investigation and treatment of adenocarcinoma of the prostate. Ann NY Acad Sci 390:110.

Byar DP (1972). Treatment of prostatic cancer: studies by the Veterans Administration Cooperative Urological Research Group (VACURG) Bull NY Acad Med 48:751.

Citrin DL, Elson P, DeWys WD (1983). Treatment of metastatic prostate cancer - an analysis of response criteria in patients with measurable soft tissue disease. Proc Am Soc Clin Oncol 2:142.

Cole P, Cramer D (1977). Diet and cancer of endocrine target organs. Cancer 40:434.

Creagen ET, Fraumeni JF (1972). Cancer mortality among American Indians, 1950-1967. J Natl Cancer Inst 49:959.

Domochowski L, Ohtsuki Y, Seman G, et al (1977). Search for oncogenic viruses in human prostate cancer. Cancer Treat Rpt 61:119.

Dunn JE (1975). Cancer epidemiology in populations of the United States - with emphasis on Hawaii and California - and Japan. Cancer Res 35:3240.

Enstrom JE, Auston DF (1977). Interpreting cancer survival rates. Science 195:847.

Ernster VL, Selvin S, Sacks ST, Austin DF, Brown SM, Winkelstein W (1978). Prostatic cancer: Mortality and incidence rates by race and social class. Am J Epidemiol 107:311.

Foti AG, Herschman H, Cooper JF (1977). Isoenzymes of acid phosphatase in normal and cancerous human prostatic tissue. Cancer Res 37:4120.

Franks IM (1973). Etiology, epidemiology and pathology of prostatic cancer. Cancer 32:1092.

Fraumeni JF, Mason TJ (1974). Cancer mortality among Chinese-Americans, 1950-1969. J Natl Cancer Inst 52:659.

Geder L, Rapp F (1980). Herpes virus and prostate carcinogenesis. Arch Androl 4:71.

Graham S, Haughey B, Marshall J, et al. (1983). Diet in the epidemiology of carcinoma of the prostate gland. J Natl Cancer Inst 70:687.

Greenwald P, Damon A, Kirmss V, et al. (1974). Physical and demographic features of men before developing cancer of the prostate. J Natl Cancer Inst 53:341.

Greenwald P, Kirmss V, Burnett WS (1979). Prostate cancer epidemiology: Widowerhood and cancer in spouses. J Natl Cancer Inst 62:1131.

Greenwald P, Kirmss V, Polan Ak, et al. (1974). Cancer of the prostate among men with benign prostatic hyperplasia. J Natl Cancer Inst 53:335.

Haenszel W, Kurihara M (1968). Studies of Japanese immigrants. I. Mortality from cancer and other diseases among Japanese in the U.S. J Natl Cancer Inst 40:43.

Heshmat MY, Kovi J, Herson J, et al. (1975). Epidemiologic association between gonorrhea and prostatic carcinoma. Urology 6:457.

Hutchinson GB (1976). Epidemiology of prostatic cancer. Semin Oncol 3:151.

Ishibe T, Usui T, Nihira H (1974). Prognostic usefulness of serum acid phosphatase levels in carcinoma of the prostate. J Urol 112:237.

Johnson DE, Scott WW, Gibbons RP, et al. (1976). Clinical significance of serum acid phosphatase levels in advanced prostatic carcinoma. Urology 8:123.

Kolonel L, Winkelstein W (1977). Cadium and prostatic carcinoma. Lancet ii, 556.

Lam KW, Li O, Li CY, et al (1973). Biochemical properties of human prostatic acid phosphatase. Clin Chem 19:483.

Lemen RA, Lee JS, Wagoner JK, Blejer HP (1976). Cancer mortality among cadmium production workers. Ann NY Acad Sci 217:273.

Mahan DE, Doctor BP (1979). A radioimmune assay for human prostatic acid phosphatase levels in prostatic disease. Clin Biochem 12:10.

Menck HR, Henderson BE, Pike MC, et al. (1975). Cancer incidence in the Mexican-American. J Natl Cancer Inst 55:531.

Moon TD, Vessella RL, Eickhoff M, Lange PH (1983). Acid phosphatase for monitoring prostatic carcinoma. Comparison of radioimmunoassay and enzymatic techniques. Urology 22:16.

Murphy GP, Reynoso G, Kenny GM, et al. (1969). Comparison of total and prostatic fraction serum acid phosphatase levels in patients with differentiated and undifferentiated prostatic carcinoma. Cancer 23:1309.

Nesbit RM, Baum WC, Mich AA (1951). Serum phosphatase determination in diagnosis of prostatic cancer. A review of 1150 cases. JAMA 145:1321.

Nesbit RM, Plumb RT (1946). Prostatic carcinoma: A follow-up on 795 patients treated prior to the endocrine era and a comparison of survival rates between these and patients treated by endocrine therapy. Surgery 20:263.

Rapp F, Geder L, Murasko D, et al. (1975). Longterm persistance of cytomegalovirus genome in cultured human cells of prostatic orign. J Virol 16:982.

Reddy BS, Cohen IA, McCoy GD, et al. (1980). Nutrition and its relationship to cancer. Adv Cancer Res 32:237.

Resnick MI (1981). Noninvasive techniques in evaluating patients with carcinoma of the prostate. Urology (suppl) 18:25.

Ries LG, Pollack ES, Young JL (1983). Cancer patient survival: Surveillance, epidemiology, and end results program, 1973-79. J Natl Cancer Inst 70:693.

Ross RK, McCurtis JW, Henderson BE, et al. (1979). Descriptive epidemiology of testicular and prostatic cancer in Los Angeles. Br J Cancer 39:284.

Rotkin ID (1977). Studies in the epidemiology of prostate cancer: Expanded sampling. Cancer Treat Rt 61:173.

Sanford EJ, Gder L, Laychock A, et al. (1977). Evidence for the association of cytomegalovirus with carcinoma of the prostate. J Urol 118:789.

Silverberg E (1980). Cancer statistics 1980. CA 30:23.

Slack MH, Mittleman A, Brady MF, et al. (1980). The importance of the stable category for chemotherapy treated patients with advanced and relapsing prostate cancer. Cancer 46:2393.

Smith JK, Lolutby LK (1968). The heterogeneity of prostatic acid phosphatase. Biochem Biophys Acta 151:607.

Stamey TA, Yang N, Hay AR, et al (1987). Prostate-specific antigen is the serum marker for adenocarcinoma of the prostate. N Engl J Med 317:909-916.

Staszewski J, Haenszel W (1965). Cancer mortality among Polish-born in the United States. J Natl Cancer Inst 35:219.

Torti FM, Aston D, Lum BL, Kohler M, Williams RD, Spaulding JT, Shortliffe L, Freiha FS (1983 a). Weekly doxorubicin in endocrine refractory carcinoma of the prostate. J Clin Oncol 1(8):477-482.

Torti FM, Bristow MR, Howes AE, Aston D, Stockdale FE, Kohler M, Brown BW, Billingham ME (1983 b). Reduced cardiotoxicity of doxorubicin delivered on a weekly schedule: assessment by endomyocardial biopsy. Ann Intern Med 99:745-749.

Torti FM, Shortliffe LD, Carter SK, Hannigan JF, Aston D, Lum BL, Williams RD, Spaulding JT, Freiha FS (1985). A randomized study of doxorubicin versus doxorubicin plus cisplatin in endocrine-unresponsive metastatic prostatic carcinoma. Cancer 56:2580-2586.

Veterans Administration Cooperative Urological Research Group: Treatment and survival of patients with cancer of the prostate. Surg Gynecol Obstet 124:1011, 1967

Vihko P, Lukkarinen O, Kontluri M, et al. (1981). Effectiveness of radioimmunoassay of human prostate-specific acid phosphatase in the diagnosis and follow-up of therapy in prostatic carcinoma. Cancer Res 41:1180.

Wynder EL, Mabuchi K, Whitmore WF (1971). Epidemiology of cancer of the prostate. Cancer 28:344.

Yam LT (1974). Clinical significance of the human acid phosphatase: A review. Am J Med 56:604.

Uro-Oncology: Current Status
and Future Trends, pages 187–200
© 1990 Wiley-Liss, Inc.

WEEKLY CHEMOTHERAPEUTIC REGIMEN IN METASTATIC PROSTATE
CANCER

Konrad B u r k

Department Medical Oncology,
FARMITALIA Freiburg (FRG)

Androgen dependency of the prostate gland was already
established at the end of the previous century. WHITE
reported, in 1895, on the removal of an obstruction
caused by adenoma of the prostate (BPH) using bilateral
orchiectomy (1).

Castration leads to a decrease in the serum testosterone
level of over 90%; the remaining 10% of the total amount
of androgen are synthesized in the adrenal gland. The
concept of androgen deprivation during treatment of BPH
was transferred to treatment of prostate carcinoma by
HUGGINS and HODGES in 1941 (2). Since androgen
deprivation has been introduced into treatment of
prostate carcinoma, it is known that some prostate
carcinoma do not react primarily to an androgen
withdrawl, and that, in a large number of cases, a
hormone independence can develop, after contrasexual
therapy and even temporary remission of the clinical
picture (3).

There are two hypotheses which attempt to explain this
mechanism: The adaption mechanism supported by LABRIE
states that an incomplete androgen deprivation may cause
hormone sesitive cells to become hormone insensitive,
with time. The second, and more favored hypothesis from
ISAACS is based upon a selection model in which the

tumor is primarily heterogenous and comprises of both
hormone sensitive and hormone insensitive cells (4).
Both of these types of cells are present in unequal
amounts at the beginning of the tumor. Whether a
prostate carcinoma is hormone sensitive, depends upon
the number of hormone sensitive cells in relation to the
number of hormone insensitive cells. Androgen withdrawl
results in inhibition of the growth of the hormone
sensitive cells. In contrast, the hormone insensitive
cells continue to reproduce and overwhelm the hormone
dependent cells. The tumor becomes hormone resistant and
requires a systemic cytostatic therapy.

The locigal conclusion, which results from the
recognition that prostate carcinoma is heterogenous,
would be an early combination of hormone and
chemotherapy (4).

The following monosubstances are known for their
objective effectiveness, when applied to the cytostatic
therapy of prostate carcinoma: ADRIAMYCIN, CISPLATIN,
CYTOXAN, METHOTREXAT, MITOMYCIN, and, to some extent,
5-FLUOROURACIL (5).

However, none of these substances was capable of
complete healing in any of the studies carried out up to
date. Treatment was simply palliative.

One of the difficulties of the cytostatic treatment of
prostate carcinoma is due to the low rate of cell
division of adenocarcinoma cells. Since most
cytostatics, with the exception of CISPLATIN, work
during the phase of cell division, only very few cells
can be destroyed in tumors having low proliferation
rates per therapy cycle.

Approximately 44% of the cells proliferate in an average
embryonic carcinoma. The natural death rate lies by
approximately 41%. If a chemotherapy lowers the rate of
cell division by more than 10%, then the natural death
rate of the tumor cells will dominate, and result in a
reduction of the tumor mass.

In contrast, only 2,9% of the cells of a typical adenocarcinoma proliferate daily; 2% die. Without influencing the natural death rate, cytostatis, in this case the rate of cell proliferation, must be decreased by at least 30%.
Otherwise the tumor will continue to grow, even if at a slower rate (4).

The effectiveness of cytostatic treatment can only be improved when either the usual cytostatics are applied more frequently than the 3-4 week rhythm, or, if the number of cells killed is raised by addition of a drug, which works independent of cycles or increases the natural death rate of the tumor cells. A combination of more frequent dosages of a cytostatic, along with CISPLATIN or TNF is feasible. However, no studies are known describing such a combined therapy.

Pharmacokinetic studies, carried out by SPETH, have shown that the plasma concentration was at a level of 592 +/- 112 ng/ml five minutes after the weekly injection of EPIRUBICIN. The elimination curve was biphasic, having a half-life of 9.6 +/- 1,8 minutes and 18,2 +/- 5,1 hours. The main metabolite, EPIRUBICINOL, which is also cytostatically active, could still be observed 3 days after injection. A significant accumulation of EPIRUBICINOL could not be observed after 8 injections at one week intervals.

In two patients EPIRUBICIN could be found in tumor tissue up to 7 days subsequent to the last injection. The cellular concentration of EPIRUBICIN was 100-fold higher than the plasma concentration and on the eighth day, after the last injection, it still had a value of 190 +/- 66 ng/10^9 cells (6).

In a Phase-I-study using EPIRUBICIN, it could be shown that using a fraction of the total application each week, the weekly dose intensity could be increased without also increasing the toxicity. Five patients received 20 mg/m2, 8 patients received 30 mg/m2, 11 patients 35 mg/m2, 6 patients 40 mg/m2, and 11 patients 45 mg/m2. The dosage was not increased in individual patients. If a toxicity of degree 3 or 4 was observed, the treatment was to be interrupted and than to be continued then with a lower dosage.

In 3 of the 11 patients receiving the highest dosage (45 mg/m2) toxicity of grade 3 and 4 concerning the number of neutrophils was observed. This effect was completely reversed on day 28. The influence upon both thrombocytes, as well as hemoglobin was negative. Nausea in grade 1 and 2 was observed, independent of dosage. Grades 1 and 2 of alopecia were seen only at dosages above 35 mg/m2 (7).

In a publication from 1983, TORTI reports on the endomyocardial biopsies in patients which received DOXORUBICIN weekly, or every 3 weeks at rates of 20mg/m2 and 60 mg/m2, respectively. Patients, who were treated weekly, received 70,5% of the intended dosage, whereas patients, who were treated every three weeks, received only 61,7% of the intended dosage of ADRIAMYCIN. 7,3% of the biopsies originating from the weekly treatment arm showed heavy myocardial damages of grades 2 and 3. In comparison, 31,9% of the patients receiving treatment every 3 weeks, showed damages to the same extent. No patient, who was treated weekly, showed any clinically relevant congestive heart failure (CHF) whereas, in the other treatment arm, 13% of the patients had clinical CHF and, with an average dose of 405 mg/m2 KOF, showed an average biopsy score or 3 (8).

TORTI's results were confirmed in the following studies using EPIRUBICIN. BECHER was able to show that, in patients with mammary carcinoma, the left ventricular ejection fraction (LVEF) remained unchanged following weekly application and constant dose intensity, whereas patients, who received 60 mg EPIRUBICIN every three weeks, showed a decrease of the LVEF of 10%, which did not, however, fall within the pathological range (9).

A weekly regime is not the same as a low dose regime, since the dose intensity remains unchanged in weekly regimes. In this case, the total dosage which is to be administered, is split into weekly intervals. In contrast, the dose intensity is lowered in low dose therapy.

Over 1000 patients have been treated weekly with ADRIAMYCIN, and the effectivity of the weekly scheme is entirely comparable with the scheme in which ADRIAMYCIN was applied every 3 weeks. This is especially true for breast carcinoma and for non small cell lung carcinoma (8).

One can assume that a weekly scheme is clearly superior in its effectivity, in tumors with a low proliferation rate, as well as toxicity rate in comparison to the conventional scheme. The reasons for this lie in the facts that, firstly, the dose intensity remains unchanged over a weekly regime; secondly, there is the belief that more frequent application of a cytostatic to slow growing tumors (i.e. such as adenocarcinoma) having a proliferation rate of 2,9%/day effect more cells in a proliferation phase than those treated every 3 weeks.

Presently, few studies have been published describing weekly schemes where prostate carcinoma has been cytostatically treated, if one excludes the work describing the use of estramastine phosphate, which is given dayly.

In the Journal of Clin. Oncology in 1983, TORTI reported that 25 patients, with hormone refractive prostate carcinoma were treated with DOXORUBICIN at a weekly dose of 20 mg/m2. The average age of the patients was 70 years. The performance status was significantly lowered in 80% of the patients. Despite the negative selection of the patients, the treatment was generally well tolerated. Only in 2 of the 368 cycles could leukocyte depressions of 1700 and 1500, respectively, be determined. Four patients had a thrombocyte reduction of under 100.000, one being as low as 35.000.

Gastrointestinal toxicity was minimal. Alopecia grade 1 was also no problem for the patients. CHF could not be observed during the entire study. There was also no dosage limiting stomatitis.

Twelve patients had 19 bidimensionally measureable metastases. 4 of the 12 patients (33%) showed an objective remission in 8 of the 19 metastases (42%). The total remission rate was 84%, according to NPCP criteria (10).

If one applies the usual EORTC criteria, then only 33% partial remissions remain. The average time up to progression was 23 weeks. 8 patients had remission times of longer than 6 months and could not be distinguished from the other patients. The average survival rate was 41 weeks for the entire group. 67% of the patients experienced pain relief and in 50% of the cases, the performance status increased more than 20% (10).

In the same year, ROBINSON reported, at an EORTC meeting, that 16 patients having hormone refractory symptomatic prostate carcinoma were treated weekly with 10 mg/m2 body surface ADRIAMYCIN. 11 of the 16 patients (68%) attained a reduction of pain from the treatment, as well as an improvement of performance status. An objective remission could not be obtained with this scheme. There were 2 progressions during the observation time.

ROBINSON could not determine any hematological toxicity in his patients. He compares the effect of a low dose therapy with the effectiveness of a hypophyseal irradiation (11).

In 1987 in the Scand. J. of Urology Nephrology a report appeared by Ms.Fossa concerning 22 patients with hormone resistant metastatic prostate carcinoma which were treated with 20 mg ADRIAMYCIN/ week total dosage.

Six of the 21 patients, which could be evaluated, showed subjective improvement. The average survival time for these patients lay at 8,5 months. In 10 of the 21 cases, there was a reduction of alkaline phosphatase, and, in 7 of 21 cases, a reduction of prostate phosphatase.

Generally, the toxicity was very low. However, one case

resulted in irreversible thrombocytopenia after 3 cycles of ADRIAMYCIN at 20 mg/week (12).

In a pilot study, which was carried out at the University of Marburg in 1984, a random comparison was made with a combination of 5-FU, ADRIAMYCIN, MITOMYCIN (MMC) vs 5-FU, EPIRUBICIN, and MMC vs the weekly fractionated application of EPIRUBICIN as a monosubstance (FAM vs FEM vs EPI weekly). It could be shown that the weekly administration of EPIRUBICIN was as effective as any of the combination schemes. However, the weekly scheme was clearly superior with respect to toxicity, since no myelotixicity, gastrointestinal toxicity, as well as cardiotoxicity could be observed here (13).

On the basis of these results, we began in the autumn of 1984 to treat patients having hormone refractive prostate carcinoma, which were progressive during ESTRACYT® treatment, with EPIRUBICIN at 25 mg/m2 each week. Patient recruiting was terminated in December 1986 with 60 patients. Both the Universities of Marburg and Frankfurt took part in these studies. EPIRUBICIN was applied up until progression. The average age of the patients was 65 (48-83). All patients had local advanced prostate carcinoma with metastases; 22% of the patients had visceral metastases; all patients were dependent upon pain relievers. The phosphatases (either alakaline or acidic phosphatase, or both) were elevated in all patients.
55 patients could be evaluated for response and toxicity. Therapy was well tolerated. 87% of the patients did not complain of side effects, 5% had nausea grade 1, 4% has alopecia grades 1 and 2. In a further 4% of the patients, a leukocyte depression of grade 2 was found. Although some of the patients received a cumulative dosage (up to 3000 mg/m2) which exceeded the cumulative maximum dosage (1000 mg/m2) no CHF could be diagnosed in any patient.

Most patients felt no pain 2-3 weeks after therapy began. 87% of the patients felt a subjective improvement and simultaneously an improved performance status. Thus, treatment not only lead to a reduction of pain, but also enabled bed-ridden patients to become capable of taking care of themselves.

The objective response rate was evaluated 12 weeks after therapy commenced. A partial ojective remission was found in 36% of the patients, according to the EORTC criteria, by means of bone scintigraphs, lung x-rays, ultrasound, urographs, and a normalization of the phosphatase values.

In a further 16% of the patients, a decrease in phosphatases of over 50% was found, which still did not fall into the normal range. With respect to other parameters, these patient had a reduction of the metastatis above 25%, which lay, however, under 50%. This result was evaluated as a minimum response and is not within the realms of the EORTC criteria. The reason that no change patients are categorized into the 2 groups is due to the fact that those patients with a phosphatase reduction of more than 50% lived far longer than those patients whose phosphatase values remained essentially unchanged during treatment.

29% of the patients experienced no change in the metastases status (= NC) after treatment with EPIRUBICIN, and in 18% of the patients, a further progression of the clinical symptoms could be determined after already 12 weeks.

After an observation period averaging 24 months (18-46), only 15 of the 55 patients remained alive (11 of 20 PR; 4 of 9 MR). The median survival time in the PR group has not yet been determined, since more than half of the patients are still alive. Patients with a minimal response have a median survival time of 23 months, whereas patients with NC or PD have median survival times of 7 and 4 months, respectively. The total survival time was median 12 months for all patients. The time up to progression was generally only 4-8 weeks shorter than the time up to death caused by the disease (14).

A team from Hamburg could confirm our results in 35 patients, with respect to both subjective and objective response rates. However, the average observation time of one year for these patients is still too short a time to draw conclusions concerning survival times (personal communication Prof. Becker, PD Hubmann).

In 33 patients, which were treated with 20 mg/m2 EPIRUBICIN for 6 months, RÜBBEN observed an objective progression rate of 49% which can be explained by the fact that, after this time, a large portion of the patiens, which were stable for 3 months, began to show progression. Treatment was generally well tolerated. 4 patients displayed grades 1 and 2 of alopecia, and in 1 patient leukopenia of grade 1 was observed (15).

At the University of Sienna, 8 patients with metastasized prostate carcinoma, which were progressive during hormonal treatment, were treated with 30 mg/m2 EPIRUBICIN weekly for 6 weeks. FRANCHINI observed a partial remission in 4 of the 8 patients; in the other 4 patients the disease was brought to a halt. Six of the 8 patients had a significantly reduced need of analgetics. After therapy had been discontinued, there was a rise in serum marker, as well as an increased need for analgetics in most patients within 4 weeks (16).

JONES reported a study in 1987 in which 33 patients with prostate carcinoma and measureable disease were treated with 12,5 mg EPIRUBICIN/week. The average age of the patients was 66 years (50-83). The performance status of thepatients was generally slightly decreased (58% WHO Performance Status I).

The toxicity in this scheme was low, as expected. In one case, there was leukopenia grade 1; there was one other case of thrombopenia, grade 1. A total of an average of 13 cycles (4-62) of complete dosages were administered. A dose reduction was not required. An objective response rate was only observed in 12% of the cases. The subjective response rate was significantly higher (17).

DISCUSSION

The objective evaluation of the response rate of a tumor
using a particular therapy for prostate carcinoma is
relatively difficult because 70-80% of the patients do
not have measureable lesions. Osseous metastases and
laboratory parameters can be evaluated, but not
measured. Moreover, it is known that visceral
metastases, if even measureable, behave differently than
osseous metastases. Visceral lesions, such as those
found in mammary carcinoma, are more readily treated
with chemotherapy than bone metastases. Furthermore, it
generally takes too long to measure changes within the
bone. In this manner, mixed responses are found using
bone scintigraphs or x-rays of the skeleton; that is,
one or several metastases become smaller or disappear,
however, new metastates are discovered elsewhere.

Therefore, the time to progression of the tumor or until
death are the most important parameters in judging
objective success in hormone refractory prostate
carcinoma. On the other hand, subjective success of a
therapy is important to the patient. One can try to
objectivize the subjective state of health of the
patients with the aid of a self-assessment form. Further
objective parameters include the use of analgetics and
the general health of the patients using either the
KARNOFSKY scale or ECOG/WHO criteria. In this manner,
judgement of the effectiveness of certain medications
using 2-dimensional lesions exclusively, is too one-
sided for prostate carcinoma, since this is only
applicable to a small number of patients, and does not
take other important parameters into consideration.

A weekly scheme cannot be compared to a low dose scheme.
When a weekly scheme is applied, the dose intensity per
time is not decreased, but rather, the total dose
required for the cycle is partitioned into weekly
intervals. In contrast, in the low dose scheme, the
entire dosage is reduced and additionally administered
at weekly intervals.

The weekly application of a cytostatic leads, when the dose intensity in unchanged, to a significantly lower toxicity than the application of the same dosage of a medicament in intervals of 3-4 weeks.

In carcinoma types with relatively slow proliferation rates, such as prostate carcinoma, the weekly fractionation of the total dosage for the cycle apparantly leads to better results than the conventional application intervals. The recovery rate of 36% for EPIRUBICIN reported by us after 12 weeks, could be confirmed in 2 other centers in the F.R.G., as well as in Sienna (31-50%). This also essentially correlates to the results that TORTI achieved with ADRIAMYCIN. The objective PR rates resulting from the weekly regime are significantly higher than those PR rates found with NPCP studies (ca. 12%) as reported by MURPHY.

The objective recovery rates described by the NPCP fall only into the same niveau as the results from the weekly scheme, when the no change cases are included. The results of the low dose scheme using either ADRIAMYCIN or EPIRUBICIN are, in contrast, disapointing, but can be explained by the decreased dose intensity.

Since the recovery rates, as well as the toxicity of both ADRIAMYCIN and EPIRUBICIN are comparable, using a weekly fractionation, one could assume that there is no difference as to which substance is administered. This is only true under certain conditions since the cumulative maximum dosage - with respect to cardiotoxicity - is 500 mg/m2 for ADRIAMYCIN and 1000 mg/m2 for EPIRUBICIN. This cumulative maximum dosage is reached after 0,5 years with ADRIAMYCIN and after 1 year with EPIRUBICIN when the dose intensity remains unchanged. This becomes significant when patients, which respond to treatment, live longer than one year. The average survival time for the total group is 12 months. TORTI could show, using myocardial biopsies, that a weekly fractionation of anthracyclines reduces the risk of cardiomyopathy, but does not eliminate it completely.

The average increase in life expectancy of 5 months found for the total group of patients, in comparison to historical control groups, requires verification using random studies such as the EPI weekly vs the BEST SUPPORTIVE CARE. Furthermore, one has to determine whether a continual administration of a cytostatic up until progression is better than interruption of therapy after objective response. Whether the combination of a weekly application of EPIRUBICIN with, for example, CISPLATIN every 3 weeks, as well as simultaneous hormone therapy, can have a curative effect upon virginal metastasized prostate carcinoma remains to be seen.

SUMMARY

1. A weekly fractionation of EPIRUBICIN at an unchanged dose intensity leads to a significant decrease in toxicity.

2. The weekly administration of 25 mg/m2 EPIRUBICIN is effective in treating hormone refractory prostate carcinoma and completely fulfills the requirements for palliation.

REFERENCES

1)   WHITE, J.W.
     The results of double castration in hypertrophy of the prostate.
     Trans.Amer.Surg.Ass. 22, 103 (1895).

2) HUGGINS, C. et al.
    Studies on prostatic cancer. The effect of
    castration of estrogen and of androgen injection on
    serum phosphatase in metastatic cancer of the
    prostate.
    Cancer Res. 1, 293-297 (1941).

3) BYAR, D.P. et al.
    The veterans administration cooperative urological
    research groups' studies of cancer of the prostate.
    Cancer 32, 1126-1130 (1973).

4) ISAACS, J.T.
    New principles in the management of metastatic
    prostatic cancer. In: Das Prostatakarzinom zwischen
    Hormontherapie und Zytostase.
    Medical trends, Solingen, 5-27 (1986).

5) MURPHY, G.P. et al.
    Current status of the National Prostatic Cancer
    Project, Treatment Protocols.
    In: Controlled clinical trials in urologic
    oncology, Raven Press, New York, 13 (1984).

6) SPETH, P.A.J. et al.
    Cellular and plasma pharmacokinetics of weekly 20
    mg 4'-EPI-Adriamycin bolus injection in patients
    with advanced breast carcinoma.
    Cancer Chemother. and Pharmacol. 18, 78-82 (1986).

7) SNYDER, R. et al.
    Phase I study of EPIRUBICIN given on a weekly
    schedule.
    Cancer Treatment Reports 71, 273-276 (1987).

8) TORTI, F.M. et al.
    Reduced cardiotoxicity of DOXORUBCIN delivered on a
    weekly schedule.
    Anuals of Int. Med. 99, 745-749 (1983).

9) BECHER, R. et al.
    Randomisierte Studie mit EPIRUBICIN und
    CYCLOPHOSPHAMID beim fortgeschrittenen
    Mammakarzinom.
    Deutscher Krebskongreß, Frankfurt/M. 1988.

10) TORTI, F.M. et al.
Weekly DOXORUBICIN in endocrine refractory
carcinoma of the prostate.
J.Clin.Oncol. 1, 477-482 (1983).

11) ROBINSON, M.R.G. et al.
Weekly low dose ADRIAMYCIN in advanced disseminated
carcinoma of the prostate: A palliative approach.
In: Controlled clinical trials in urologic
oncology, Raven Press, New York, 187 (1984).

12) FOSSA, S.D. et al.
Weekly low dose ADRIAMYCIN in hormone-resistant
metastatic cancer of the prostate.
Scand.J.Urol.Nephrol. 21, 13-16 (1987).

13) BURK, K. et al.
A new concept of chemotherapy for hormone resistant
progressive carcinma of the prostate, 4'-EPI-
Doxorubicin 40 mg weekly.
Poster presentation: American Urological
Association, May 1987, Anaheim/California.

14) BURK, K. et al.
Weekly EPIRUBICIN in patients with hormone
refractory prostatic cancer.
A two years follow up.
International Symposium on therapeutic progress in
Urological Cancers, Alan R. Liss, in press.

15) RÜBBEN, H. et al.
Chemotherapie des symptomatischen metastasierenden
hormonrefraktären Prostatakarzinoms durch
wöchentliche EPIRUBICIN-Applikation.
Urologe B, im Druck (1988).

16) FRANCHINI, G. et al.
Chemotherapy of advanced prostatic cancer with
EPIRUBICIN.
Eur. J. Cancer Clin. Oncol. 23 (8), 1240 (1987).

17) JONES, W.G. et al.
EORTC Phase II study of low-dose weekly EPIRUBICIN
in metastatic prostate cancer.
Cancer Treatm. Rep. 71, 1317-1318 (1987).

Uro-Oncology: Current Status
and Future Trends, pages 201–225
© 1990 Wiley-Liss, Inc.

SYSTEMIC TREATMENT FOR RENAL CELL CARCINOMA: AN
OVERVIEW

David A. Swanson, M.D.

Department of Urology, The University of Texas
M. D. Anderson Cancer Center, 1515 Holcombe
Boulevard, Houston, Texas   77030

INTRODUCTION

The management of metastatic renal cell carcinoma remains
one of the most important problems in urologic oncology today.
Because these tumors commonly show no early pathognomonic
clinical signs or symptoms, the diagnosis is often made late in the
course of the disease when the tumors have had ample time to grow
large or become locally invasive. A large number of patients have
metastatic disease, not only because metastases are already present
at the time of diagnosis in about one third, but also because there is
such a high late-relapse rate following radical nephrectomy for
patients without recognized metastases at presentation.

Traditional systemic treatment for renal cell carcinoma has
been largely ineffective to date. This is due in part to the
ineffectiveness of our antitumor agents both singly and in
combination and, perhaps, the inefficiency of our delivery systems
as well. Further, preclinical data confirm the heterogeneity of cell
populations in any primary or secondary neoplasm, which helps to
explain why we see such diversity in cell-surface properties,
antigenicity, immunogenicity, growth rate, karyotype, sensitivity to
various cytotoxic drugs, and even the ability to invade and
metastasize (Fidler and Balch, 1987). This concept of biologic
heterogeneity has important implications for why our therapeutic
strategies in the past have not worked consistently and why a basic
understanding of cancer biology is essential for future success in
preventing or eradicating cancer metastasis.

This report briefly reviews past experience with systemic treatment for renal cell carcinoma, which can be summarized by saying we still have no therapy with proven, consistent efficacy. It tries to avoid duplicating material available in other reviews and focuses instead on new directions and the rationale behind them. Current knowledge suggests that future therapeutic strategies will offer more hope and, possibly, be even dramatically better.

FOUNDATIONS OF THERAPY

Animal Models

The development of the nude mouse has allowed the establishment of in vivo models for various human tumors. Although human renal cell carcinoma was first successfully transplanted into the nude mouse in the mid-1970s, this system has been used to answer important clinical questions only relatively recently. NMRI nu/nu mice were shown to accept consistently human renal cell carcinoma xenografts that were identical with the original tumor in morphology and chromosomal modes, and usually in DNA content per cell as well (Otto et al., 1984c). Using this model, Otto et al. (1984b) demonstrated that tumor growth could be decreased in response to various doses of vinblastine sulfate and that the response was dose dependent. More recently, this group of investigators demonstrated that NMRI mice pretreated with cyclosporin A could also accept xenogeneic transplants of human renal cell carcinoma (Otto et al., 1987). They concluded that although the thymus-aplastic mouse tumor model was in many respects superior to the immunocompetent animal treated with immunosuppressive agents, the easier experimental conditions and reduced costs of the latter made it a practical tumor model.

Although human tumors grown in nude mice maintain their original morphologic and biochemical characteristics, human renal cell carcinoma cells transplanted subcutaneously in the nude mouse recipient rarely metastasize, regardless of their degree of malignancy in the original (donor) patient. It has recently been demonstrated, however, that the growth rate and incidence of cancer metastasis can be influenced by the nature of the cell line and by the site of innoculation in athymic BALB/c nude mice (Naito et al., 1986; Naito et al., 1987; Fidler et al., 1989). Thus, by manipulating the variables, a consistently high incidence of metastasis can be generated in the nude mouse model.

The nude mouse model once again affirms that metastatic ability is heterogeneous and that metastasis is regulated by tumor and host interactions. It is not a random process, and these interactions can be studied. Appropriate animal models permit us to understand better the biology of metastasis, plan better therapeutic strategies, test specific therapeutic agents, and predict outcome.

Prognostic Information

It is essential when comparing results of treatment within the same institution or between institutions to know that all patients within each treatment group had tumors likely to display similar clinical behavior. In the past, prognosis has been based primarily on surgical stage and sometimes on nuclear grading. Robson's staging system has been the most popular in the United States, and clearly predicts behavior (Robson et al., 1969). Stage as a prognostic variable by itself is not sufficient for our needs, however, because tumors within any given stage, even stage I or stage IV, exhibit diverse patterns of behavior and widely different long-term results. Histologic grade correlates with clinical behavior, but too crudely to be helpful, except, perhaps, at the extremes of the grading spectrum or in combination with stage (Fuhrman et al., 1982).

Flow cytometry has added another prognostic tool for renal cell carcinoma (Bennington and Mayall, 1983; Otto et al., 1984a). Using this technique on paraffin-embedded tissue permits archival material to be studied and then correlated with follow-up clinical information. A number of investigators have now reported that ploidy and DNA content correlate with nuclear grade and stage (Kloppel et al., 1986; Ljungberg et al., 1986a; Rainwater et al., 1987). Abnormal ploidy tends to correlate with increasing grade and stage, although this relationship is not perfect. Further, although the tumor's ploidy does not predict the outcome for any given patient, Ljungberg et al. (1986a) reported that among 55 patients presenting with nonmetastatic renal cell carcinoma, 33 survived, 32 of whom had diploid neoplasms. In contrast, all 22 patients who had aneuploid tumors died of disease.

The heterogenity of tumors is confirmed once again when we look at DNA content. For example, even among oncocytic tumors, which are known to be associated with an excellent prognosis, 11% of grade I tumors and 24% of grade II tumors demonstrated a distinct aneuploid peak in the DNA histogram (Rainwater et al., 1986). Both diploid and aneuploid primary tumors do metastasize, although the site and number of metastases may vary according to the ploidy of the primary tumor (Ljungberg et al., 1988). When the primary tumor and the metastatic lesion do not have the same DNA content, Ljungberg et al. (1986b) report that the clinical course of the patient is more dependent on the DNA content of the metastatic lesion than on that of the primary tumor. Among 32 patients with metastatic renal cell carcinoma, the primary tumors of 15 had a diploid/near-diploid pattern and of 17, an aneuploid DNA pattern; no correlation could be found between DNA content and survival time. When these tumors metastasized, 10 patients showed a diploid/near-diploid DNA pattern in the metastases and survived a mean of 31.1 months; 22 patients had aneuploid metastases and survived a mean of only 11.5 months ($\underline{P}$=.004). Likewise, among 7 patients whose metastatic tumors contained a diploid or near-diploid DNA content, 1 died, 2 were alive with disease, and 4 were free of disease after a solitary metastasis was excised, whereas all 7 patients with aneuploid metastases—even if solitary—died quickly (Ljungberg et al., 1986c).

This ability to estimate prognosis led Baisch et al. (1986) to formulate a malignancy index based on Robson's stage, nuclear grade, and findings on flow cytometry. Using this malignancy index, they were able to correctly predict outcome in 91% of 55 patients with renal cell carcinoma. These data, together with information that clinical course in patients with other genitourinary malignancies such as prostate cancer correlates with DNA ploidy, should make us wonder whether it is now essential that we know the DNA content of all tumors studied when we try to compare the results of treatment (Winkler et al., 1988). Clearly, a comparison of treatment regimens when one treatment was administered to a patient population that had all diploid tumors and the second treatment was directed to patients with all aneuploid tumors would almost certainly lead to an erroneous conclusion. Even if DNA content is not yet useful for predicting the clinical outcome of a single patient, it may now be appropriate to insist it be included when variables in any patient population are being analyzed.

TRADITIONAL SYSTEMIC TREATMENT

Hormonal Therapy

Interest in hormonal therapy for renal cell carcinoma may have originated with the observation that renal cortical tumors can be produced in Syrian golden hamsters by administering estrogen, and induction can be blocked by progestins or testosterone. Bloom was the first to champion the efficacy of progestins and androgens when he reported an objective response rate of 16% in 80 patients with metastatic renal cell carcinoma whom he had treated (Bloom, 1973). Other reports have cited similar response rates for a variety of combinations of hormones. However, Hrushesky and Murphy's review (1977) noted that the objective response rate was less than 2% in over 400 patients treated with progestins and/or androgens between 1971 and 1976, probably because stricter response criteria had been imposed. An excellent recent review concluded that the reported incidence of cytosol receptors for estrogen, progestin, androgen, and glucocorticoids varied widely, and that there was no correlation between receptor status and rate of response to treatment or subsequent relapse rate (Bojar, 1984). Further, a prospective randomized study of 136 consecutive patients who had no clinical evidence of distant metastases after radical nephrectomy compared treatment with 500 mg adjuvant medroxyprogesterone acetate 3 times a week for 1 year to no treatment and demonstrated no significant difference in the median interval free of disease and no correlation among receptors, relapses, and treatment, although the rate of complications in the long-term hormonal therapy group was significant (Pizzocaro et al., 1987).

Today, few data support the use of hormonal therapy to achieve objective responses in patients with advanced renal cell carcinoma, although it is probably fair to say that a substantial number of patients with advanced renal cell carcinoma obtain a subjective reponse to hormonal administration and feel better. Whether this subjective response is sufficient to justify the risk of side effects and complications of therapy must be decided by each clinician.

Chemotherapy

Major reviews of cytotoxic chemotherapy for renal cell carcinoma have all failed to identify a single drug or combination of drugs that is consistently active against this disease (Hrushesky and Murphy, 1977; Cockburn and de Vere White, 1984; Yagoda, 1989). Although sporadic reports cite specific agents or combinations of agents as eliciting response in more than the traditional 5% to 10% of patients, such conclusions are usually based on a limited number of patients, and patient selection factors undoubtedly play a major role. Subsequent testing has invariably failed to confirm promising early results of any cytotoxic agent(s) for renal cell carcinoma. The litany of negative results already so well documented in the literature will not be repeated here.

Obviously, the search for an effective chemotherapeutic agent continues at many institutions with clinical trials of phase I agents or combinations of well-tested cytotoxic drugs. The extent of our previous failures, however, is such as to make most investigators very skeptical that a new cytotoxic drug or

combination of cytotoxic drugs will be found that is effective
enough to have a major impact on this disease. Instead, perhaps,
chemotherapy will make some contribution by changing our delivery
strategies--alternating noncross-reactive regimens or employing
arterial infusion or chemoembolization. Alternating regimens of
drugs have been shown to be more effective than standard regimens
for patients with advanced Hodgkin's disease or nonseminomatous
germ cell tumors of the testis (Santoro et al., 1982; Logothetis et
al., 1985). Kato et al. (1981) have reported using transcatheter
arterial chemoembolization of renal cell carcinoma with
microencapsulated mitomycin C, a technique that has demonstrated
some apparent advantage for patients with other malignancies that
are only marginally responsive to cytotoxic agents.

Even newer delivery strategies offer exciting potentials. The
first of these is infusing colony-stimulating factors, molecularly
cloned recombinant proteins that control the proliferation of
granulocytes and macrophages. These glycoproteins have been
shown to increase leukocyte counts, thus permitting patients to
receive full doses of antitumor agents on time according to protocol
design or to recover more quickly from chemotherapy-induced
neutropenia. That this technique is clinically feasible was recently
demonstrated with patients who had transitional cell carcinoma of
the urothelium, were treated with M-VAC chemotherapy
(methotrexate, vinblastine, adriamycin, cisplatin), and subsequently
received recombinant human granulocyte colony-stimulating factor
(Gabrilove et al., 1988).

Using circadian rhythms in the timing of cancer drug therapy
is a second innovative delivery strategy. Chronobiology, the study
of the time structure of life, demonstrates that all organisms
possess intrinsic circadian rhythms that govern all biologic
processes. Preclinical data have clearly shown that the time of day
when anticancer drugs are administered has a significant effect on
their toxicity. Normal tissues show predictable rhythmic variations
in susceptibility to the toxic effects of chemotherapy during the
circadian cycle; malignant tissues do too, but to a lesser extent.
The toxicity of at least 11 commonly used anticancer drugs has been
shown to depend on the time of day it is administered (Hrushesky,
1985). For example, adriamycin is most toxic in the rat late in the
animal's daily activity cycle, and cisplatin is most toxic near the
rat's awakening. This concept has now been applied to human
cancers, and a pilot clinical study of patients with metastatic renal
cell carcinoma who received continuous, long-term infusion of 5-
fluoro-2-deoxyuridine (FUDR) in time-specific infusion shapes was
recently reported (von Roemeling et al., 1988). In treating 19
patients who had progressive disease, these authors used an

implanted pump programmed so that 68% of the daily dose of FUDR was administered between 3 and 9 p.m. The incidence of treatment delays and dose reductions owing to drug toxicity was significantly lower in these patients than in those receiving flat (continuous rate) infusion of the drug. Among 18 evaluable patients there were 1 complete response (CR), 4 partial responses (PR), and 2 minor responses. These investigators have also shown that the cure rate in BALB/C mice with Meth A-induced sarcomas treated with recombinant human tumor necrosis factor is seven times higher if treatment occurs at a time of the day associated with lowest toxicity (Hrushesky et al., 1987). These data seem to suggest that we may be able to increase the therapeutic index of a variety of agents by taking advantage of circadian rhythms.

The use of multilamellar liposomes is now well established in human medicine. Cytotoxic agents such as amphotericin B and even biologic agents can be encapsulated in liposomes with a resultant decrease in toxicity of the drugs. For example, muramyl dipeptide is a basic compound of the bacille Calmette-Guérin (BCG) cell wall and has significant macrophage-activating activity. A synthetic lipophilic analogue (MTP-PE) can be incorporated into liposomes and has demonstrated antiviral, antifungal, and antitumor activity, both when given alone and when encapsulated into liposomes (Key et al., 1982; Fidler et al., 1982). The toxicity of free MTP-PE administered intravenously is considerable, but it can be reduced at least tenfold while retaining its desired biologic activity when MTP-PE is encapsulated in liposomes. The liposomes are generally cleared from circulation by the mononuclear phagocyte system, and might therefore be a particular good vehicle for drugs effective against macrophage-associated diseases. Phase I trials have already confirmed some responses in patients with renal cell carcinoma, and a phase II trial will soon begin testing this macrophage-activating factor encapsulated in liposomes.

Finally, the concept of drug resistance needs to be considered among the newer delivery strategies. A gene has been discovered whose expression is associated with the development of multidrug-resistance in cultured cells. This gene has been called the mdr 1 gene, and its successful cloning has permitted exploration of the mechanism of multidrug-resistance in human tumors. Recently, Fojo et al. (1987) reported that normal human kidney, 6 of 8 adenocarcinomas of the kidney, and 4 cell lines derived from kidney adenocarcinomas expressed a high level of the mdr 1 mRNA. The 4 cell lines showed resistance to colchicine, adriamycin, and vinblastine, and the resistance of these kidney carcinoma cell lines to vinblastine was overcome with verapamil and quinidine, two drugs known to reverse the multidrug-resistance phenotype. These data support the hypothesis that intrinsic drug resistance in renal carcinoma may be due at least in part to the presence of the mdr 1 gene and its protein product, and that pharmacologic manipulation to reverse multidrug-resistance might make renal cell carcinoma more sensitive to agents such as adriamycin or the vinca alkaloids.

Immunotherapy

The natural history of renal cell carcinoma has long suggested that there might be important interactions between the host and tumor that invite immunologic manipulation. Attempts to treat patients by altering the host immune response date back at least to 1971, when Horn and Horn observed a good clinical response after infusing plasma from a patient cured of renal cell carcinoma into a family member with metastatic renal cell carcinoma. Since then numerous clinical trials of both passive and active immunotherapy have been reported, most showing occasional objective responses and purporting to show increased survival times. These trials have been well summarized in several excellent reviews (McCune, 1983; deKernion, 1984; Pontes and Huben, 1984).

Two of these trials deserve special mention. Active-specific immunotherapy has been investigated in Helsinki, Finland, using a soluble fraction of autologous tumor polymerized with ethylchlorformiate plus either purified protein derivative tuberculin or Candida albicans as adjuvant. Among 71 patients with advanced renal adenocarcinoma who received immunotherapy and supportive measures, 13 remain alive after a minimum of 3 years follow-up, as compared with only 3 survivors among 56 patients treated by the best possible conservative measures (Tallberg et al., 1985). The 13-year survival rate in the immunotherapy group was 18.3% and the calculated life expectancy 44.5 months, as compared with 5.4% and 19 months in the control group, a statistically highly significant difference. Lung metastases visible on chest x-ray disappeared completely in 14 and partially in 5 of 21 patients belonging to the immunotherapy group, whereas only 1 among 15 patients in the control group achieved a PR. Since the immunotherapy group of patients also received dietary supplementation with inorganic (trace-element) and organic (amino acid) complexes, the relative contributions of the specific tumor vaccination and the dietary supplements (which Dr. Tallberg considers to be of vital importance) remain unevaluable.

More recently, Kurth et al. (1987) reported on 33 patients with metastatic renal cell carcinoma who were treated monthly with an intradermal injection of autologous or allogeneic irradiated tumor cell preparation mixed with <u>Corynebacterium parvum</u> after palliative nephrectomy or excision of tumor metastases. Antitumor activity was evident in 8 patients (1 CR, 4 PRs, and 3 minor responses) for a 24% response rate. Responding patients had a median survival of 32 months, whereas the median survival of all patients was 17 months; however, the difference was not significant. No significant toxicity was observed.

In summary, most of the immunotherapy trials have demonstrated low toxicity, and there have been some responses and some reportedly lengthened survival times. Prospective randomized trials have seldom confirmed the effectiveness of any one approach, however. This should not be surprising, since the immune response is very complex and the net effect of any immunologic manipulation is unpredictable. Recruitment of active effector mechanisms might also stimulate competitive or inhibitory mechanisms. Ineffectiveness might also be due to failure to deliver activated immune products to the site of the tumor. For this reason, the future may lie in biologic therapy as opposed to immunotherapy.

BIOLOGIC THERAPY

As just discussed, immunotherapy manipulates the host immune response. Biologic therapy does, too, but it may have a better rationale since the term reflects information and an understanding of the immune response achieved relatively recently as a result of advances in molecular biology and recombinant DNA technology. Biologic response modifiers comprise immunomodulators, growth factors, cytokines (lymphokines and monokines), activated killer cells, and monoclonal antibodies; the last 3 categories have demonstrated relevance for renal cell carcinoma.

Lymphokines and monokines (the products of lymphocytes and monocytes, respectively) are hormone-like molecules produced by normal cells in response to specific stimuli; they serve as messengers, modulating immune functions and regulating production of other biologic response modifiers, and may also have direct cytotoxic effects on the tumor. Lymphokines include the interferons and interleukin 2 (IL-2); tumor-necrosis factor, interleukin 1 (IL-1), and colony-stimulating factor are monokines. Cloned molecules produced by recombinant DNA technology provide adequate quantities of these agents for clinical testing.

Immunomodulators and Growth Factors

Immunomodulators and growth factors are natural products or synthetic compounds that can enhance immune responses such as cytotoxicity of macrophages and natural killer (NK) cells against tumors. A large number of immunomodulators have been described, including BCG, C. parvum, thymosin, levamisol, tuftsin, and ampligen (mismatched double-stranded RNA). These compounds generate a nonspecific enhancement of immune response, and some have been tested in clinical trials. Growth- and differentiation-promoting molecules, exemplified by colony-stimulating factors, transferin, insulin, epidermal growth factor, phorbol esters, bombesin, and laminin, have been studied in preclinical tumor models and some human tumors, although renal cell carcinoma has not yet been one of them. It is theoretically possible to use growth and differentiating factors to cause the tumor cell to mature to a developmental stage amenable to other therapies. Bombesin is an example of a growth factor for oat cell carcinoma. By interfering with the binding of growth-, differentiation-, or metastasis-promoting substances to receptors on the tumor cell surface, they may also inhibit tumor-cell growth or seeding. Laminin is a compound that binds to receptors on certain tumor cells and appears responsible for metastases taking hold; preclinical studies suggest that the metastatic potential of the tumor cells may be reduced by competitive binding of an anti-laminin to the laminin receptor (Barsky et al., 1984).

Interferon

Interferon is a family of glycoproteins—single-chain polypeptides produced de novo by almost all nucleated cells in response to a variety of inducers. There are 3 basic types: (1) alpha (leukocyte) interferon, (2) beta (fibroblast) interferon, and (3) gamma (immune) interferon, which appears to be distinctly different from either alpha or beta interferon. The various interferons have demonstrated antiviral, antiproliferative, and immunoregulatory activity. Interferon alpha and beta are primarily antiviral, whereas interferon gamma, produced by the T cell, seems to function as an immunoregulatory molecule (Roehm and Zlotnik, 1986).

Clinical trials of interferon in the late 1970s demonstrated its activity against a variety of metastatic tumors. We began our own trials with partially purified interferon alpha in 1978, and in early 1980 began to treat patients who had metastatic renal cell carcinoma. Our initial trial demonstrated that interferon alpha was active against this disease, a finding that has been duplicated by many investigators and extended to include other varieties of interferon as well. Our experience with interferon in 274 patients with metastatic renal cell carcinoma treated and evaluated under multiple protocols has been reported (Swanson and Quesada, in press), and excellent reviews are available that summarize interferon treatment of renal cell carcinoma (Neidhart, 1986; Krown, 1987).

Recombinant alpha interferon has been tested in the most patients and has generated reported response rates up to 31% (Krown, 1987). We treated 89 patients with recombinant alpha interferon at a variety of doses and saw 2 CRs, 1 at a dose of 9 million units total daily dose and the other at 20 million units/m^2/day. Seventeen patients achieved a PR, 1 at 9 million units total daily dose, 5 at 18 million units total daily dose, and 11 at 20 millions units/m^2/day. Thus, 19 patients (21%) achieved an objective response. In addition, 21 patients (24%) had minor responses, and 22 patients (25%) exhibited no change; disease progressed in the remaining 27 patients (30%). Seventy-three patients received initial doses within what we considered to be the effective range of between 9 million units total daily dose and 20 million units/m^2/day; 19 (26%) achieved an objective response and 18 (25%) achieved a minor response (Quesada et al., 1985; Swanson and Quesada, in press). Review of the data in other series suggests that maximal response rates are achieved when interferon alpha is administered within a fairly restricted range of moderate to high doses, suggesting that interferon acts, at least in part, as a biologic response modifier (Krown, 1987).

Until recently, interferons beta and gamma have not been available in quantities sufficient for large-scale clinical trials, but preliminary experience has suggested that both of these varieties exhibit antitumor activity. In a study of recombinant interferon gamma, we treated 30 evaluable patients by both intramuscular and continuous intravenous routes. Two PRs occurred (7%), and disease progressed in 20 patients (67%). Thus, at the doses tested, we found only marginal antitumor activity from interferon gamma. Among 106 patients treated by partially purified interferon alpha and recombinant interferon alpha A, our 95% confidence intervals of response were 16% to 33%; by comparison, they were 2% to 22% for the 30 patients treated with recombinant interferon gamma ($\underline{P}$=.03).

Surprisingly, we noted 8 patients with lung metastases whose disease progressed during the interferon gamma studies, 5 of whom subsequently responded when switched to interferon alpha. Conversely, however, 1 patient who relapsed after a remission induced by interferon alpha successfully achieved a PR with

interferon gamma. These observations suggest to us that the
responsiveness of renal cell carcinoma may vary according to the
type of interferon, and that combinations of alpha and gamma
interferons may have a therapeutic advantage that goes beyond
direct synergism.

The pairing of different varieties of interferon or of
interferon plus either chemotherapy or other biologic response
modifiers is a very attractive concept. The combination of
interferon alpha or beta and interferon gamma, which are
antigenically distinct interferon species, has produced synergistic
biologic effects both in vitro and in animal models (Czarniecki et
al., 1984). Interferon gamma seems not only to share the antiviral
properties of the other two, but also can induce tumoricidal activity
in the macrophage and NK cells. It also increases the expression of
class I and class II molecules of the major histocompatibility
complex (MHC), which results in an enhanced ability of these cells
to present antigens to T cells. Although it specifically inhibits
tumor-cell replication, it also inhibits rapidly proliferating cells in
general, so that it is capable of suppressing immune responses if it is
administered at a time when lymphocyte proliferation is taking
place; this suggests that timing and dose may play a particularly
critical role in combinations employing interferon gamma. The few
clinical studies available using interferon alpha plus interferon
gamma tend to support this hypothesis. We treated 37 patients by
daily intramuscular injections of interferon alpha and interferon
gamma; toxicity was acceptable, and 4 patients (16%) achieved a PR
(Swanson and Quesada, in press). No definite clinical synergy was
evident. De Mulder et al. (1988), however, achieved a PR in 6
patients (24%) and a CR in 2 (8%) among their series of 25 evaluable
patients treated with combination alpha and gamma interferons.

It has been difficult to select cytotoxic chemotherapeutic
agents to combine with interferon because of the absence of a
chemotherapeutic agent consistently effective against renal cell
cancer. Nonetheless, several trials have been performed testing
alpha interferon plus vinblastine and alpha interferon plus BCNU
(Figlin et al., 1985; Creagan et al., 1986). No definite synergism was
noted, and toxicity seemed to be a little higher than with interferon
alone. In contrast, a randomized study of interferon alone versus
interferon plus vinblastine conducted in Europe demonstrated a
higher PR rate and a longer median survival time--but no increase in
toxicity--in responders among patients treated with interferon plus
vinblastine (Fossa et al., 1988).

Experience with various interferon protocols for patients with
metastatic renal cell carcinoma has demonstrated definite

antitumor activity, and it is now clear that the response rates for interferon exceed those reported for standard cytotoxic chemotherapy. The data appear to indicate that the best response rates occur in patients whose metastases are pulmonary and in those with a good performance status. Thus, the potential effect on results of a selection bias cannot be overemphasized. Furthermore, selection bias is only one factor making difficult a comparison of results of clinical trials within the same institution, much less from different institutions. The study groups are always heterogeneous with respect to patient characteristics, and the types of interferon, the dose schedules, and even the routes of administration are diverse. Finally, because most protocols have tested relatively small numbers of patients, the 95% confidence intervals of response are quite broad.

Based on available data, it is hard to make definitive conclusions about the efficacy of various types of interferon and their effect on survival. However, interferon seems to offer a viable alternative to cytotoxic chemotherapy as an investigative treatment for metastatic renal cell carcinoma, and future clinical trials investigating new species of interferon and synergistic combinations of interferons or interferon plus biologic therapy offer promise for even better clinical results.

Interleukin 2

IL-2 was originally described as the T-cell growth factor. Its primary biologic activity is to induce and amplify specific cytotoxic T-cell activity and nonspecific lymphokine-activated killer (LAK) and NK cell activity. It restores many observed immunodeficiencies and modulates many of the effector links in the immune system. Since the initial dramatic report of a "possible new approach to the treatment of cancer" only 2 1/2 years ago (Rosenberg et al., 1985), additional clinical testing has confirmed both the efficacy and morbidity of IL-2, with and without LAK cells, for patients with renal cell carcinoma. Among 57 evaluable patients with metastatic renal cell carcinoma, 21 of whom received IL-2 alone and 36 IL-2 plus LAK cells, 13 patients (23%) achieved a CR or a PR (Rosenberg et al., 1987). A recent update showed that the CR-plus-PR rate for 67 patients treated with IL-2 plus LAK cells was 34%, whereas it was 21% for 48 patients treated with IL-2 alone (W. M. Lineham, personal communication). Initially it appeared that the patients receiving IL-2 plus LAK cells had a higher objective response rate than those who received IL-2 alone, but preliminary results of a randomized trial using only high-dose IL-2 in nephrectomized patients do not confirm this difference.

Although the toxicity of IL-2 has become somewhat less with alternate treatment strategies such as continuous infusion (West et al., 1987; Sosman et al., 1988), the "capillary leak syndrome" remains an ominous threat and a definite deterrent to the widespread application of this therapy. Thus, it is encouraging to see objective responses in patients with renal cell carcinoma after substantially lower doses of IL-2, suggesting that much more work is needed to determine the optimal dose and treatment schedule for IL-2 (Marumo et al., 1988). Nonetheless, particularly when we consider the potential combinations that can be devised with this potent immunomodulatory molecule, we have to be very hopeful. As Dr. Durant of the Fox Chase Cancer Center in Philadelphia, Pennsylvania, observed, the data seem to reflect the successful manipulation of the cellular immune system and indicate a meaningful direction for rational and vigorous pursuit of even better understanding, bringing us, perhaps, to "the end of the beginning of the search for successful immunotherapy for cancer" (Durant, 1987).

Interferon and IL-2 are both lymphokines, whereas tumor-necrosis factor (TNF), IL-1, and colony-stimulating factor are monokines. TNF was initially detected in the sera of mice infected with BCG and injected with endotoxin. TNF, probably originating in the macrophage, induces hemorrhage and necrosis of subcutaneous murine and human tumor grafts in mice and has direct cytotoxic and cytostatic effects on a wide range of human cancer cells in vitro (Chapman et al., 1987). In animal studies, it damages blood vessels that nourish tumors and promotes tumor death, whereas in noncancerous tissue it actually plays an important role in normal angiogenesis. Clinical studies have demonstrated that TNF is tolerable, producing only constitutional symptoms. So far, however, only 1 patient among 51 with various malignancies--including renal cell carcinoma--has shown a measurable response (Chapman et al., 1987; Figlin et al., 1988).

IL-1 acts like an endogenous adjuvant, serving as a cofactor during lymphocyte activation, primarily by inducing the synthesis of other lymphokines and the activation of the resting T cell (Dinarello and Mier, 1987). IL-1 also acts as a cofactor with colony-stimulating factor in the promotion of bone-marrow precursors. It acts synergistically with TNF in a variety of biologic responses such as tumor necrosis and a local Shwartzman reaction. Colony-stimulating factor, as has already been mentioned, has the ability to augment de novo marrow generation of granulocytes and macrophages, and it can function as a macrophage-activating factor.

Activated Killer Cells

Lymphokine-activated killer cells have already been discussed in conjunction with IL-2. Further research in the field of adoptive transfer has identified tumor-infiltrating lymphocytes (TIL) that, in mice, appear to be 50 to 100 times more effective in their therapeutic potency than LAK cells (Rosenberg et al., 1986). Like LAK cells, TILs are a very heterogeneous population of cells, but predominantly cytotoxic and suppressor T cells. They are "expanded" when enzymatic digests of fresh tumor are cultured in the presence of IL-2 (Belldegrun et al., 1988). Although TILs can mediate antitumor effects in the absence of IL-2, low doses of IL-2 seem to enhance the effects of TIL. Furthermore, cyclophosphamide enhances the therapeutic benefit of TILs, but not of LAK cells, possibly eliminating suppressor cells that interfere with the effectiveness of transferred cells. Cyclophosphamide also decreases the toxicity of IL-2 in animal models. This raises the hope that effects comparable to those seen in murine models might be achieved in humans with less toxicity than high doses of IL-2 now produce.

Unfortunately, clinical investigations have not yet confirmed the efficacy of TILs in humans with metastatic cancers. Two of 12 patients (including 1 of 4 with metastatic renal cell carcinoma) have demonstrated a PR to varying doses and combinations of TIL, IL-2, and cyclophosphamide (Topalian et al., 1988). Researchers are now looking at ways to determine whether TILs are "trafficking" to tumor sites, and lymphocytes from tumor-draining lymph nodes are also being evaluated. The accumulation of lymphocytes (particularly T cells) may reflect an immunologic recognition of the neoplasm by the host, suggesting a specific function of TILs directed against antigenic determinants present on T cells. Compared to peripheral-blood lymphocytes, TILs demonstrated higher levels of IL-2 receptors and HLA-DR antigens (Belldegrun et al., 1988). The clinical utility of TILs and other activated lymphocytes undoubtedly awaits further research efforts.

Monoclonal Antibodies

Hybridoma technology, first reported in 1975 by Koehler and Milstein, permits a veritable factory to be set up to produce unlimited quantities of a specific (monoclonal) antibody. Because they can be used to regulate growth factors or to block cell-surface receptors from molecules regulating tumor growth or attachment, monoclonal antibodies are also considered biologic response modifiers. Their specificity for tumor-associated antigens or surface receptors means that monoclonal antibodies may also have a therapeutic potential in combination with radionuclides, cytotoxic drugs, or even other biologic response modifiers.

Several broad applications can be described (Bander and Klotz, 1986). In the area of cancer biology, investigators in several laboratories have produced a large number of monoclonal antibodies to kidney antigens (Scharfe et al., 1985; Bander, 1987). These monoclonal antibodies can characterize the distribution, significance, and even the function of the antigens and can be cloned and mapped on the genome.

Cancer detection and surveillance are potential, if not already realized, immunodiagnostic applications for monoclonal antibodies. Several radiolabeled monoclonal antibodies have been successfully used to radiolocalize renal cancer xenografts (Bander et al., 1984; Lange et al., 1985). Although other applications in renal cell carcinoma are still speculative, only a small extrapolation from proven technology seems necessary to imagine that monoclonal antibodies might someday have a role in diagnosis and staging through radioimmunoscintigraphy, particularly when metastases are the result of a clinically occult neoplasm. In addition, using a reliable tumor marker based on a monoclonal antibody might greatly enhance surveillance after definitive therapy, much as prostate-specific antigen has done for patients with adenocarcinoma of the prostate.

The presence or absence of tumor antigens on a given cell pathologically defines an antigenic phenotype and, using antigenic phenotypes of normal kidney cells as a reference, can characterize renal cancers at the molecular level. Antigenic expression has already identified several molecular subtypes of renal cancer. Patients with 1 of these subtypes enjoyed a 90% survival rate at 2 years, whereas patients negative for the two antigens tested belong to a phenotype that achieved only a 10% survival rate at 2 years (Bander and Klotz, 1986).

Several general strategies for treating cancer by monoclonal antibodies have been proposed: (1) immunologically destroying tumor cells, (2) targeting the antibodies to molecules that are critical for growth or differentiation of tumor cells, and (3) delivering antitumor agents (Scheinberg and Houghton, 1987). The latter is one of the most appealing strategies, perhaps the so-called magic bullet dreamed of by German bacteriologist Paul Ehrlich in the early 1900s. Monoclonal antibody activity has been studied in very few solid tumors, but early clinical trials are underway for some, particularly melanoma and colorectal and renal cancers

(Bander, 1987).

In one trial, 1 of 9 patients receiving unlabeled F23 monoclonal antibody achieved a PR, and 2 mixed responses occurred among the 20 patients who received ^{131}I-mAb F23 (Real et al., 1987). Also, Chiou et al. (1988) have directed an A6H monoclonal antibody labeled with iodine-131 to a human renal cell carcinoma xenograft in mice. The ^{131}I-labeled A6H-treated mice developed smaller tumors and achieved a survival rate statistically higher than that of the control groups.

Although many technical problems in immunoreactivity, stability, and pharmacokinetics remain, new technology once again offers hope for solving some of these problems (Bander, 1987). For example, it is now possible to make human monoclonal antibodies, which should eliminate any potential adverse effects from administering foreign proteins such as mouse monoclonal antibodies. Also, hybrid monoclonal antibodies, in which each of the two combining sites binds to a different antigen, might permit production of a monoclonal antibody that binds to a cancer antigen as well as to a toxin. Finally, gene cloning techniques are being combined with hybridoma technology to produce chimeras and even to transplant genes. As the technology expands, what might be accomplished in this area seems limited only by our imagination.

FUTURE CONSIDERATIONS

Certain areas seem ripe for further laboratory research. Several recent papers have reported on chromosomal rearrangements in sporadic (nonhereditary) adult renal cell carcinoma. Kovacs et al. (1987) found changes in chromosome 3 in 22 of 25 patients studied. There was either the loss of the entire chromosome, deletion of the shorter arm, or a deletion/translocation. Because a change in the 3p14 band was the first detectable chromosome change in both familial and sporadic renal cell carcinoma, these investigators hypothesize that such a change may mark renal cell carcinoma and may be the initiating cytogenetic event in its development. Similarly, using restriction fragment-length polymorphism analysis, Zbar et al. (1987) found nonrandom DNA sequence deletion between 3p14 and 3p21 in all 11 patients evaluated. Karyotype analysis has also shown a nonrandom deletion at 3p in small-cell lung carcinoma. By analogy to retinoblastoma, the authors speculate that molecular analysis of the 3p region should ultimately disclose a null mutation at 1 3p allele associated with loss of the wild-type allele. A gene located on 3p might be involved in the origin or evolution of renal cell carcinoma and small-cell carcinoma of the lung.

In addition to the changes already described in chromosome 3, a translocation between chromosome 5 and the short arm of 3 was involved in 12 of 25 patients (Kovacs et al., 1987). The cellular oncogene fms is on 5q, and c-fms was found in 4 of 9 renal cell carcinomas, whereas it was otherwise rare or weak except in Hodgkin's disease, chronic myelogenous leukemia, or breast cancer (Slamon et al., 1984). The viral oncogene (v-fms) of the McDonough strain of feline sarcoma virus encodes an integral transmembrane glycoprotein with biochemical and topologic properties of known cell-surface receptors (Sherr et al., 1985). They have determined that the murine c-fms proto-oncogene product and the CFS-1 (a macrophage growth factor) receptor are related, and possibly identical, molecules.

In a series of papers from the University of Nijmegen in the Netherlands, c-onc fes/fps was found in some fresh renal cell carcinomas and all xenografts of human renal cell carcinomas in nu/nu mice, and that c-fur, located just upstream, encodes a protein with transmembrane domain that resembles class II MHC antigens and may have a recognition function (Karthaus et al., 1986; Karthaus et al., 1987). Thus, the concepts of molecular genetics and proto-oncogenes, combined with the technology of monoclonal antibodies, give rise to speculation that genes and gene products may be manipulated some day either to prevent or to alter the course of renal cancers. In vitro studies have already shown that introducing antibodies specific for proto-oncogene products into cells can reverse the phenotype transformation (Drebin et al., 1985; Feramisco et al., 1985).

In the area of clinical research, chronotherapy, liposome delivery, and the multi-drug resistant genes seem potentially fruitful. Particularly exciting, though, is the testing of multiple combinations of biologic agents suggested by our current understanding of their mechanisms of action. For instance, murine tumors that express class I MHC molecules are more responsive to IL-2. There is known to be a down-regulation of human leukocyte antigen (HLA) class I loci in human tumors, which may help explain why some human tumors are insensitive to IL-2. This suggests that pretreatment with interferon alpha or gamma, or with TNF alpha-- all known to increase HLA expression--may increase the response of human tumors to IL-2 (Weber et al., 1987).

Such strategies for producing synergistic responses are currently being tested in a variety of clinical protocols: IL-2 plus gamma interferon, IL-2 plus alpha interferon, TNF plus alpha or gamma interferon, LAK cells and TILs plus IL-2. It is obvious that a large number of permutations exists, and that clinical confirmation of preclinical studies and speculative strategies is required.

CONCLUSION

Traditional systemic treatment of metastatic renal cell carcinoma has been largely unsuccessful. Because of dramatic new technology, however, biologic therapy has been developed and preliminary data are promising. Its clinical relevance and ultimate effect on disease control are largely unproved, if not untested. Nonetheless, considering where we've been, and having found the past wanting in terms of controlling advanced renal cell carcinoma, most investigators are optimistic that we are closer than ever to having effective systemic therapy for renal cell carcinoma.

REFERENCES

Baisch H, Otto U, Kloppel G (1986). Malignancy index based on flow cytometry and histology for renal cell carcinomas and its correlation to prognosis. Cytometry 7:200-204.

Bander NH (1987). Monoclonal antibodies: State of the art. J Urol 137:603-612.

Bander NH, Klotz LH (1986). Monoclonal antibodies and tumor antigens. In Graham SD (ed): "Urologic Oncology," New York: Raven Press, pp 1-22.

Bander NH, Welt S, Houghton AN, Lloyd KO, Grando R, Yeh S, Whitmore WF, Vaughan ED, Old LJ (1984). Radionuclide imaging of human renal cancer with labeled monoclonal antibodies. American College of Surgeons 1984 Surgical Forum 35:652-655.

Barsky SH, Rao CN, Williams JE, Liotta LA (1984). Laminin molecular domains which alter metastasis in a murine model. J Clin Invest 74:843-848.

Belldegrun A, Muul LM, Rosenberg SA (1988). Interleukin 2 expanded tumor-infiltrating lymphocytes in human renal cell cancer: Isolation, characterization, and antitumor activity. Cancer Res 48:206-214.

Bennington JL, Mayall BH (1983). DNA cytometry on four-micrometer sections of paraffin-embedded human renal adenocarcinomas and adenomas. Cytometry 4:31-39.

Bloom HJG (1973). Hormone-induced and spontaneous regression of metastatic renal cancer. Cancer 32:1066-1071.

Bojar H (1984). Hormone responsiveness of renal cancer. World J Urol 2:92-98.

Chapman PB, Lester TJ, Casper ES, Gabrilove JL, Wong GY,

Kempin SJ, Gold PJ, Welt S, Warren RS, Starnes HF, Sherwin SA, Old LJ, Oettgen HF (1987). Clinical pharmacology of recombinant human tumor necrosis factor in patients with advanced cancer. J Clin Oncol 5:1942-1951.

Chiou RK, Vessella RL, Limas C, Shafer RB, Elson MK, Arfman EW, Lange PH (1988). Monoclonal antibody-targeted radiotherapy of renal cell carcinoma using a nude mouse model. Cancer 61:1766-1775.

Cockburn AG, de Vere White R (1984). Chemotherapy of advanced renal adenocarcinoma. World J Urol 2:136-141.

Creagan ET, Kovach JS, Long HJ, Richardson RL (1986). Phase I study of recombinant leukocyte A human interferon combined with BCNU in selected patients with advanced cancer. J Clin Oncol 4:408-413.

Czarniecki CW, Fennie CW, Powers DB, Estell DA (1984). Synergistic antiviral and antiproliferative activities of Escherichia coli-derived human alpha, beta, and gamma interferons. J Virol 49:490-496.

deKernion JB (1984). Immunotherapy of renal cell carcinoma. In Kurth KH, Debruyne FMJ, Schroeder FH, Splinter TAW, Wagener TDJ (eds): "Progress and Controversies in Oncological Urology," New York: Alan R. Liss, pp 409-421.

de Mulder PHM, Debruyne FMJ, Geboers ADH, Strijk S, Damsma O (1988). Recombinant (r) alpha- and gamma interferon (IFN) in the treatment of advanced renal cell carcinoma (RCC) (abstract). J Urol 139:294A.

Dinarello CA, Mier JW (1987). Lymphokines. N Engl J Med 317:940-945.

Drebin JA, Link VC, Stern DF, Weinberg RA, Greene MI (1985). Down-modulation of an oncogene protein product and reversion of the transformed phenotype by monoclonal antibodies. Cell 41:695-706.

Durant JR (1987). Immunotherapy of cancer. N Engl J Med 316:939-940.

Feramisco JR, Clark R, Wong G, Arnheim N, Milley R, McCormich F (1985). Transient reversion of ras oncogene-induced cell transformation by antibodies specific for amino acid 12 of ras protein. Nature 314:639-642.

Fidler IJ, Balch CM (1987). The biology of cancer metastasis and implications for therapy. Curr Probl Surg 24:129-209.

Fidler IJ, Naito S, von Eschenbach AC (1989). The biologic heterogeneity of metastatic renal cell carcinoma. In Johnson DE, Logothetis CJ, von Eschenbach AC (eds): "Systemic Therapy for Genitourinary Cancers," Chicago: Year Book Medical Publishers (in press).

Fidler IJ, Sone S, Fogler WE, Smith D, Braun DG, Tarcsay L, Gisler RH, Schroit AJ (1982). Efficacy of liposomes containing a lipophilic muramyl dipeptide derivative for activating the tumoricidal properties of alveolar macrophages in vivo. J Biol Response Mod 1:43-55.

Figlin RA, deKernion JB, Maldazys J, Sarna G (1985). Treatment of renal cell carcinoma with (human leukocyte) interferon and vinblastine in combination: A phase I-II trial. Cancer Treat Rep 69:263-267.

Figlin R, deKernion J, Sarna G, Moldawer N, Saks S (1988). Phase II study of recombinant tumor necrosis factor (rTNF) in patients with metastatic renal cell carcinoma (RCCa) and malignant melanoma (MM) (abstract). Proceedings of the American Society of Clinical Oncology 7:169.

Fojo AT, Shen DW, Mickley LA, Pastan I, Gottesman MM (1987). Intrinsic drug resistance in human kidney cancer is associated with expression of a human multidrug-resistance gene. J Clin Oncol 5:1922-1927.

Fossa S, Cavalli F, Otto U, Bauer HW, Oberling JM, Achtnich U, Stein G, Holdener EE (1988). Randomized study of Roferon-A (IFN) with or without vinblastine (VLB) in advanced or metastatic renal cell cancer (RCC) (abstract). Proceedings of the American Society of Clinical Oncology 7:118.

Fuhrman SA, Lasky LC, Limas C (1982). Prognostic significance of morphologic parameters in renal cell carcinoma. Am J Surg Pathol 6:655-663.

Gabrilove JL, Jakubowski A, Scher H, Sternberg C, Wong G, Grous J, Yagoda A, Fain K, Moore MAS, Clarkson B, Oettgen H, Alton K, Welte K, Souza L (1988). Effect of granulocyte colony-stimulating factor on neutropenia and associated morbidity due to chemotherapy for transitional-cell carcinoma of the urothelium. N Engl J Med 318:1414-1422.

Hrushesky WJM (1985). Circadian timing of cancer chemotherapy. Science 228:73-75.

Hrushesky WJ, Murphy GP (1977). Current status of the therapy of advanced renal carcinoma. J Surg Oncol 9:277-288.

Hrushesky WJ, Nygaard SD, Young J (1987). Timing may be a critical factor in drug therapy. Cancer Treat Rep 71:1321.

Karthaus HJ, Bussemakers MJ, Schalken JA, Kurth KH, Feitz WF, Debruyne FM, Bloemers HP, Ven de Ven WJ (1987). Expression of proto-oncogenes in xenografts of human renal cell carcinomas. Urol Res 15:349-353.

Karthaus HF, Schalken JA, Feitz WF, Debruyne FM, de Haan PT, Bloemers HP, Van de Ven WJ (1986). Expression of the human fes cellular oncogene in renal cell tumors. Urol Res 14:123-127.

Kato T, Nemoto R, Mori H, Takahashi M, Tamakawa Y (1981). Transcatheter arterial chemoembolization of renal cell carcinoma with microencapsulated mitomycin C. J Urol 125:19-24.

Key ME, Talmadge JE, Fogler WE, Bucana C, Fidler IJ (1982).

Isolation of tumoricidal macrophages from lung melanoma metastases of mice treated systemically with liposomes containing a lipophilic derivative of muramyl dipeptide. JNCI 69:1189-1198.

Kloppel G, Knofel WT, Baisch H, Otto U (1986). Prognosis of renal cell carcinoma related to nuclear grade, DNA content and Robson stage. Eur Urol 12:426-431.

Kovacs G, Szucs S, DeRiese W, Baumgartel H (1987). Specific chromosome aberration in human renal cell carcinoma. Int J Cancer 40:171-178.

Krown SE (1987). Interferon treatment of renal cell carcinoma: Current status and future prospects. Cancer 59:647-651.

Kurth KH, Marquet R, Zwartendijk J, Warnaar SO (1987). Autologous anticancer antigen preparation for specific immunotherapy in advanced renal cell carcinoma. Eur Urol 13:103-109.

Lange PH, Vessella RL, Chiou RW, Elson MK, Moon TD, Palme D, Shafer RK (1985). Monoclonal antibodies in human renal cell carcinoma and their use in radioimmune localization and therapy of tumor xenografts. Surgery 98:143-149.

Ljungberg B, Forsslund G, Stenling R, Zetterberg A (1986a). Prognostic significance of the DNA content in renal cell carcinoma. J Urol 135:422-426.

Ljungberg B, Stenling R, Roos G (1986b). DNA content and prognosis in renal cell carcinoma: A comparison between primary tumors and metastases. Cancer 57:2346-2350.

Ljungberg B, Stenling R, Roos G (1986c). Prognostic value of deoxyribonucleic acid content in metastatic renal cell carcinoma. J Urol 136:801-804.

Ljungberg B, Stenling R, Roos G (1988). Tumor spread and DNA content in human renal cell carcinoma. Cancer Res 48:3161-3162.

Logothetis CJ, Samuels ML, Selig D, Swanson D, Johnson DE, von Eschenbach AC (1985). Improved survival with cyclic chemotherapy for nonseminomatous germ cell tumors of the testis. J Clin Oncol 3:326-335.

Marumo K, Masaaki T, Deguchi N, Baba S, Jitsukawa S, Hata M, Tazaki H (1988). Anti-cancer effects of human recombinant interleukin2 against advanced urological cancer (abstract). Proceedings of the American Society of Clinical Oncology 139:283A.

McCune CS (1983). Immunologic therapies of kidney carcinoma. Semin Oncol 10:431-436.

Naito S, von Eschenbach AC, Fidler IJ (1987). Diferent growth pattern and biologic behavior of human renal cell carcinoma implanted into different organs of nude mice. JNCI 78:377-385.

Naito S, von Eschenbach AC, Giavazzi R, Fidler IJ (1986). Growth and metastasis of tumor cells isolated from a human renal cell carcinoma implanted into diferent organs of nude mice. Cancer Res 46:4109-4115.

Neidhart JA (1986). Interferon therapy for the treatment of renal cancer. Cancer 57:1696-1699.

Otto U, Baisch H, Huland H, Kloppel G (1984a). Tumor cell deoxyribonucleic acid content and prognosis in human renal cell carcinoma. J Urol 132:237-239.

Otto U, Huland H, Baisch H, Kloppel G (1984b). Transplantation of human renal cell carcinioma into NMRI nu/nu mice. II. Evaluation of response to vinblastine sulfate monotherapy. J Urol 131:134-138.

Otto U, Huland HHH, Kloppel G, Baisch H (1987). Xenogenic transplantation of human bladder- and renal-cell carcinoma into NMRI mice treated with cyclosporin A and into NMRI nu/nu mice. Urol Int 42:1-5.

Otto U, Kloppel G, Baisch H (1984c). Transplantation of human renal cell carcinoma into NMRI nu/nu mice. I Reliability of an experimental tumor model. J Urol 131:130-133.

Pizzocaro G, Piva L, DiFronzo G, Giongo A, Cozzoli A, Dormia E, Minervini S, Zanollo A, Fontanella U, Longo G, Maggioni A (1987). Adjuvant medroxyprogesterone acetate to radical nephrectomy in renal cancer: 5-year results of a prospective randomized study. J Urol 138:1379-1381.

Pontes JE, Huben RP (1984). Immunotherapy of renal cell carcinoma. World J Urol 2:142-145.

Quesada JR, Rios A, Swanson D, Trown P, Gutterman JU (1985). Antitumor activity of recombinant-derived interferon alpha in metastatic renal cell carcinoma. J Clin Oncol 3:1522-1528.

Rainwater LM, Farrow GM, Lieber MM (1986). Flow cytometry of renal oncocytoma: Common occurrence of deoxyribonucleic acid polyploidy and aneuploidy. J Urol 135:1167-1171.

Rainwater LM, Hosaka Y, Farrow GM, Lieber MM (1987). Well differentiated clear cell renal carcinoma: Significance of nuclear deoxyribonucleic acid patterns studied by flow cytometry. J Urol 137:15-20.

Real FX, Bander NH, Yeh S, Cordon-Cardo C, Lloyd KO, Welt S, Wong G, Old LJ, Oettgen HF (1987). Monoclonal antibody F23: Radiolocalization and phase I study in patients with renal cell carcinoma (abstract). Proceedings of the American Society of Clinical Oncology 6:240A.

Robson CJ, Churchill BM, Anderson W (1969). The results of radical nephrectomy for renal cell carcinoma. J Urol 101:297-301.

Roehm NW, Zlotnik A (1986). Lymphokines. In Graham SD Jr (ed): "Urologic Oncology," New York: Raven Press, pp 23-33.

Rosenberg SA, Lotze MT, Muul LM, Leitman S, Chang AE, Ettinghausen SE, Matory YL, Skibber JM, Shiloni E, Vetto JT,

Seipp CA, Simpson C, Reichert CM (1985). Observations on the systemic administration of autologous lymphokine-activated killer cells and recombinant interleukin-2 to patients with metastatic cancer. N Engl J Med 313:1485-1492.

Rosenberg SA, Spiess P, Lafreniere R (1986). A new approach to the adoptive immunotherapy of cancer with tumor-infiltrating lymphocytes. Science 233:1318-1321.

Santoro A, Bonadonna G, Bonfante V, Balagussa P (1982). Alternating drug combinations in the treatment of advanced Hodgkin's disease. N Engl J Med 306:770-775.

Scharfe T, Becht E, Kaltwasser R, Thuroff JW, Jacobi GH, Hohenfellner R (1985). Tumor-specific monoclonal antibodies for renal cell carcinoma. Eur Urol 11:117-120.

Scheinberg DA, Houghton AN (1987). Current status of antitumor therapy with monoclonal antibodies. Oncology 1:31-40.

Sherr CJ, Rettenmier CW, Sacca R, Roussel MF, Look AT, Stanley ER (1985). The c-fms proto-oncogene product is related to the receptor for the mononuclear phagocyte growth factor, CSF-1. Cell 41:665-676.

Slamon DJ, deKernion JB, Verma IM, Cline MJ (1984). Expression of cellular oncogenes in human malignancies. Science 224:256-262.

Sosman JA, Kohler PC, Hank J, Moore KH, Bechhofer R, Storer B, Sondel PM (1988). Repetitive weekly cycles of recombinant human interleukin-2: Responses of renal carcinoma with acceptable toxicity. JNCI 80:60-63.

Swanson DA, Quesada JR (in press). Interferon therapy for metastatic renal cell carcinoma. Semin Surg Oncol.

Tallberg T, Tykka H, Mahlberg K, Halttunen P, Lehtonen T, Kalima T, Sarna S (1985). Active specific immunotherapy with supportive measures in the treatment of palliatively nephrectomized, renal adenocarcinoma patients. Eur Urol 11:233-243.

Topalian SL, Solomon D, Avis FP, Chang AE, Freerksen DL, Linehan WB, Lotze MT, Robertson CN, Seipp CA, Simon P, Simpson CG, Rosenberg SA (1988). Immunotherapy of patients with advanced cancer using tumor-infiltrating lymphocytes and recombinant interleukin-2: A pilot study. J Clin Oncol 6:839-853.

von Roemeling R, Rabatin JT, Fraley EE, Hrushesky WJM (1988). Progressive metastatic renal cell carcinoma controlled by continuous 5-fluoro-2-deoxyuridine infusion. J Urol 139:259-262.

Weber JS, Jay G, Tanaka K, Rosenberg SA (1987). Immunotherapy of a murine tumor with interleukin 2: Increased sensitivity after MHC class I gene transfection. J Exp Med 166:1716-1733.

West WH, Tauer KW, Yannelli JR, Marshall GD, Orr DW, Thurman GB, Oldham RK (1987). Constant-infusion recombinant interleukin-2 in adoptive immunotherapy of advanced cancer N Engl J Med 316:898-905.

Winkler HZ, Rainwater LM, Myers RP, Zincke H, Farrow GM,

Therneau TM, Nativ O, Raz Y, Hosaka Y, Boyle ET, Lieber MM (1988). Prognostic significance of DNA ploidy in stage C and D1 prostate cancer (abstract). J Urol 139:337A.

Yagoda A (1989). New cytotoxic single-agent therapy for renal cell carcinoma. In Johnson DE, Logothetis CJ, von Eschenbach AC (eds): "Systemic Therapy for Genitourinary Cancers," Chicago: Year Book Medical Publishers, in press.

Zbar B, Brauch H, Talmadge C, Linehan M (1987). Loss of alleles of loci on short arm of chromosome 3 in renal cell carcinoma. Nature 327:721-724.

Uro-Oncology: Current Status
and Future Trends, pages 227–241
© 1990 Wiley-Liss, Inc.

PHASE II CYTOTOXIC CHEMOTHERAPY TRIALS IN RENAL CELL
CARCINOMA: 1983-1988

Alan Yagoda

Solid Tumor Service, Department of Medicine,
Memorial Sloan-Kettering Cancer Center, New
York, New York 10021

INTRODUCTION

Hormonal and cytotoxic investigational and standard
agents used singly (Table 1) evaluated prior to 1983 demonstrated little, if any, significant antitumor activity
(Hrushesky and Murphy, 1977; Harris, 1983). Additionally,
combination regimens of these drugs were no more efficacious than any single component, and overall objective
tumor regression (complete [CR] and partial [PR] remission)
was observed in 0-10%. Remission rates with hormones have
also been disappointing: 9% of 477 progesterone, 8% of 115
androgen treated cases, and 6% of 162 anti-androgen treated
cases (Harris, 1983). Although many studies reported
higher response rates when the categories of minor response
(MR) and stable disease (STAB) were used, definitions of
these response categories varied. In some studies they
were defined as tumor regression of <50% or of <25% with
tumor progression of 25% or 50%. While spontaneous
regression of metastases following nephrectomy has been
observed, the incidence ranges from 0.4% in 1,348 cases
(DeKernion et al., 1980) to 24% in 69 cases (Oliver, 1987).
It would be best that the response category STAB not be
included in reported remission rates since there exists, at
present, no accurate biochemical or immunological
diagnostic technique to document small changes in the
growth rate of renal cell carcinoma. In fact, the
experience of many investigators in this field suggests
that a remission rate of ≤10%-15% may simply represent
"background noise"; albeit, for the responding patient, the
response rate is 100% and tumor regression can be

TABLE 1. Some Cytotoxic Agents for Renal Cell Carcinoma
Evaluated Prior to 1983

Actinomycin-D	Bleomycin	Carmustine
Chlorozotocin	Cisplatin	Dacarbazine
Dianhydrogalactitol	Doxorubicin	Fluorouracil
Fluoxidine	Hydroxyurea	Hexamethylmelamine
Mercaptopurine	Methotrexate	Mitomycin-C
Semustine	Vinblastine	Vincristine

beneficial in selected cases. Generally, patient selection
for protocol entry also was inconsistent with some patients
having a large tumor burden, a poor Karnofsky or ECOG
Performance Status, or a history of extensive prior therapy
with irradiation and/or chemotherapy. Such exposure to
other cytotoxic agents may significantly alter tumor
sensitivity to a subsequent cytotoxic drug because of the
presence in renal cell carcinoma of the multi-drug resistant gene, mdr-1 (Fojo et al., 1987). The definitions of
study parameters to measure response differed too. Many
older studies did not require the selection of patients
with bidimensionally measurable soft tissue lesions--a
mandatory component of Phase II trials in order to obtain a
clear end-point for response evaluation. Thus, many pre-
1983 trials not only employed less strict response and
patient selection criteria but permitted entry of those
with osseous and other unidimensional/nonevaluable lesions.

Since 1983, there have been many new Phase II trials
in renal cell carcinoma. While some have re-explored older
standard and investigational agents administered in
different dosages and schedules, the majority have evaluated new investigational drugs. This paper summarizes
results of such trials in adequately treated cases during
the past five years.

RESULTS

Between 1983 and 1988, there have been >35 agents
evaluated singly and in combination with radio-sensitizers
or with biologics. Again, since these drugs have shown
little evidence of significant anti-tumor activity when
used as part of multi-drug regimens, such combinations have

TABLE 2. New Agents: 1983-1988 (Abbreviation; NSC number)

Acivicin	(AT-125;	163501)
L-Alanosine	(L-ALANO;	153353)
Aminothiadiazole	(A-TDA;	4728)
Amsacrine	(AMSA;	24992)
5-Aza-2-deoxycytidine	(DAC;	127716)
Bisantrene	(ADAH;	337766)
Carboplatin	(CBDCA;	241240)
4'-Demethoxydaunorubicin	(DMDR:	256439)
4'-Deoxydoxorubicin	(DXDX;	267469)
10-Deazaaminopterin	(10-DAAM;	none)
Diaziquone	(AZQ;	182986)
Dibromodulcitol	(DBD;	104800)
Doxifluridine	(FUDR;	27640)
Elliptinium	(ELLIP;	none)
4'-Epiadriamycin	(EpiDOX;	256942)
Fludarabine	(2-FLAMP;	312887)
Gallium Nitrate	(GaN;	15200)
Ifosfamide	(IFOS;	109724)
Lonidamine	(LONID;	none)
Menogaril	(7-OMEN	269148)
Mitoguazone	(MGBG;	32946)
Mitoxantrone	(DHAD;	301739)
N-methylformamide	(NMF;	3051)
PCNU	(PCNU;	95466)
Piperazinedione	(ICRF-187;	135758)
Sparfosic acid	(PALA;	224131)
Spirogermanium	(SPIROG;	192965)
Streptozotocin	(STZ;	85998)
Taxol	(Taxol;	125973)
Teniposide	(VM-26	122619)
Tetrahydropyranyldoxoribicin	(THP-DOX;	none)
Triglycidylurazole	(TGU;	332488)
Trimetrexate	(TMTX;	249008)
Vinblastine	(VLB;	49842)

not been reviewed. Combining single-agent data from these 1983- 1988 trials with those using the same agent before 1983 results in <10% responses in 1829 cases which illustrates the continued non-responsiveness of renal cell carcinoma to presently available therapeutic options.

Little efficacy was found with the anthracyclines, DMDR (idarubicin), DXDX (esorubicin), EpiDOX (epirubicin)

and 4'-)-tetrahydropyranyl-doxorubicin (THP-DOX), and with
the anthracenediones, ADAH (bisantrene) and DHAD
(mitoxantrone). In two post-1983 ADAH studies (Evans et
al., 1985; Elson et al., 1987), 4 responses were described
in 46 cases given either 180 mg/m2 weekly for three consecutive doses Q6W or 260 mg/m2 Q4W. Overall, there have been
6 (6%) remissions in 109 cases, 87 of whom were unpretreated. In four studies with DHAD given weekly in doses of 5
mg/m2 or Q3W in doses of 12-30 mg/m2, there was only one
remission in 137 patients (Taylor et al., 1984; Gams et
al., 1986; Van Oosterom et al., 1984; Oliver, 1987). In
four DXDX trials (Van Oosterom et al., 1986; Kish et al.,
1986; Braich et al., 1986; Carlson et al., 1987), 2% of 99
adequately treated cases responded, both having had no
prior therapy. The usual dose was 25-30 mg/m2 Q3-4W. No
response was observed in 19 cases each given DMDR (Scher et
al., 1985) and EpiDOX (Benedetto et al., 1983) Q3W. THP-
DOX was given in two schedules of either 30-50 mg/m2 Q3W or
20-40 mg/m2 days 1, 2, and 3 Q3-4W, and produced one PR in
16 cases (de Vassal et al., 1987). Another intercalating
agent, AMSA, 90-160 mg/m2 Q3-4W, yielded 2 responses in 103
cases (Amrein et al., 1983; Earhart et al., 1983). Combining these results with two prior AMSA trials, the overall
rate is 1.7% in 140 cases, 61 of whom had no prior cytotoxic agents. Menogaril, 200mg/m2 Q4W, demonstrated no
activity in 14 cases (Long et al., 1988).

Many alkylating agents, or those functioning as such,
continued to be evaluated. In three studies of AZQ (Hansen
et al., 1984; Decker et al., 1986; Stephens et al., 1986),
2% of 99 cases responded. The doses employed were 27-40
mg/m2 Q3-4W and 20 mg/m2 QW for four consecutive weeks.
Overall, 88 cases had no prior cytotoxic therapy. Brubaker
et al. (1986a; 1986b) found remission in 9.6% of 31 cases
given 180 mg/m2 PO of DBD (mitolactol) QD for ten days Q4W,
but none occurred with ICRF-187. One of 16 patients responded to IFOS + mesna (DeForges et al., 1987) 3000 mg/m2
QD for two days Q4W, and when these data are combined with
a pre-1983 study, there were 2/27 (7.4%) remissions which
included 23 unpretreated cases. The nitrosoureas, PCNU (a
chlorethyl piperidyl derivative) and streptozotocin (a
naturally occurring nitrosourea), exhibited no significant
anti-tumor activity. In 79 cases given 75-100 mg/m2 Q6W of
PCNU (Harvey et al., 1984; Elson et al., 1987), and in 18

given 500 mg/m2 QD for five days of STZ Q4W (Licht et al., 1987), only 1 patient each had a remission: 15 patients, respectively, had no prior therapy. CBDCA was ineffective, 0/19, in standard (450 mg/m2 Q4W) and calculated doses to renal function (Tait et al., 1988). TGU, a new triepoxide alkylating agent, also was inactive with no response in 30 cases (Bruntsch et al., 1986; Wagner et al., 1987).

Elliptinium, in daily doses of 800-1000 mg/m2 for five consecutive days Q4W, induced remission in 5 of 46 (11%) patients, 35 of whom were unpretreated (Sternberg et al., 1985; Caille et al., 1985) while spirogermanium was inactive in 60 cases, 27 of whom were unpretreated (Schulman et al., 1984; Saiers et al., 1987). The usual SPIROG dose was 80-120 mg/m2 TIW for two weeks.

The podophyllin and vinca alkaloid derivatives continued to be evaluated. In five studies of vinblastine by continous infusion (VLB-CI) of 1.4-1.9 mg/m2 QD for five consecutive days Q3-4W (Zeffren et al., 1984; Kuebler et al., 1984; Tannock et al., 1985; Crivellari et al., 1987; Elson et al., 1988), 5 (7.8%) of 64 patients responded--a rate similar to standard weekly VLB administration. In two recent VM-26 studies of 60 mg/m2 QD for five consecutive days or 100 mg/m2 QW, Q3-4W, 4 (4.8%) of 83 cases responded (Pfeifle et al., 1986; Oishi et al., 1987).

Trials of various antimetabolites, purine and pyrimidine antagonists, and antifols have shown these compounds to be relatively ineffective too, except possibly for FUDR given in a chronobiological schedule. Hrushesky et al. (1987) described 6 (33%) responses in 18 patients with FUDR 0.25 mg/kg/day continuously infused intra-arterially for 14 days QM with doses adjusted to the time of day, 68% of the daily dose administered between 1500 and 2100 hours. The total FUDR dosage was significantly higher than the standard evenly distributed dose. Further trials of this chronobiologically administered schedule has been initiated by other investigators. The polyamine inhibitor MGBG, and the L-glutamine antagonist acivicin, demonstrated marginal antitumor activity. In four MGBG trials prior to 1983, 7 (7.5%) of 93 adequately treated patients responded to 400-900 mg/m2 QW and in a more recent study (Knight et al., 1983), only 4 (4.6%) of 87 responded. AT-125 induced one (4%) remission in 27 cases (Elson et al., 1988). Two purine biosynthesis inhibitors, L-alanosine which blocks

adenylsuccinate synthetase and aminothiadiazole which
inhibits inosine monophosphate dehydrogenase, induced 1
(3%) of 36 and of 46 (2%) remissions, respectively (Elson
et al., 1988). DAC, a new deaza-cytidine derivative, was
inactive in 12 cases administered 75 mg/m2 Q8H for one day
Q5W (Abele et al., 1987). Fludarabine was evaluated in 45
patients, none of whom responded, as a continuous five-day
infusion Q3-4W in a dose of 25-30 mg/m2 (Balducci et al.,
1987; Shevrin et al., 1988). PALA in a daily schedule of
1500 mg/m2 for five consecutive days Q3W and in a weekly
dose of 3750-4500 mg/m2 produced 2/66 (3%) responses
(Natale et al., 1982; Earhart et al., 1983), 30 of whom had
had no prior cytotoxic chemotherapy. There was no activity
with NMF in 27 patients given 800-1000 mg/m2 QD for five
consecutive days Q4W (Sternberg et al., 1986; Silva et al.,
1986), 24 of whom were unpretreated. The antifols, 10-DAAM
and TMTX, induced no remission in 12 and 14 cases, respectively (Scher et al., 1984; Sternberg et al., 1988).

Gallium nitrate was evaluated in a continuous daily
infusion in doses of 100-200 mg/m2 for seven consecutive
days Q3W (Schwartz et al., 1984) and in a bolus Q2W dosage
of 700 mg/m2 (Vugrin et al., 1987). Overall, none of 35
patients, 32 of whom had no prior therapy, obtained a
response. Taxol, 250 mg/m2 by continuous infusion, was
administered to 18 patients without producing tumor
regression (Einzig et al., 1988). Lonidamine, an anti-
spermatocytic agent which is also an antimitochondrial
poison, induced 2 (8%) responses in 25 cases given a daily
dose of 450 mg PO (Weinerman et al., 1986). Of note, Thill
et al. (1988) have demonstrated a synergistic effect of the
combination of two anti-mitochondrial agents, LONID and
deoxycycline, in a human renal carcinoma cell line, and
this combination deserves clinical examination.

Cytotoxic drugs have also been combined with immunological agents, particularly interferon. Although response
with alpha interferon has varied from <10% to >40% (Harris,
1983; Krown, 1985), the overall rate is, at best, 13-18% in
selected patients, mostly those with minimal visceral
(non-osseous and hepatic) disease. High doses of 30-100
Mum^2 QW was no more effective than 3-6 Mum^2 TIW (Muss et
al., 1987; Krown, 1985; Eisenhauer et al., 1987).
Additionally, there is no evidence in prospectively
randomized trials that interferon combined with VLB (Figlin
et al., 1985; Fossa et al., 1986; Niedhart et al., 1987;

TABLE 3. Results (±95% Confidence Intervals) of 71 Phase
II Trials for Renal Cell Carcinoma: 1983-1987

Drug	No. Trials	No. Adequate	% CR + PR	
ADAH	4	109	6	(∓7)
AMSA	4	140	1	(±2)
A-TDA	1	46	2	(±10)
AT-125	1	27	4	(±15)
AZQ	4	119	2	(±3)
CBDCA	1	19	0	(±15)
10-DAAM	1	14	0	(±20)
DAC	1	12	0	(±21)
DBD	2	44	9	(±9)
DHAD	4	137	1	(±2)
DMDR	1	19	0	(±15)
DXDX	4	78	3	(±4)
EpiDOX	1	19	0	(±15)
ELLIP	2	46	11	(±9)
2-FLAMP	2	45	0	(±2)
FUDR	1	18	33	(±22)
GaN	2	35	0	(±9)
ICRF-187	1	40	0	(±5)
IFOS	2	27	7	(±10)
L-ALANO	1	36	3	(±12)
LONDID	1	25	8	(±11)
7-OMEN	1	14	0	(±20)
MGBG	5	180	6	(±4)
NMF	2	27	0	(±11)
PALA	2	66	3	(±4)
PCNU	2	79	1	(±2)
SPIROG	2	62	0	(±3)
STZ	1	18	6	(±11)
Taxol	1	18	0	(±15)
TGU	2	30	0	(±10)
THP-DOX	1	16	6	(±12)
TMTX	1	14	0	(±20)
VM-26	3	96	4	(±1)
VLB-CI	5	99	8	(±5)
Coumarin + cimetidine	2	55	26	(±12)

Schorngel et al., 1987) was more efficacious than either
agent used singly. Similar findings were noted with inter-

feron and ADM (Muss et al., 1985), and with cyclophosphamide (Wadler et al., 1987).

Another immunological approach was reported by
Marshall and colleagues (1987) who used coumarin
(1,2-benzopyrone, a warfarin derivative) in combination
with cimetidine. Although the former drug may possess a
direct cytotoxic effect upon tumor cells, as well as
inhibiting tumorigenesis, it also modulates the immune
system, possibly by augmenting NK activity. Of 42
evaluable patients with renal cell carcinoma, 29 unpretreated and 41 with measurable disease, 3 achieved CR and
11 a PR (33%) to 100 mg PO daily of coumarin and 300 mg QID
of cimetidine which was started on day 15. CR lasted 4+,
9.5 and 9.5+ months, and the median response duration for
PR was 5 months, range 4-21+. Of note, all response
occurred in the 31 nephrectomized cases compared to none in
14 non-nephrectomized cases. However, another phase II
study (Herrmann et al., 1988) in 15 patients given a
similar schedule, 12 of whom had had a nephrectomy, found
no evidence of tumor regression. Randomized trials have
been undertaken to further evaluate these two agents.
Addition- ally, a phase I of coumarin has also been started
with doses >3 gms PO daily.

Lastly, cytotoxic agents have been combined with
radiosensitizers. Both misonidazole + cyclophosphamide
(Glover et al., 1986), and metronidazole + mitomycin-C
(Stewart et al, 1987) produced significant toxicity with
little evidence of synergy in limited trials in 31 (1 PR)
and 12 (3 PR) cases, respectively.

CONCLUSION

Little indication for the development of effective
multidrug regimens is forthcoming from these 41 trials in
1825 patients, except possibly for FUDR and coumarin +
cimetidine, both of which still need confirmatory trials.
In fact, one wonders if the 0-10% remission incidence with
these single agents reflects "background noise" or even an
indirect effect on tumor destruction by immunological
modulation by cytotoxic agents. Until the natural defense
mechanism inherent to renal tissue, both normal and tumor
cells, mdr-1, can be overcome, cytotoxic agents probably
will remain ineffective (Fojo et al., 1987). The role of
monoclonal antibodies becomes of importance not only for

diagnoses, prognosis, and cytogenicity, but also as
vehicles when cytotoxic agents are attached to monoclonal
antibodies to deliver high membrane and possibly persistent
intracellular drug concentrations (Bander, 1987). The
finding of a selected portion of the proximal tubule as
origin of almost all renal cell carcinomas should lead to
the development of more specifically directed agents to
this segment (Bander et al., submitted). Uro-2, URO-3, and
URO-4 monoclonal antibodies are prime candidates for
clinical study (Cordon-Cardo et al., 1984), as are URO-10
and URO-8 which delineate a proximal tubular progenitor
cell (Bander et al., submitted). The past experience is
bleak; the future bright.

REFERENCES

Abele R, Clavel M, Dodion P, Bruntsch U, Gundersen S, Smyth
    J, Renard J, van Glabbeke M, Pinedo HW (1987). The
    EORTC Early Clinical Trials Cooperative Group experience
    with 5-aza-2'-deoxycytidine (NSC 127716) in patients
    with colo-rectal, head and neck, renal carcinomas and
    malignant melanomas. Eur J Cancer Clin Oncol 23:1921-
    1924.
Amrein PC, Coleman M, Richards F, Poulin EF, Berkowitz I,
    Kennedy BJ, Green M, Herschktopf R, Rafla S (1983).
    Phase II study of amsacrine in metastatic renal cell
    carcinoma. Cancer Treat Rep 67:1043-1044.
Balducci L, Blumenstein B, Von Hoff DD, Davis M, Hynes HE,
    Bukowski RM, Crawford ED (1987). Evaluation of fludara-
    bine phosphate in renal cell carcinoma: a Southwest
    Oncology Group study. Cancer Treat Rep 71:543-544.
Bander NH (1987). Monoclonal antibodies: state of the
    art. J Urol 137:603-612.
Bander NH, Finstad CL, Cordon-Cardo C, Ramsawak RD, Vaughan
    ED, Whitmore WF, Oettgen HF, Melamed MR, Old LJ (submitt-
    ed). Mouse monoclonal antibody defines a specific region
    of the human proximal tubule and major subsets of renal
    cell carcinomas.
Benedetto P, Ahmed T, Yagoda A, Needles B, Watson RC
    (1983). Phase II trial of 4'epiadriamycin in advanced
    hypernephroma. Amer J Clin Oncol 6:553-554.
Braich TA, Salmon SE, Robertone A, Alberts DS, Jones SE,
    Miller JP, Garewal HS (1986). Phase II trial of eso-
    rubicin (4' deoxydoxorubicin) in cancers of the breast,
    colon, kidney, lung, and melanoma. Invest New Drugs 4:
    269-274.

Brubaker LH, Vogel CL, Einhorn LH, Birch R (1986a). Treatment of advanced adenocarcinoma of the kidney with ICRF-187: a Southeastern Cancer Study Group trial. Cancer Treat Rep 70:915-916.

Brubaker LH, Nelson MO, Birch R, Williams S (1986b). Treatment of advanced adenocarcinoma of the kidney with mitolactol: a Southeastern Cancer Study Group trial. Cancer Treat Rep 70:305-306.

Bruntsch U, Dodion P, Huinink WWT-B, Hansen HH, Pinedo HM, Hansen M, Renard J, van Glabbeke M (1986). Primary resistance of renal adenocarcinoma to 1,2,4-triglycidyl-urazol (TGU, NSC 332488), a new triexpoxide cytostatic agent: a Phase II study of the EORTC Early Clinical Trials group. Eur J Clin Oncol 22:697-699.

Caille P, Mondesir JM, Droz JP, Kerbrat P, Goodman A, Ducret JP, Theodore C, Spielman M, Rouesse J, Amiels JL (1985). Phase II trial of elliptinium in advanced renal cell carcinoma. Cancer Treat Rep 69:901-902.

Carlson RW, Williams RD, Billingham ME, Kohler M, Torti F (1987). Phase II trial of esorubicin in the treatment of metastatic carcinoma of the kidney: a study of the Northern California Oncology Group. Cancer Treat Rep 71:767-768.

Cordon-Cardo C, Bander NH, Fradet Y, Finstad CL, Whitmore WF, Lloyd KO, Oettgen HF, Melamed MR, Old LJ (1984). Immunoanatomic dissection of the human urinary tract by monoclonal antibodies. J Histochem Cytochem 32:1035-1040.

Crivellari D, Tumolo S, Frustaci S, Galligioni E, Figoli F, Re GL, Veronesi A, Monfardini S (1987). Phase II study of five-day continuous infusion of vinblastine in patients with metastatic renal-cell carcinoma. Amer J Clin Oncol 10:231-233.

Decker DA, Kish J, Al-Sarraf M, Goldfarb S (1986). Phase II clinical evaluation of AZQ in renal cell carcinoma. Amer J Clin Oncol 9:126-128.

De Forges A, Droz JP, Ghosn M, Theodore C (1987). Phase II trial of ifosfamide/mesna in metastatic adult renal carcinoma. Cancer Treat Rep 71:1103.

DeKernion JB, Berry D (1980). The diagnosis and treatment of renal cell carcinoma. Cancer 45:1947-1953.

De Vassal F, Misset JL, Brienza S, Musset M, Despax R, Machover D, Goldschmidt E, Ribaud P, Mathe G (1987). A phase II trial of 4'-0-tetrahydropyranyl-adriamycin (THP-ADM) in advanced solid tumors. Invest New Drugs (abstract 947)5:123.

Earhart RH, Elson PJ, Rosenthal SN, Hahn RG, Slayton RE (1983). PALA and AMSA for renal cell carcinoma. Amer J Clin Oncol 5:555-560.

Einzig AJ, Gorowski E, Sasloff, Wiernik PH (1988). Phase II trial of taxol in patients (pts) with renal cell carcinoma. Proc Amer Assoc Cancer Res (abstract 884)29: 222.

Eisenhauer EA, Silver HK , Venner PM, Thirlwell MP, Weinerman B, Coppin CML (1987). Phase II study of high dose weekly intravenous human lymphoblastoid interferon in renal cell carcinoma. Brit J Cancer 55:541-542.

Elson PJ, Earhart RH, Kvols LK, Spiegel R, Keller AM, Kies MS, Davis TE, Stevens C, Gumas L, Trump DL (1987). Phase II studies of PCNU and bisantrene in advanced renal cell carcinoma. Cancer Treat Rep 71:331-332.

Elson PJ, Kvols LK, Vogl SE, Glover DJ, Hahn RG, Trump DL, Carbone PP, Earle JD, Davis TF (1988). Phase II trial of 5-day vinblastine infusion (NSC 49842), 1-alanosine (NSC 153353), acivicin (NSC 163501), and aminothia-diazole (NSC 4728) in patients with recurrent or metastatic renal cell carcinoma. Invest New Drugs 6:97-103.

Evans WK, Shepherd FA, Blackstein ME, Soba O, Taylor D (1985). Phase II evaluation of bisantrene in patients with patients with advanced renal cell carcinoma. Cancer Treat Rep 69:727-728.

Figlin RA, DeKernion JB, Maldazys J, Sarna G (1985). Treatment of renal cell carcinoma with alpha human leuco-cyte interferon and vinblastine in combination: a Phase I-II trial. Cancer Treat Rep 69:263-265.

Fojo AT, Shen DW, Mickley LA, Pastan I, Gottesman MM (1987). Intrinsic drug resistance in human kidney cancer is associated with expression of a human multidrug-resistance gene. J Clin Oncol 5:1922-1927.

Fossa SD, Cavalli F, Otto U, Bauer HW, Oberling JM, Achtnich U, Stein G, Holdener EF (1988). Randomized study of roferon-A (IFN) with or without vinblastine (VLB) in advanced metastatic renal cell cancer (RCC). Proc Amer Soc Clin Oncol (abstract 453)7:118.

Gams RA, Nelson O, Birch R (1986). Phase II evaluation of mitoxantrone in advanced renal cell carcinoma: a South-eastern Cancer Study Group trial. Cancer Treat Rep 70: 921-922.

Glover D, Trump D, Kvols L, Elson P, Vogl S (1986). Phase II trial of misonidazole (MISO) and cyclophosphamide (CYC) in metastatic renal cell carcinoma. Intern J

Radiat Oncol Biol Phys 12:1405-1408.

Hansen M, Gallmeier WM, Vermorken J, Holdener E, Hansen HH, Renard J, Rosenzweig M (1984). Phase II trial of diaziquone in advanced renal adenocarcinoma. Cancer Treat Rep 68:1055-1056.

Harris DT (1983). Hormonal therapy and chemotherapy for renal-cell carcinoma. Semin Oncol 10:422-430.

Harvey JH, Smith FP, Bowers MW, Neefe JR, Butler TP, Gullo JJ, Schertz G, Lokey J, Schein PS, Woolley PV (1984). Phase II trial of PCNU in advanced renal cell carcinoma and malignant mesothelioma. Cancer Treat Rep 68:1049-1050.

Herrmann R, Egri T, Manegold C, Matthiessen W (1988). Coumarin and cimetidine in the treatment of metastatic renal cell carcinoma. Proc Amer Soc Clin Oncol (abstract 505)7:131.

Hrushesky WJ, Murphy GP (1977). Current status of therapy for advanced renal cell carcinoma. J Surg Oncol 9: 277-288.

Hrushesky WJM, Roemeling R, Rabatin J, Fraley E (1987). Continuous FUDR infusion is effective in progressive renal cell cancer (RCC). Proc Amer Soc Clin Oncol (abstract 425)6:108.

Kish J, Ensley J, Tapazoglou E, Al-Sarraf M (1986). Phase II evaluation of deoxydoxorubicin for patients with advanced and recurrent renal cell cancer. Proc Amer Soc Clin Oncol (abstract 411)5:106.

Knight WA, Drehlichman A, Fabian C, Bukowski RM (1983). Mitoguazone in advanced renal carcinoma: a phase II trial of the Southwest Oncology Group. Cancer Treat Rep 67:1139-1140.

Krown SE (1985). Therapeutic options in renal cell carcinoma. Semin Oncol (suppl 5)4:13-17.

Kuebler JP, Hogan TF, Trump DL, Bryan GT (1984). Phase II study of continuous 5-day vinblastine infusion in renal adenocarcinoma. Cancer Treat Rep 68:925-926.

Licht JD, Garnick MC (1987). Phase II trial of streptozotocin in the treatment of advanced renal cell carcinoma. Cancer Treat Rep 71:97-98.

Long Hd, Hauge MD, Therneau TM, Buchner JC, Frytak S, Hahn RG (1988). Phase II evaluation of menogaril in patients with advanced hypernephroma. Proc Amer Soc Clin Oncol (abstract 493)7: 128.

Marshall ME, Mendelsohn L, Butler K, Riley L, Cantrell J, Wiseman C, Taylor R, Macdonald JS (1987). Treatment of metastatic renal cell carcinoma with coumarin (1,2-

benzopyrone) and cimetidine: a pilot study. J Clin Oncol 5:8622-866.

Muss HB, Welander C, Caponera M, Reavis K, Cruz JM, Cooper R, Jackson DV, Richards F, Stuart JJ, Spurr CL, White DR, Zekan PJ, Cappizzi RL (1985). Interferon and doxorubicin in renal cell carcinoma. Cancer Treat Rep 69:721-722.

Muss HB, Costanzi JJ, Leavitt R, Williams RD, Kempf RA, Pollard R, Ozer H, Zekan PJ, Grunberg SM, Mitchell MS, Caponera M, Gavigan M, Ernst ML, Venturi C, Greiner J, Spiegel RJ (1987). Recombinant alfa interferon in renal cell carcinoma: a randomized trial of two routes of administration. J Clin Oncol 5:286-291. Natale RB, Yagoda A, Kelsen DP, Gralla RJ, Watson RC (1982). Phase II trial of PALA in hypernephroma and urinary bladder cancer. Cancer Treat Rep 66:2091-2092.

Neidhart J, Harris J, Tuttle R (1987). A randomized study of Wellferon (WFN) with or without vinblastine (Vlb) in advanced renal cancer. Proc Amer Soc Clin Oncol (abstract 935)6:239.

Oishi N, Berenberg J, Blumenstein BA, Johnson K, Rivkin SE, Bukowski RM, O'Bryan RM, Stephens RL, Quagliana J, Saiers JH, Crawford ED (1987). Teniposide in metastatic renal and bladder cancer: a Southwest Oncology Group study. Cancer Treat Rep 71:1307-1308.

Oliver RTD (1987). Unexplained spontaneous regression and its relevance to the clinical behavior of renal cell carcinoma and its response to interferon. Proc Amer Soc Clin Oncol (abstract 383)6:98.

Pfiefle D, Renter N, Hahn R, Hilton JU, North Central Cancer Treatment Group (1984). Phase II trial of VM-26 in advanced measurable renal cell carcinoma. Proc Amer Soc Clin Oncol (abstract C-634)3:162.

Saiers JH, Slavik M, Stephens RL, Crawford ED (1987). Therapy for advanced renal cell cancer with spirogermanium: a Southwest Oncology Group study. Cancer Treat Rep 71:207-208.

Scher HI, Yagoda A, Ahmed T, Hollander P, Watson RC (1984). Phase II trial of 10-deaza-aminopterin for advanced hypernephroma. Anticancer Res 4:409-410.

Scher HI, Yagoda A, Ahmed T, Budman D, Sordillo P, Watson RC (1985). Phase II trial of 4-demethoxydaunorubicin for advanced hypernephroma. Cancer Chemother Pharmacol 14: 79-80.

Schornagel J, Verwey J, Huinink WT-B, Klijn J, de Mulder P, Van Deijk W, Roozendaal K, Kok T, Veenhof C, Van Benthem B, Berkel J, Van Oosterom AT (1987). Phase II study of recombinant interferon alpha-2 (IFN) and vinblastine (Vlb) in advanced renal carcinoma (RCC). Proc Amer Soc Clin Oncol (abstract 417)6:106.

Schulman P, Davis RB, Rafla S, Green M, Henderson E (1984). Phase II trial of spirogermanium in advanced renal cell carcinoma: a Cancer and Leukemia Group B study. Cancer Treat Rep 68:1305-1306.

Schwartz S, Yagoda A, Watson RC (1984). Phase I-II trial of gallium nitrate for advanced hypernephroma. Anticancer Res 4:317-318.

Shevrin DH, Lad TE, Kilton LJ, Cobleigh MA, Vogelzang N, Blough RR, Weidner LL (1988). Phase II trial of fludarabine phosphate in advanced renal cell cancer. Proc Amer Soc Clin Oncol (abstract 477)7:124.

Silva H, Abrams J, Olver I, Eisenberger M, Tchekmedyian NS, Leavitt R, Van Echo D, Aisner J (1986). Phase II trial of n-methylformamide (NMF) in patients with unresectable or recurrent renal cell carcinoma. Proc Amer Soc Clin Oncol (abstract 416) 5:107.

Stephens RL, Kirby R, Crawford ED, Bukowski R, Rivkin SE, O'Bryan RM (1986). High dose AZQ in renal cancer: a Southwest Oncology Group phase II study. Invest New Drugs 4:57-59.

Stewart DJ, Futter N, Irvine A, Danjoux C, Moors D (1987). Mitomycin-C and metronidazole in the treatment of advanced renal cell carcinoma. Amer J Clin Oncol 10: 520-522.

Sternberg C, Yagoda A, Ahmed T, Hollander P (1985). Phase II trial of elliptinium in advanced renal cell carcinoma and carcinoma of the breast. Anticancer Res 5:415-418.

Sternberg C, Yagoda A, Scher HI, Hollander P (1986). Phase II trial of n-methylformamide in renal cancer. Cancer Treat Rep 70:681-682.

Sternberg C, Yagoda A, Scher HI, Bosl G, Dershaw D, Rosado K, Houston C, Rosenbluth R, Vinceguerra V, Boselli B (1988). Phase II trial of trimetrexate in patients with advanced renal cell carcinoma. Proc Amer Assoc Cancer Res (abstract 815)29:205.

Tait N, Abrams J, Egorin MJ, Cohen AE, Eisenberger M (1988). Phase II carboplatin (CBDCA) for metastatic renal cell cancer with a standard dose (SD) and a calculated dose (CD) according to renal function. Proc Amer Soc Clin Oncol (abstract 484)7:125.

Tannock IF, Evans WK (1985). Failure of 5-day infusion in the treatment of patients with renal cell carcinoma. Cancer Treat Rep 69:227-228.

Taylor SA, Von Hoff DD, Baker LH, Balcerzak SP (1984). Phase II clinical trial of mitoxantrone in patients with advanced renal cell carcinoma: a Southwest Oncology Group study. Cancer Treat Rep 68:919-920.

Thill JR, Bennett CJ, Riggs CE, Williams RD, Clamon GH (1988). Effects of the anti-mitochondrial agents lonidamine and deoxycyline against 786-0 human renal carcinoma cells. Proc Amer Assoc Cancer Res (abstract 1282)29:322.

Van Oosterom AT, Fossa SD, Pizzocaro G, Bergerat JP, BOno AV, De Pauw M, Sylvester R (1984). Mitoxantrone in advanced renal cancer: a phase II study in previously untreated patients from the EORTC Genito-urinary Tract Cancer Cooperative Group. Eur J Cancer Clin Oncol 20: 1239-1241.

Van Oosterom AT, Bono AV, Kaye SB, Splinter TAW, Calciatti A, Fossa SD, DePauw M, Sylvester R (1987). 4' Deoxy-doxorubicin in advanced renal cancer: a phase II study in previously untreated patients from the EORTC Genito-urinary Tract Cancer Cooperative Group. Eur J Cancer Clin Oncol 22:1531-1532.

Vugrin D, Einhorn LH, Birch R (1987). Phase II trial of gallium nitrate in patients with metastatic renal carcinoma. Proc Amer Assoc Cancer Res (abstract 806)28: 203.

Wadler S, Einzig A, Dutcher JP, Ciobanu N, Landau L, Wiernik PH (1987). Phase II trial of recombinant alpha 2b interferon (IFN) and low dose cyclophosphamide (CY) in advanced melanoma and renal cell carcinoma. Proc Amer Soc Clin Oncol (abstract 969) 6:246.

Wagner H, Possinger K, Bremer K, Donhujsen-Ant R, Peukert M, Queisser W (1987). Phase II trial of 1,2,4-tri-gly-cidylurazol in patients with metastasized renal cell car-cinoma. Cancer Treat Rep 71:209-210.

Weinerman BH, Eisenhauer EA, Besner JG, Besner JG, Coppin CM, Stewart D, Band PR (1986). Phase II study of lonid-amine in patients with metastatic renal cell carcinoma: a National Cancer Institute of Canada Clinical Trials Group study. Cancer Treat Rep 70:751-753.

Zeffren J, Yagoda A, Kelsen D, Winn R (1984). Phase I-II trial of a 5-day continuous infusion of vinblastine sulfate. Anticancer Res 4:411-414.

Uro-Oncology: Current Status
and Future Trends, pages 243–255
© 1990 Wiley-Liss, Inc.

NEW PROSPECTS IN THE MANAGEMENT OF METASTATIC RENAL CELL
CARCINOMA. EXPERIMENTAL AND CLINICAL DATA

Frans M.J. Debruyne, Mart P.H. Franssen, Anton J.M.C.
Beniers, Jack A. Schalken, Pieter H.M. de Mulder
Department of Urology (F.M.J.D., M.P.H.F., A.J.M.C.B.,
J.A.S.) and Department of Medical Oncology
(P.H.M.d.M), University Hospital Nijmegen, The
Netherlands

Renal cell carcinoma is the most common tumor in
adults. Surgery may only have a curative intention if the
disease is local and not penetrating beyond the capsula
(Pt1 and pT2). However, patients have few therapeutic
options once the disease has become metastatic. Approximately 25-40% of the patients have metastatic disease at the
time of diagnosis (Richie and Chisholm, 1983). Furthermore
metastases will develop in a majority of untreated patients
within one year after discovery. Once the disease has
become metastatic their remain few therapeutic options.
Radio-, chemo- and hormonal therapy have failed to improve
the overall survival. The median survival of those patients
is 6 to 12 months (McDonald, 1982). Spontaneous regression
of metastases after tumor nephrectomy is less than 1%
(Montie et al., 1977). In view of the unusual natural
history of the tumor, such as spontaneous regression and
the dormant state of especially pulmonary metastases followed by a rapid growth phase, an interaction between the
host and the tumor has been suggested. Against this background immunotherapy has been proposed and applied especially with the aim to induce immune stimulation of the host
resulting in regressions of the tumor and its metastases.
This approach is currently addressed as treatment with
Biological Response Modifiers (BRMs). Interferon (IFN) and
Tumor Necrosis Factor (TNF) are the BRMs we will describe
in this chapter, discussing both experimental and clinical
data of these substances and their combinations.

Interferons are a group of naturally occuring proteins
with potent antiviral, antiproliferative and immuno-

modulatory properties such as activation of natural killer cells, macrophages, the increased expression of tumor associated antigens and the modulation of class I and II antigens. On the basis of their antigenic properties a division is made into 3 main groups. The alpha-IFNs are a group of closely related proteins with approximately 75% homology in their amino acid sequences. They are produced by macrophages and leucocytes upon exposure to virus particles and compete with the same receptor as bêta-IFN. Gamma-IFN is the product of a single gene and produced by activated T-lymphocytes and natural killer cells (Wagstaff and Melief, 1987). Tumor Necrosis Factor (TNF) is also produced by macrophages. It has direct cytotoxic activity against tumor cells (Haranaka and Satomi, 1981) but also induces a host mediated factor which contributes to the antitumor effects, especially in relation to T-cells (Gresser et al., 1986).

PRECLINICAL STUDIES

Preclinical studies have been performed in our laboratory with five different renal cell carcinoma xenografts. After original subcutaneous transplantation of small tumor pieces (2 mm^3) in both flanks of Balb-C nu/nu mice, the tumors were passaged every four weeks. Single cell suspensions of these tumors were used for the in vitro tests in which the antiproliferative effects of alpha-IFN, gamma-IFN and TNF as single agents and in combination were measured using a soft agar colony forming assay. (Verheyen et al., 1985). Drugs were administered as a single application on day 1 and colony formation was followed during four weeks in which growth was measured using temporal growth curves (Feitz et al., 1986).

Single drug studies

Determination of optimal plating densities for analysis of colony fromation according to the temporal growth curves revealed a concentration of 1x10^5 cells per dish for all tumor lines. Single drug tests were performed using 1,500, 15,000 or 150,000 IU IFN/ml and 300, 3,000 or 30,000 IU TNF/ml. These tests showed differences in the responsiveness of the different lines towards the drugs. Inhibition of colony formation appeared to be dose dependent

although differences in sensitiveness between the doses of
15,000 and 150,000 IU IFN/ml or 3,000 and 30,000 IU TNF/ml
was very small. All tumors showed sensitivity for alpha-IFN
of which two appeared to be very sensitive for this drug
for which a single dose of 1,500 IU/ml resulted in a
percentage survival of only 35% or less as compared to the
untreated growth control. Gamma-IFN showed antiproliferative efficacy in only two of the lines (RC-43 and NU-12).
Maximum antiproliferative efficacy of 1,500 IU/ml of this
BRM resulted in a percentage survival fraction of 30%. This
dose, however, inhibited colony formation for only 5-10% in
three of the lines and rising the gamma-IFN concentration
to 15,000 or 150,000 IU/ml did not substantially rise inhibition of colony formation. TNF as single drug was effective in all lines and percentage survival after a single
application of 300 IU TNF/ml appeared to be 100% for the
least sensitive line (RC-43) and 25% for the most sensitive
line (HAM-III). Higher doses of TNF resulted in substantial
inhibition of colony formation of the RC-43 line as well.

Combination drug tests

        Because IFNs and TNF can act synergistically (Hubbel
et al., 1987; Salmon et al., 1987) IFN concentrations of
1,500 IU IFN/ml were used for the combination tests. The
TNF concentration used was 3,000 IU/ml because the single
drug tests showed that one of the lines (RC-43) was insensitive for a TNF concentration of 300 IU/ml.

        The results of the combination tests are shown in
Figures 1a+b, and 2a-c and are summarized in Table 1 which
shows the percentage survival values for the combination
tests as well as those for the single drug tests.

Figure 1a shows the in vitro colony forming capacity of the
RC-43 tumor cells when treated with different combinations
of the BRMs. Calculated according to Valeriote and Lin
(1975), synergistic effects were found for all different
combinations on RC-43. The number of colonies in the alpha-
gamma-IFN combination rising hardly above $HgCl_2$ cytotoxic
control level. The most effective combination appears to be
that of alpha-IFN with TNF in which colony formation equals
that of the cytotoxic control. The combination of gamma-IFN
with TNF, however, proves to be less effective for this
tumor since it gives rise to about 20% survival as compared
to the growth control.

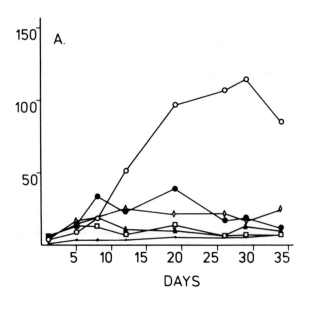

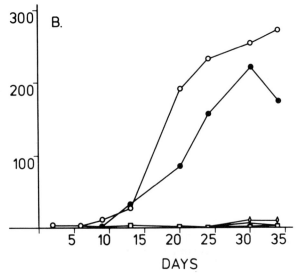

Figure 1a+b. Effect of combinations of IFN-alpha (1,500 IU/ml), IFN-gamma (1,500 Iu/ml) and TNF (3,000 IU/ml) on colony formations of A: RC-43, and B: NC-65 renal tumor xenograft cells in soft agar after application of a single dose of the drugs. o——o = growth control; •——• = cyto-

toxic growth control (100 g HgCl$_2$/ml) (small black dots);
•——• = IFN-alpha/IFN-gamma (large black dots); ▫——▫ =
IFN-alpha/TNF; ◇——◇ = IFN-gamma/TNF.

Figure 1b, in which the in vitro colony formation of
NC-65 renal carcinoma cells is shown after treatment with
different combinations of the tested BRMs, shows a rather
high survival percentage of these cells with the drug
combination of alpha-IFN/gamma-IFN as compared to the RC-43
cells. The most effective treatment of these tumor cells,
however, also appears to be the combinations of alpha-IFN
and TNF. Furthermore, the drug combination of gamma-IFN and
TNF appears to have a similar effect because the number of
formed colonies is only 1% of the number of colonies formed
in the growth control.

Figure 2A shows the in vitro colony forming capacity
of NU-12 renal tumor cells. Al tested combinations appear
to have highly antiproliferative effects on the cells. A
10% survival value is measured for the combination of
alpha- and gamma-IFN. All other combinations, i.e. the
combinations with TNF coincide and give rise to only a 4%
survival fraction as compared to the growth control.

Figure 2b, in which the in vitro colony formation of
HAM-II renal carcinoma cells is shown after treatment with
the tested BRMs, shows a rather high survival percentage of
these cells with the drug combinations of alpha-IFN and
gamma-IFN. However, because of the low activities of the
tested concentrations as shown in the single drug studies,
this combination nevertheless results in a synergistic
antiproliferative efficacy against the tumor cells as do
the other tested combinations which, as found for the NU-12
colony formation of the cells.

Figure 2c and Table 1 show that also for the HAM-III
line all combinations tested act synergistic antiproliferative on colony formation of these tumor cells.

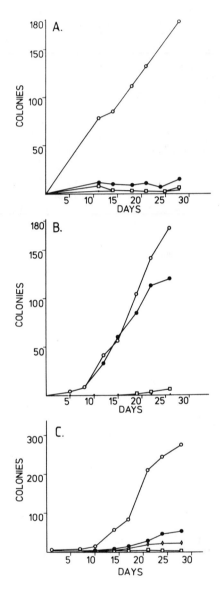

Figure 2a-c. Effects of combinations of IFN-alpha (1,500 IU/ml), IFN-gamma (1,500 IU/ml) and TNF (3,000 IU/ml) on colony formation of A: NU-12, B: HAM-II, and C: HAM-III renal tumor xenograft cells in soft agar after application of a single dose of the drugs. The combinations of IFN-alpha/TNF and IFN-gamma/TNF in a A and B all coincide. o———o = growth control; •——• = cytotoxic growth control (100 g HgCl$_2$/ml) (small black dots); •——• = IFN-alpha/IFN-gamma (large black dots); □——□ = IFN-alpha/TNF; ◇——◇ = IFN-gamma/TNF.

TABLE 1. Percentage survival after drug therapy.

Drug Combinations	RC-43 % surv.	NC-65 % surv.	NU-12 % surv.	HAM-II % surv.	HAM-III % surv.
Alpha-IFN	25	70	55	85	35
Gamma-IFN	45	90	30	90	95
TNF	55	75	40	35	25
Alpha-/gamma-IFN	3	65	10	70	20
Alpha-IFN/TNF	0	0	3	3	0
Gamma-IFN/TNF	20	2	4	3	8

Percentage survival of RC-43, NC-65, NU-12, HAM-II and HAM-III renal tumor xenograft cells after growth in soft agar and application of a single dose of different combinations of IFN-alpha, IFN-gamma and TNF as compared to the untreated control. IFN concentrations used were 1,500 IU/ml and TNF concentration was 3,000 IU/ml.

CLINICAL STUDIES

In view of the synergistic activity of IFN-alpha and IFN-gamma based on both (own) experimental data and other observations (Czarnicki et al., 1984) we studied the efficacy of the combination of an escalating dose r-IFN-alpha (6 µg/m^2 = 2x10^6 U/m^2 starting dose) and a fixed low dose of r-IFN-gamma (100 µg/m^2 = 2x10^6/m^2) two times weekly s.c. in patients with proven progressive metastatic renal cell carcinoma. After 8 weeks of treatment the dose of r-IFN-alpha was escalated with 6 µg/m^2 until the maximum tolerated dose (MTD).

A total of 32 patients (21 males and 11 females) has been entered in this study. The mean age was 57.2 years (35-74 years). The majority of the patients had metastatic spread in soft tissue (lungs, liver, and lymph nodes) with the lungs as predominant site (84%). Noteworthy is that 55% of the 11 females were under 50 years of age in contrast to only 10% of the 21 males. Of the 32 patients 29 had undergone neprectomy prior to the start of treatment. The time to documented progression after neprectomy varies for 1 to 53 months (median 8 months). The median Karnofski performance status index was 90 (70-100).

Twenty-nine patients were evaluable for response. One patient was ineligible due to spontaneous regression after tumor nephrectomy. Two other patients were early withdrawn from the study due to toxicity. These 2 patients stopped before 8 weeks of treatment, both due to dose adjustment resistent severe subjective complaints and the latter also because of therapy resistent dyspepsia. At time of off-study also progressive disease was established in both patients. The overall response rate was 28% (best obtained objective response according to WHO criteria). Two patients (7%) had a complete remission (CR), 6 patients (21%) had a partial response (PR), 5 patients (17%) showed stable disease (SD), and 16 patients (55%) developed progressive disease despite combined IFN treatment. The median response for PR was 14 months (8-16 months). One CR is still ongoing (24+ months). The other patient with CR recently progressed after 22 months of therapy (abdominal metastases). The median time to response for PR was 24 weeks (18-36 weeks). The 2 CRs had a median time to response of 24 and 28 weeks respectively. The median time to a first sign of regression was 12 weeks (4-16 weeks). Remarkable was the observation that 5 initially not responding patients eventually developed a partial or complete remission after the dose of IFN-alpha was escalated.

Side effects were evaluated according to the WHO toxicity grading system. The highest observed grade in each patient was recorded.

Subjectively, all patients showed periods op drug fever (100%). The majority of patients showed fatigue/weakness (97%), anorexia (87%), and nausea and/or vomiting (71%). Diarrhea was scored in 45% of the patients, and dry mouth and/or mucositis in 42%. Neurological abnormalities were observed in 35% (mild periferal neuropathy). Furthermore, cutaneous symptoms were observed in 29% and mild alopecia in 19% of the patients. All subjective symptoms were mild (grade I) or moderate (grade II)in the majority of the patients.

Objectively, hematological disorders were encountered rather frequently. We observed anemia in 52% of the patients, leukopenia in 39% and thrombocytopenia in 6% (mostly mild, grade I toxicity). In one patient grade IV leukocytopenia (nadir: 0.6x10/l) developed with concomitant septicemia. IFN treatment was stopped immediately and patient recovered after proper therapy. Erythrocyte sedimentation rate (ESR) was disturbed in 78% of all patients. Kidney function disorders occured in 23% of the patients (creatinine serum level). It seems, however, likely that part of these "side effects" are due to the tumor itself or its metastases. Anemia and ESR disturbances were frequently encountered before start of IFN treatment.

In a subsequent study 25 patients were treated with a starting dose r-IFN-alpha of 24 $\mu g/m^2$ and a fixed low dose of r-IFN-gamma (100 $\mu g/m^2$). The patient characteristics of this group were comparable with the first group. Twenty-one patients are evaluable for response, 2 are ineligible and 2 stopped treatment within 8 weeks due to excessive toxicity. A CR was found in 4 (19%), a PR in 1 (5%), SD in 4 (19%) patients, and in 12 (57%) a PD. The overall response of this second group was 24%. The median time to response was 12 weeks (4-12 weeks). The higher starting dose of r-IFN-alpha seems to induce a more rapid response.

The 12% CR (6 CRs on 50 for response evaluable patients) for the 2 studies is a remarkable finding and might indicate a possible positive effect of r-IFN-gamma when combined with an optimal dose of r-IFN- alpha. A randomized study is needed to answer this question more definitely and is currently undertaken by the EORTC GU co-operative group.

DISCUSSION

Preclinical studies

Our experimental results show that all tumors demonstrate in vitro sensitivity for alpha-IFN, gamma-IFN, and TNF. A dose dependent inhibition of colony formation was evident when treated with the BRMs in direct exhibition to a single dose of the drugs. Sensitivities of the lines to the drugs, however, show distinct differences.

The most effective drug combination for all tumor lines was the combination of alpha-IFN (1,500 IU/ml) and TNF (3,000 IU/ml) resulting in a percentage survival of 0% for the RC-43, NC-65 and HAM-III line and of only 3% of the NU-12 and HAM-II lines as compared to the growth control.

In summary our findings demonstrate that the five xenografts show distinct but different in vitro sensitivities towards alpha-IFN, gamma-IFN and TNF. Most sensitive are the RC-43 and NU-12 xenografts which appear to be sensitive for all three BRMs. Least sensitive are the NC-65 and HAM-II xenografts which are only moderately sensitive for alpha-IFN and TNF but shows no or hardly any sensitivity towards gamma-IFN. Almost all tested combinations of the tested BRMs showed synergistic antiproliferative effects against colony formation of the five tumors. Most effective was the combination alpha-IFN (1,500 IU/ml)/TNF (3,000 IU/ml).

Clinical studies

Since the first report that a partially purified human alpha-IFN preparation could induce the regression of metastatic RCC numerous therapeutic trials have been conducted to assess the efficacy of various alpha-IFN preparations. Most studies provided evidence for modest but reproducible antitumor activity in advanced RCC. Pooled data indicate a response rate of 15% with the best response in the intermediate dose range ($15-75\times10^6$ IU/wk) (Krown, 1986). The responses in the low and high dose range were significantly lower. These observations are suggestive for the existence of a bell shape relation between the dose and response. Our own observations with an escalating dose of r-IFN-alpha in combination with a fixed dose r-IFN-gamma two times weekly s.c. indicate also the existence of a dose response relationship.

So far no definite superior regime i.e. cyclic, continuous, 2 or 3 times weekly nor a "best" route of administration i.e. subcutaneous, intramuscular, intravenous had been found. It is well recognized that bone lesions, central nervous system localization and the primary tumor rarely respond to this type of treatment. Furthermore, large tumor masses are less likely to regress than limited disease. Localization especially susceptible for response are those in the lungs (Muss, 1988). Final conclusion in this respect should be made with caution in view of eligibility criteria used in the different trials such as prior nephrectomy, performance status, etc.

The experience with IFN-gamma monotherapy is still very limited. In a recent phase I-II study poor response data were reported (Garnick et al., 1988). Little is known about the optimal dose, schedule and route of IFN-gamma administration.

As demonstrated in our study the experimentally and clinically suggested synergistic effect of IFN-alpha and IFN-gamma is also benificial for patients with metastatic renal cell carcinoma. This has also been documented in a few other studies (Quesada et al., 1988). The regimen used in our study was reasonably well tolerated.

From our data as well as from data already published it is clear that patients with soft tissue metastases, limited metastatic tumor load and good performance status are more likely to respond to therapy with BRMs. Furthermore there is an indication that prior tumor nephrectomy enhances the efficacy of IFN-therapy although this suggestion has to be confirmed by further clinical (comparative) studies. These studies are also needed to establish more exactly the future role of BRMs in the management of metastatic renal cell carcinoma. Questions with regard to dose, schedule, route of administration, etc. are still open. Furthermore a variety of questions concerning their antiproliferative as well as their immunostimulating capacities remain to be answered. This demands a further in dept research of many unknown factors which will define the direction of future developments.

Recently the first clinical results of lymphokine activated killer cells and recombinant Interleukin-2 in advanced renal cell carcinoma have been published (Roosenberg et al., 1987). This form of therapy as well as other new approaches using Tumor Infiltrating Lymphocytes (TIL therapy) indicate the future direction in which BRMs will be used. Likewise, other combinations of BRMs such as Il-2 with r-IFN-alpha, and r-IFN-gamma or TNF-alpha with IFN-gamma are currently tested. Although progress is slow it is likely that BRM therapy will play an increasing role in the management of advanced and metastatic renal cell carcinoma.

REFERENCES

Czarnicki CW, Fennie CW, Powers DB, Estell DA (1984). Synergistic antiviral and antiproliferative activities of E. Coli derived, human alpha, beta and gamma interferon. J Virol 49: 490-495.

Feitz WFJ, Verheyen RHM, Kirkels WJ, Vooijs GP, Debruyne FMJ, Herman CJ (1986). Dynamics of human renal tumor colony growth in vitro. Urol Res 14: 109-112.

Garnick MB, Reich SD, Maxwell B, Coval-Goldsmith S, Richie JP, Rudnick SA (1988). Phase I-II study of recombinant Interferon-gamma in advanced renal cell carcinoma. J Urol 139: 251-255.

Gresser K, Belardelli F, Tavernier J, Fiers W, Podo F, Federico M, Carpinelli G, Duvillard P, Prade M, Maury C, Bandu MT, Maunoury MT (1986). Anti-tumor effects of interferon in mice injected with interferon-sensitive and interferon-resistant Friend leukemia cells. V. Comparisons with the action of tumor necrosis factor. Int J Cancer 38: 771-778.

Haranaka K, Satomi N (1981). Cytotoxic activity of tumor necrosis factor (TNF) on human cancer cell in vitro. Jpn J Exp Med 51: 191-194.

Hubbel HR, Craft JA, Leibowitz PJ, Gillespie DH (1987). Synergistic antiproliferative effect of recombinant alpha-interferon with recombinant gamma-interferon. J Biol Resp Modif 6: 141-153.

Krown SE (1986). Interferon treatment of renal cell carcinoma. Current status and future prospects. Cancer 46: 4315-4329.

McDonald MW (1982). Current therapy for renal cell carcinoma. J Urol 127: 211-217.

Montie JE, Stuwart BH, Straffon RA, Banowsky LHW, Hewitt CB, Montague DK (1977). The role of adjunctive nephrectomy in patients with metastatic renal cell carcinoma. J Urol 117: 272-275.

Muss HB (1988). Interferon therapy of metastatic renal cell cancer. Sem Surg Oncol 4: 199-203.

Quesada JR, Evans L, Saks SR (1988). Recombinant interferon alpha and gamma in combination as treatment for metastatic renal cell carcinoma. J Biol Resp Mod 7: 234-239.

Richie AWS, Chisholm DG (1983). The natural history of renal cell carcinoma. Semin Oncol 10: 390-400.

Roosenberg SA, Lotze MT, Muul LM, Chang AE, Avis FP, Leitman S, Linekam WM, Robertson CN, Lee RE, Rubin JT, Seipp CA, Simpson CG, White DE (1987). A progress report on the treatment of 157 patients with advanced cancer using lymphokine activated killer cells and interleukin-2 or high dose interleukine-2 alone. N Engl J Med 316: 889-897.

Salmon SE, Young L, Scuderi P, Clark B (1987). Antineoplastic effects of tumor necrosis factor in combination with gamma-interferon on tumor biopsies in clonogenic assay. J Clin Oncol 5: 1816.1821.

Valeriote F, Lin H (1975). Synergistic interaction of anticancer agents: a cellular perspecitve. Cancer Chemother Rep 59: 895-900.

Verheyen RHM, Feitz WFJ, Beck JLM, Debruyne FMJ, Vooijs GP, Kenemans P, Herman CJ (1985). Cell DNA content - correlation with clonogenicity in the human tumor cloning system (HTCS). Int J Cancer 35: 653-657.

Wagstaff J, Melief KJ (1987). In Pinedo HM, Longo DL, Chabner BA (eds): "Cancer Chemotherapy and Biological Response Modifiers," Annual 9, Amsterdam: Elseviers Science Publishers BV, pp. 432.

Uro-Oncology: Current Status
and Future Trends, pages 257–262
© 1990 Wiley-Liss, Inc.

CYCLIC INTERFERON GAMMA APPLICATION IN PATIENTS WITH RENAL CELL CARCINOMA

J.W. Grups, H.G.W. Frohmüller

Department of Urology, School of Medicine, University of Würzburg, Josef-Schneider-Str. 2, 8700 Würzburg, FRG

Introduction

Complete surgical removal of the kidney together with the adrenal gland and the adjacent lymph nodes is still regarded as the only curative treatment in localized renal cell carcinoma (RCC). However, distant metastases are present in up to 30% of patients with RCC at the time of diagnosis. In another 50% of the patients, in whom no metastases can be demonstrated initially, tumor progression occurs in subsequent years.

Therefore an effort was undertaken to evaluate whether the course of the disease can be affected by cyclic immunotherapy with recombinant human interferon (rHu-IFN) gamma. Studies published in recent years demonstrated that human interferon (IFN) or other "biological response modifiers" can produce promising results. It has not been clarified as yet, however, what regime of treatment and which dosage of interferon is especially suitable for treating patients with metastasised RCC (1).

From our own experience with long term IFN-alfa-application we are aware of the fact that this form of treatment does not result in a permanent immunological stimulation. As published previously the NK cell activity was augmented only for a short period of time despite continuing IFN-alfa-application (2). This was the reason why we decided to use repeated short term IFN gamma-medication.

Patients and methods

Between June 1986 and April 1988, 14 patients, who suffered from metastasised renal cell carcinoma, were treated systemically with cyclic rHu-IFN gamma applications.

In order to evaluate the immunological effects of this treatment its influence on lymphocytes and their subpopulations of the peripheral venous blood was examined. The amount of T- and B-lymphocytes, T-helper- and T-suppressor- cells, monocytes and NK- cells was determined by flow cytometry after labeling them with monoclonal antibodies.

The determination of the spontaneous cellular cytotoxicity was carried out with a ^{51}Cr-releasing assay. Suspension cells of the permanent cell line K 562 were used as target cells.

In 12 of these 14 patients treated with IFN gamma, tumor nephrectomy had been performed prior to treatment. In two patients surgical removal of the tumor was not feasible because of their poor general condition. In four patients the metastases had been verified histologically by biopsy. In the other ten patients the metastatic spreading was verified by means of CT, ultrasonography or x-ray of the chest. With one exception none of the 14 patients had received prior radiotherapy, chemotherapy or hormonal treatment.

After extensive information and written consent the patients received daily intramuscular injections of 0.25 mg rHu- IFN gamma over a period of eight days as a standard dosage.

Interferon was provided by Boehringer Co., Ingelheim, FRG. It had a 98 % degree of purity and a specific activity of 2×10^{7} IU/mg protein. Following the eight-day administration of IFN there was a treatment-free interval of three to four weeks followed by repeated eight-day IFN gamma cycles. In some patients, up to 11 IFN cycles were administered.

Results

In the analysis of the various lymphocyte subpopulations before, during and after systemic treatment with rHu IFN gamma it became clear that the ratio of the T4 population (T-helper cells) to the T8 population (T-suppressor cells) was significantly changed for a short period of time. Whereas a T4/T8 ratio of 3:1 could be detected prior to treatment, the proportion of T-helper cells rose significantly eight hours after the beginning of treatment, so that a T4/T8 ratio of 9:1 resulted. In the subsequent period the number of helper cells fell roughly to pretherapeutic levels. The curve of the T4/T8 ratio is shown graphically on fig. 1.

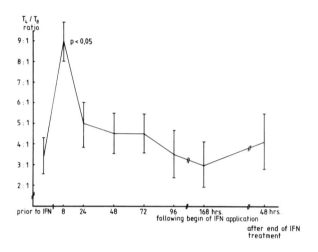

Figure 1: T4/T8 ratio during treatment with IFN gamma.

Concerning the other lymphocyte subpopulations investigated in this study no significant alteration was noted.

The brief shift of the T4/T8 ratio from about 3:1 to 9:1 during the systemic treatment with rHu IFN gamma can be interpreted as a manifestation of immunological stimulation.

The NK cell activity could be stimulated in all 14 patients by treatment with rHu IFN gamma. A loss of NK cell activity was demonstrable initially after eight hours; this was followed by a significant rise of NK cell activity above the initial pretherapeutic levels. The maximum cytolytic activity of the NK cells was attained usually on the seventh day. The NK cell activity during various consecutive treatment cycles is shown on fig. 2. It becomes evident that the NK cells could be stimulated in all consecutive treatment cycles. This was statistically significant in each case (p0.01).

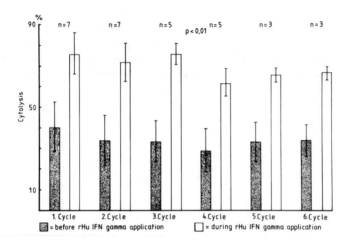

Figure 2: NK cell activity during various cycles of treatment with rHu IFN gamma.

The effectiveness of treatment could be appraised in 10 of the 14 patients. In the other 4 patients the duration of treatment was inadequate for various reasons.

A partial tumor remission could be attained in three out of those ten patients who could be evaluated. A stable disease could be arrived at another two patients. In 5 patients a progression of the disease was noticed.

Patient	Metastases	IFN-Cycles	Result	Duration
1	Lungs	11	PR	18 months
2	Bones	9	PR	10 months
3	Lungs	5	PR	4 months
4	Bones	8	SD	14 months
5	Lungs	8	SD	8 months
6	Lungs	10	Progression	---
7	Bones	8	Progression	---
8	Lungs/Bones	8	Progression	---
9	Lungs	6	Progression	---
10	Lungs	5	Progression	---

Table 1: Results of cyclic treatment with rHu IFN gamma

Two patients died of causes unconnected with IFN gamma application after the first treatment cycle. One of these patients died of an acute hemorrhage from an aortic aneurysm and the other patient suffered a fatal pulmonary embolism 28 days after the end of the first IFN treatment cycle.

During systemic treatment with rHu-IFN gamma so-called "influenza like symptoms" occured in all patients. Fever (up to 39.5° C), occasional shivering and limb pain were the most frequent clinical symptoms. The laboratory tests showed no essential alterations apart from leucocytopenia. The flu-like symptoms became apparent about two hours after the i.m. injection of IFN gamma. They reached their maximum about four to five hours later and regressed within several hours. After the end of IFN treatment, leukocyte levels rose again and normalized completely in all patients. A rHu-IFN gamma-dependent change of liver tests was not observed. Superficial thrombosis in the legs occured in two patients.

Discussion

Since a connection between immune reactivity and the further clinical progress of the renal cell carcinoma might exist (3), the alterations of the immunological parameters can be interpreted as manifestation of a stimulated immune response. Owing to the repeatedly inducible immune stimulation the concept of cyclic rHu IFN gamma administration appears to be a better form of treatment than long-term continuous IFN administration. Theoretically, NK precursor cells are converted into mature and cytolytically active NK cells in these recurrent immunostimulations, thus leading to intensified tumor defence (4).

In view of the advanced tumor stage and the poor prognosis of the patients treated in this study, for which promising methods of therapy were otherwise not available, the present results are encouraging. However, since complete tumor remission could not be attainded, it becomes evident that at present the cyclic application of IFN gamma appears to be a palliative therapeutic concept only.

Literature

1. Interferon therapy for the treatment of renal cancer. Neidhart, J.A.
   Cancer 57: 1696-1699 (1986)

2. Immunological findings in patients with superficial bladder cancer during human alpha-2 interferon treatment.
   Grups J.W., Frohmüller H.G.W., Ackermann R.
   Urol. int. 40: 301-306 (1985)

3. Studies on the immune status of patients with renal adeno-carcinoma.
   Brosman S., Hausman M., Shaks S.J.
   J. Urol. 114: 375-380 (1975).

4. Studies on the mechanism of natural killer cell-mediated cytotoxicity.
   Wrigth S.C., Bonavida B.
   J. Immunol. 133: 3415-3423 (1984)

Uro-Oncology: Current Status
and Future Trends, pages 263–273
© 1990 Wiley-Liss, Inc.

ANTI-TUMOR EFFECTS OF INTERLEUKIN2 AGAINST RENAL CELL
CARCINOMA. IN VITRO STUDY AND CLINICAL APPLICATION.

Ken Marumo and Hiroshi Tazaki

Department of Urology, School of Medicine, Keio
University, Tokyo, 160 Japan

INTRODUCTION

     Renal cell carcinoma(RCC) is one of the most insensi-
tive urologic tumors to either radiotherapy or anticancer
chemotherapy. The past several years have shown that inter-
feron(IFN) is the agent of greatest promise in treating advanced RCC. Reports have shown, however, that the effectiveness of IFN is limited; its response rates range from 5
to 26 percent(Quesada et al., 1983; deKernion et al., 1983;
Marumo et al., 1984). On the other hand, interleukin2(IL2),
discovered as a T-cell growth factor(Morgan et al., 1976) is
a lymphokine produced by helper T-lymphocytes. Recent advances in the characterization of this lymphokine have shown
that IL2 is necessary for the continuous proliferation of
cytotoxic T-lymphocytes(Dennert, 1979) and natural killer
(NK) cells(Domzig et al., 1983). It also induces lymphokine-activated killer(LAK) cells(Grimm et al., 1982), which
have proven to be cytotoxic to NK-resistant solid tumor
cells. Here we describe the antitumor effects of IL2
against RCC in vitro, which were studied in order to determine optimum mode of administration, and show safety and
efficacy of low-dose IL2 in 12 patients with advanced RCC.

MATERIALS AND METHODS

     IL2 and gamma-IFN: The recombinant human IL2 and re-
combinant human gamma-IFN had been produced by Biogen, Inc.
(Switzerland) and were provided by Shionogi Pharmaceutical
Company(Osaka, Japan). The titer of IL2 was expressed in

accordance with the titer of Jurkat IL2 standard received
from the Biological Response Modifiers Programme(NCI).

Lymphocyte separation: Human peripheral mononuclear
cells were isolated by Ficoll-Hypaque sedimentation from
heparinized venous blood. Peripheral blood lymphocytes(PBL)
were used after eliminating adherent monocytes by incubating
cells two times in a plastic tissue culture plate at 37°C
for 30 minutes.

Tumor cells: The human myeloid cell line, K562, human
renal carcinoma cell line, KU-2 and CaKi 1, Burkitt lymphoma
cell line, Daudi, and freshly prepared renal carcinoma cells
obtained from surgical specimens from 4 patients with RCC,
as previously described(Marumo et al., 1987), were used as
target cells of cell-mediated cytotoxicity test.

Cytotoxicity test: Cell-mediated cytotoxicity was determined by four-hour ^{51}Cr-release assay as previously de-
scribed(Marumo et al., 1987).

Analysis of PBL surface antigen: The expression of
lymphocyte subpopulations and IL2 receptor on cell surfaces
were determined using fluorescein isothiocyanate(FITC)-
labeled monoclonal antibodies(MoAb) and flow cytometer(Ortho
Spectrum III, Ortho Diagnostic System Inc., Westwood, MA).
The FITC-conjugated MoAb against Leu 2(suppressor/cytotoxic
T cells), Leu 3(helper/inducer T cells), Leu 4(pan T cells),
Leu 7(NK cells), Leu 11(NK cells), Leu HLA-DR(Ia analogue),
and Anti-IL2 receptor(human IL2 receptor)(Becton Dickinson
Monoclonal Center Inc., Mountain Views, CA) were used to
stain the PBL.

Patient selection: IL2 therapy was initiated in 12
consecutive patients with advanced RCC(Table 1), during the
period from March 1986 to June 1987. All patients received
nephrectomy; and all were treated for a minimum of two weeks
after previous therapy was discontinued.

Administration of interleukin 2: Two-hour intravenous
drip infusions containing $5x10^5$U of IL2 were given twice
daily while the patients were hospitalized, but, after at
least 28 days of this mode of administration, subcutaneous
injection of IL2 at a dose of $1x10^6$U was given six days a
week on a outpatient basis.

Response criteria: Clinical response was evaluated using response criteria adopted by Japan Society for Cancer Therapy. Complete response was defined as disappearance of all known disease. Partial response was 50 percent or greater decrease in the product of diameters(width x length) in measurable lesions. No lesion could have progressed nor any new lesion appear. No change was defined as less than 50 percent decrease or less than 25 percent increase for at least four weeks in measurable lesion. Progressive disease was defined as an increase of at least 25 percent in measurable lesion or appearance of new lesion.

Statistical analysis: The results were compared using Student t (paired t) test. A p value less than 0.05 was considered statistically significant.

TABLE 1. Characteristics of patients treated with IL2

Case	Age	Sex	Metastases	PS*
1. I.S.	65	M	Lung,bone,lymphnodes	3
2. E.Y.	62	M	Lung,bone	4
3. I.Y.	62	M	Bone	3
4. K.M.	55	M	Lung	0
5. S.M.	68	M	Bone	4
6. O.S.	75	M	Lung,bone,brain	4
7. O.T.	67	M	Liver	4
8. T.S.	55	M	Lung	0
9. W.Y.	62	M	Lung,colon	1
10. I.T.	29	F	Lymphnodes	2
11. S.M.	59	M	Lung,liver	1
12. A.S.	73	M	Lung,mediastinum	1

*PS=ECOG performance status

RESULTS

Enhancement of cytotoxicity by IL2 in vitro: Dose-dependent effects of IL2 on lymphocyte-mediated cytotoxicity were investigated using CaKi 1, KU-2, and K562 lines as target cells. When PBL were incubated with 100 U/ml of IL2 for 72 hours, cytotoxicity was increased significantly rising from 5.5 percent to 38.3 percent(p less than 0.01) against CaKi 1, from 8.9 percent to 61.7 percent(p less than 0.001) against KU-2, and from 46.7 to 74.2 percent(p less than 0.01) against K562(Fig. 1). IL2 increased cytotoxicity against renal carcinoma cell lines, which are less suscepti- ble to NK cells than K562 line, by approximately seven- fold. Even at such low concentration as 4 U/ml, the cytotoxicity was significantly enhanced against KU-2(p less than 0.01).

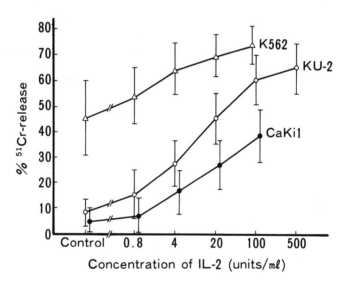

FIGURE 1. Concentration-dependent effects of IL2 on lympho- cyte-mediated cytotoxicity against CaKi 1, KU-2, and K562. PBL from 8 different healthy donors were incubated with 0.8, 4, 8, 20, 100, and 500 U/ml of IL2 for 72 hours. Control indicated lymphocytes were incubated with complete medium for 72 hours. Effector/target cell ratio was 50:1.

A comparison was made between the NK activating effects of IL2 and gamma-IFN. Gamma-IFN was used at a concentration of 400 IU/ml, which was found to be the optimum concentra- tion, as well no significant difference between the cyto- toxicity of that PBL exposed to gamma-IFN for 24 hours and that exposed for 48 hours(Marumo et al., 1987). On the ba-

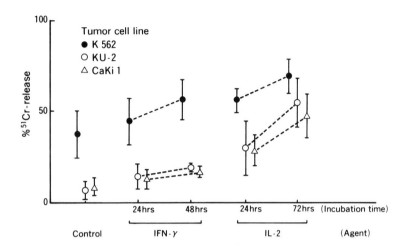

FIGURE 2. Effects of IL2 and gamma-IFN on lymphocyte-mediated cytotoxicity against CaKi 1, KU-2, and K562. PBL from 6 different healthy donors were incubated with 100 U/ml of IL2, and 400 IU/ml of gamma-IFN. Control in the absence of any reagents but medium for 72 hours. Effector/target cell ratio was 50:1.

TABLE 2. Effects of IL2 and gamma-IFN on lymphocyte-mediated cytotoxicity against fresh renal carcinoma cells, separated from surgical specimens from 4 different patients. Effector/target cell ratio was 50:1.

Stimulation of PBL		%^{51}Cr-release
Control		7.0 ± 2.9
Gamma-IFN	400 IU/ml	21.6 ± 2.5
IL2	4 U/ml	21.3 ± 2.9
	100 U/ml	53.0 ± 2.5

(Mean ± S.D.)

sis of these data,respective incubation time with IL2 and
gamma-IFN used to compare the activating effect in these two
agents was 24 hours and 72 hours for IL2 and 24 hours and 48
hours for gamma-IFN. IL2 induced significantly greater
cytotoxicity against CaKi 1 and KU-2 than did gamma-IFN(Fig.
2). The effects of these lymphokines on cytotoxic reactions
were also shown to be time-dependent.

The cytotoxicity against freshly prepared renal carcinoma cells was 7.0 percent in the control PBL, indicating
that these solid tumor cells were resistant to NK cells.
PBL were incubated with 4 U/ml and 100 U/ml of IL2 for 72
hours, and incubated with 400 IU/ml of gamma-IFN for 48
hours. One hundred U/ml of IL2 augmented cytotoxicity from
7.0 percent to 53.0 percent(p less than 0.001). A concentration of only 4 U/ml of IL2 induced the same level of
cytotoxicity of gamma-IFN(Table 2).

Serum IL2 level after intravenous drip infusions: We
used radioimmunoassay to make multiple serum measurements of
IL2 before and after two-hour intravenous drip infusions

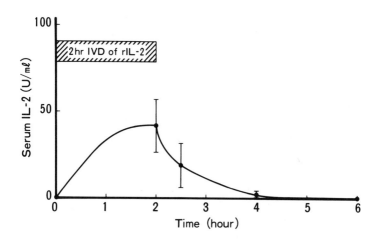

FIGURE 3. Serum IL2 level before and after two-hour intravenous drip infusions containing 5×10^5 units of IL2 in four
patients(Mean ± S.D.).

containing 5×10^5 U of IL2 were administered to 4 patients.
Serum IL2 level went up to 42 U/ml by the end of the drip
infusion, but fell to 19 U/ml within 30 minutes, and 2 U/ml
within 2 hours. IL2 was no longer detectable in the serum
6 hours after the end of the drip infusion(Fig. 3).

    Immunological effects of IL2 in patients: NK cell ac-
tivity against K562 cells was increased 20 percent or more
in 8 of 12 patients 2 weeks after initiation of IL2 therapy,
and in 8 of 10 patients 4 weeks after the therapy was
started(Fig. 4). LAK cell activity against Daudi cells was
increased 40 percent or more in all 8 patients tested 4
weeks after the start of the therapy(Fig. 5).

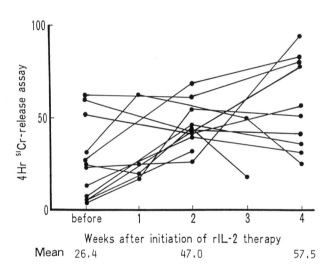

FIGURE 4. NK cell activity against K562 target cells before
and after initiation of IL2 therapy. Effector/target cell
ratio was 20:1.

    Peripheral blood lymphocyte count increased 20 percent
or more in 10 of 12 patients in 2 weeks, and in 8 of 10 patients in 4 weeks. IL2 receptor positive cells and HLA-DR
positive cells in PBL were significantly increased by administration of IL2. There were no significant changes in Leu
2, 3, 4, 7 or 11 positive cells, however.

Side effects of IL2 therapy: Adverse effects due to IL2 include fever over 38°C after injection of IL2(6/12), chill(4/12), fatigue(5/12), nausea and vomiting(2/12), anorexia(5/12), headache(1/12), and elevation of serum GOT level(3/12). Eosinophilia was observed in all patients by administration of IL2. All of these side effects were transient on discontinuation of the therapy. The dosage used here did not produce pulmonary edema and other serious adverse effects.

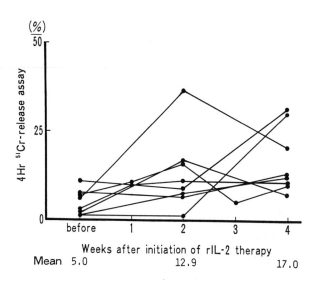

FIGURE 5. LAK cell activity against Daudi target cells before and after initiation of IL2 therapy. Effector/target cell ratio was 20:1.

Tumor regression: Patients were treated with IL2 for periods from 3 weeks to more than 16 months. In one patient, because of eosinophilia with a ratio of up to 74 percent, and in another patient, because of his request, the therapy was stopped in 3 weeks. In these two patients, disease was stable for more than 4 weeks. Three patients achieved complete response; seven, no change; and two, progressive disease(Table 3). Case 4, who had multiple pulmpnary metastases, achieved complete response 13 weeks after the therapy started. The patient is disease-free for more than 10 months. Case 8, who had multiple pulmonary metastases, achieved complete response 16 weeks after the tharapy started, and the patient has remained disease-free for more than 5 months. Case 12 had metastases in the lung and mediastinum. In the ninth post-therapeutic week, partial response was achieved. During the treatment on a outpatient basis, the tumor decreased in size progressively, and complete response was achieved 10 months after initiation of the therapy. Details of the patients are described in a literature(Marumo et al., 1988).

TABLE 3. Results of IL2 therapy for advanced renal cell carcinoma

Case	IL2 therapy		Response[*] (months)
	Duration (days)	Doses ($\times 10^6$ units)	
1	33	33	PD
2	85	52	NC
3	21	21	NC
4	56	56	CR(10+)
5	39	39	NC
6	21	21	NC
7	80	80	NC
8	198	167	CR(5+)
9	492	640	NC
10	81	67	NC
11	56	56	PD
12	343	293	CR(1+)

[*]CR=complete response, PR=partial response, NC=no change, PD=progressive disease

DISCUSSION

Possible treatment modes with IL2 include its systemic administration and combination of adoptive immunotherapy and systemic administration of IL2. Rosenberg and his colleagues have recently reported promising results using combination therapy of adoptive immunotherapy with systemic administration of IL2, and systemic administration of high doses of IL2(Rosenberg et al., 1987) against variety of advanced malignant disease. They isolated large number of

lymphocytes from inidividual patients, cultured them with IL2
to generate LAK cells, and then infused these LAK cells
intravenously. This method is superb, but requires too much
effort to treat each patient to make it practical on a large
scale. Large doses of IL2, on the other hand, cause serious
side effects. The potimum mode of systemic administration
of IL2 should be thus established.

In order to determine mode of administration for clinical application, antitumor effects of IL2 against RCC was
investigated, these effects with those of gamma-IFN were
compared. The results showed that PBL, cultured in IL2 developed the ability to kill renal carcinoma cell lines and
freshly prepared renal carcinoma cells, and that this so-
called LAK cell activity, induced by IL2, exceeded the degree of NK cell activity enhanced by gamma-IFN. LAK cells,
induced by the systemic administration of IL2 to patients
with RCC, are thus expected to kill renal carcinoma cells
which are resistant to IFN-therapy. The results further
suggest that the serum levels of IL2 should be maintained
over 4 U/ml to generate LAK cells when this agent is administered to patients. We thus chose daily multiple repeated
doses for inpatients. To prevent withdrawal from the therapy as a result of intolerable adverse effects, daily dose
was set at 1×10^6 U.

The results of serum measurements of IL2 indicated that
serum IL2 concentration, which is able to activate lymphocytes of patients, is maintained daily nearly 8 hours by repeated intravenous drip infusions. We demonstrated that IL2
increased lymphocyte-mediated cytotoxicity, specifically,
NK cell activity and LAK cell activity in patients with advanced RCC, and brought about an increase in number of
lymphocytes and IL2 receptor- and HLA-DR antigen-positive
cells, which are indicated to be activated lymphocytes.

We concluded that low-dose IL2 administered to patients
with advanced RCC activated immunity of the patients, and
has a safety and potential antitumor effects in selected
patients.

REFERENCES

deKernion J B, Sarna G, Figlin R, Lindner A, Smith R B
    (1983). The treatment of renal cell carcinoma with human

leukocyte alpha-interferon. J. Urol. 130: 1063-1066.

Dennert G (1979). Cytolytic and proliferative activity of a permanent T killer cell line. Nature 277: 476-477.

Domzig W, Stadler B M, Herberman R B (1983). Interleukin 2 dependence of human natural killer (NK) cell activity. J. Immunol. 130: 1970-1973.

Grimm E A, Mazumder A, Zang H Z, Rosenberg S A (1982). Lymphokine-activated killer cell phenomenon. Lysis of natural killer-resistant fresh solid tumor cells by inter-leuki 2-activated autologous human peripheral blood lymphocytes. J. Exp. Med. 155: 1825-1841.

Marumo K, Murai M, Hayakawa M, Tazaki H (1984). Human lymphoblastoid interferon therapy for advanced renal cell carcinoma. Urology 24: 567-571.

Marumo K, Ueno M, Muraki J, Baba S, Tazaki H (1987). Augmentation of cell-mediated cytotoxicity against renal carcinoma cells by recombinant interleukin 2. Urology 30: 327-332.

Marumo K, Muraki J, Ueno M, Tachibana M, Deguchi N, Baba S, Jitsukawa S, Hata M, Tazaki H (1988). An immunological study of human recombinant interleukin 2(IL2) in patients with advanced renal cell carcinoma by low-dose IL2. Urology in press.

Morgan D A, Ruscetti F W, Gallo R (1976). Selective in vitro growth of T-lymphocytes from normal human bone marrows. Science 193: 1007-1008.

Quesada J R, Swanson D A, Trindada A, Gutterman J U (1983). Renal cell carcinoma: Antitumor effects of leukocyte interferon. Cancer Res. 43: 940-947.

Rosenberg S A, Lotze M T, Muul L M, Chang A E, Avis F P, Leitman S, Linehan W M, Robertson C N, Lee R E, Robin J T, Seipp C A, Simpson C G, White D E (1987). A progress report on the treatment of 157 patients with advanced cancer using lymphokine-activated killer cells and interleukin-2 or high-dose interleukin-2 alone. N. Engl. J. Med. 316: 889-897.

Uro-Oncology: Current Status
and Future Trends, pages 275–282
© 1990 Wiley-Liss, Inc.

RECOMBINANT ALPHA-2 OR GAMMA INTERFERON IN THE TREATMENT OF METASTATIC RENAL CELL CARCINOMA: RESULTS OF TWO PHASE II/III TRIALS

Ullrich Otto, Andreas W. Schneider, Stefan Conrad and Herbert Klosterhalfen

UNIVERSITY OF HAMBURG, DEPARTMENT OF UROLOGY

Martinistr. 52, 2000 Hamburg 20, WEST GERMANY

INTRODUCTION

The problem in the treatment of renal cell carcinoma (RCC) is characterized by the facts that 40 % of all patients show evidence of metastatic disease at time of diagnosis, that at least 50 % of all patients with stage I- III RCC treated by nephrectomy develop metastases and die of their disease within the next five years and that additional 30 % die of metastatic disease later on (1). No effective cytostatic, radiation or endocrine therapy is available for patients with metastatic RCC. In 1983, QUESEDA et al. (2) and DeKERNION et al. (3) reported promising results about human leucocyte alpha-Interferon (IFN) therapy in patients with metastatic RCC.

We could demonstrate in previous studies that transplantation of human RCC into NMRI nu/nu mice is a reliable experimental model especially for the evaluation of new therapeutic drugs. Our experimental data with recombinant alpha-2- or gamma-IFN in human RCC demonstrated a high antitumor activity. Response rates could be improved by the combination of different lymphokines (e.g. alpha-2- + gamma-IFN or alpha-2-IFN plus vinblastine). Data of the flowcytometry measurements showed a strong cytotoxic effect. Best results using alpha-2-IFN were obtained at intermediate doses and fractioned intramuscular administration while in gamma-IFN, intravenous fractioned application of low doses was superior to all other regimens (4).

Based on these preclinical data obtained in the nude mouse model, we performed two clinical phase II/III studies to evaluate the efficacy, safety, and toxicity of recombinant IFN alpha-2a alone or in combination with vinblastine and of recombinant IFN-gamma in patients with histological proven metastatic RCC.

MATERIAL AND METHODS

Alpha-2a-Interferon study

The study was designed as a prospective, randomized clinical phase III trial. Patients with histological proven RCC, who showed at least one measurable metastase with proven progression within 4 weeks before therapy, were included into the study. Nephrectomy had to be performed at least one month prior to therapy. Patient's eligibility criteria included an upper age limit of 75 years, an ECOG-Zubrod index of 0-2 and an estimated life expectancy of at least 6 months.

Recombinant alpha-2a-Interferon (Hoffmann-LaRoche, West-Germany) used had an antiviral activity of 1.3-2.9×10^8 U/mg and a purification of more than 95 %.

Patients received 18×10^6 U r-alpha-2a-IFN i.m. 3 x/week every week alone or in combination with vinblastine 0,1 mg/kg i.v. every third week.

Tumor response and toxicity were evaluated every 6 weeks and graded according to WHO criteria.

Gamma-Interferon study

The study was designed as a prospective, nonrandomized clinical phase II trial. Patient's eligibility criteria included histological proven RCC with a history of nephrectomy, at least one measurable metastase, age between 16 and 75 years and an estimated life expectancy of at least 4 months.

Recombinant gamma-IFN (Biogen Research Corp., USA) had an antiviral activity of 1.2-2.4×10^7 U/mg and a degree of purification of more than 95 %. The protocol of the IFN gamma study included intermittent low dose therapy ($100 \ \mu g/m^2$ r-IFN gamma i.v. over 4 hours 3 x/week every other week) with a switch to continuous high doses ($500 \ \mu g/m^2$ r-IFN gamma i.v. over 24 hours 5 x/week every other week) for patients with stable or progressive disease.

Tumor response and toxicity were measured at monthly intervals and classified according to WHO-criteria.

Table 1. Patient Characteristics

	alpha-IFN	gamma-IFN
sex		
male	26	15
female	10	7
age		
mean	55	56
range	38 - 73	43 - 71
pretreatment		
nephrectomy	36	22
chemotherapy	7	3
hormonetherapy	1	1
radiotherapy	3	2
performance status		
0	23	8
1	11	8
2	2	6
3	0	0
4	0	0
site of metastase		
lung only	19	7
bone only	4	3
liver only	6	1
others and multiple	7	11

RESULTS

Alpha-2a-Interferon study

Patient criteria:
Of the 36 patients included into the study 27 received alpha-2a-IFN monotherapy and 9 patients were treated in addition with vinblastine. Patient criteria are listed in table 1.

Response:
8 of the 36 patients showed an objective tumor response with a response rate of 26 % including 1 complete remission (CR) and 7 partial remissions (PR) (see table 2).

Table 2. Tumor response to Interferon-(IFN)-treatment (according to WHO-criteria)

response to	n	CR	PR	SD	PD	NE
alpha-Interferon						
alpha-IFN-monotherapy	27	-	24 %	43 %	33 %	6
alpha-IFN and vinblastine	9	11 %	22 %	33 %	33 %	-
alpha-IFN overall	36	3 %	23 %	40 %	33 %	6
gamma-Interferon						
gamma-IFN 100 ug/m^2	22	9 %	23 %	23 %	45 %	-
additional gamma-IFN 500 ug/m^2	10	10 %	-	70 %	20 %	-
gamma-IFN overall	22	13 %	23 %	32 %	32 %	-

Survival:
Patients with an objective tumor response to therapy or achieving a stable disease (SD) under therapy showed a significantly longer survival than those with progressive disease (PD) (figure 1 and table 3).

Toxicity:
Toxicity included fever, chills and flu-like symptoms in almost all of the patients. Anemia requiring transfusions was common (see table 4).

Table 3. Survival (in month from start of therapy)

alpha-IFN	CR	PR	SD	PD
median	32+	15	20	7
range		(6-26)	(3-28)	(3-20+)
gamma-IFN	CR	PR	SD	PD
median	12+	39	38	4
range	(11+ -17)	(12-45+)	(3-49+)	(3-6)

Gamma-Interferon study

Patient criteria:
Of the 22 patients treated with gamma-IFN, all received low-dose therapy and 10 out of 15 with SD and PD were treated with additional high dose therapy.

Response:
There were 2 CR and 5 PR to low-dose therapy with one additional CR after switch to high-dose treat ment. The overall response rate was 36 % (see table 2).

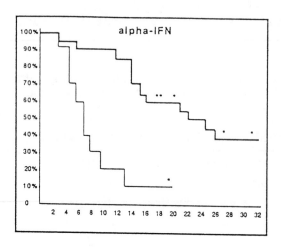

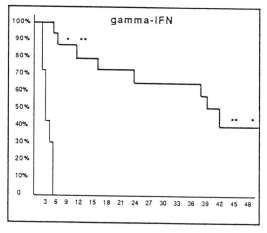

Figure 1. Survival of responders (CR+PR+SD) versus non-responders (PD)
(-- = responders, -- = non-responders. Survival in month from start of therapy to death. indicate patient alive 6-88)

Survival:
Survival of responders and patients with SD was significantly longer than in PD (figure 1 and table 3)

Toxicity:
Toxicity was mild to moderate and included fever, chills and flu-like symptoms in almost all of the patients (see table 4)

DISCUSSION

In two clinical phase II/III studies we could demonstrate that alpha-2-IFN alone or in combination with vinblastine as well as gamma-IFN is effective in the treatment of metastatic RCC. The objective response rate was 26 % for alpha-2-IFN and 36 % for gamma-IFN on a low-dose schedule. Furthermore we could demonstrate that patients responding to therapy or showing a stable disease had a significantly higher probability of survival compared to the non-responders. Patients with good performance status and metastases limited to the lung were those who responded best to therapy.

The toxicity of alpha-2-IFN treatment was mostly mild to moderate with the necessity of dose reduction in 40 % while in gamma-IFN treatment no dose reduction was necessary. Therapy in both schedules could be performed on an outpatient basis.

In conclusion, alpha-2- and gamma-IFN treatment seems to be beneficial for at least a selected group of patients with metastatic RCC.

Table 4. Toxicity of Interferon (IFN)-therapy

	alpha-IFN	gamma-IFN
fever	94.5 %	100.0 %
flu-like symptoms	83.3 %	100.0 %
weight-loss (>10 %)	66.7 %	22.7 %
fatigue	38.8 %	27.3 %
hematotoxicity		
anemia requiring transfusions	38.8 %	18.1 %
leuco- and/or thrombocytopenia	36.1 %	36.8 %
hepatotoxicity, enzyme elevation of SGOT, SGPT, AP, gGT and/or LDH	36.1 %	27.3 %
headache	11.1 %	-
hair-loss	8.7 %	-
neurological disorders	8.7 %	-

References

1. Robson CJ, Churchill BM, Anderson W. The results of radical nephrectomy for renal cell carcinoma. J. Urol. 101: 297-301 (1968)

2. Queseda JR, Swanson DA,Trindade A, Gutterman JU. Renal cell carcinoma: antitumor effects of leucocyte Interferon. Cancer Res. 43: 940-947 (1983)

3. DeKernion B, Sarna G, Figlin R, Lindner A, Smith RB. The treatment of renal cell carcinoma with human leucocyte alpha-Interferon. J. Urol 130: 1063-1066 (1983)

4. Otto U, Huland H, Baisch H, Klöppel G, Schneider A, Denkhaus H. Influence of r-IFN alpha-2, r-IFN alpha plus vinblastine and r-IFN gamma on human renal cell carcinoma after transplantation into NMRI nu/nu mice. In: Stewart WE, Schellekens H (eds.) The biology of the Interferon system 1985, pp 383-387. Amsterdam, New York, Oxford 1986

Uro-Oncology: Current Status
and Future Trends, pages 283–293
© 1990 Wiley-Liss, Inc.

OVERVIEW: TREATMENT OF LOCAL REGIONAL DISEASE

John P. Donohue, M.D.

Indiana University
Medical Center
        Urology, 926 W. Michigan St.,
UH A112, Indianapolis, IN   46223

Nonseminomatous germ cell tumor is an extraordinary tumor in terms of demonstrating the impact of regional lymphadenectomy on survival. Over the years, many series have shown that node-positive (pathologic stage II patients) can still be cured with local measures in excess of 50% of the time. There are a variety of anatomical considerations that make testicular lymphatic drainage predictable. These relate to features of anatomic descent of the gonad and its associated lymphatics. A number of topographic studies have supported the regional deposition of metastatic disease, and we have a good understanding of this. More importantly, there are biologic considerations that probably lend to the opportunity for cure with testis cancer patients with surgery alone. Many patients will have teratomatous elements which have somewhat lower metastatic potential. What is fascinating, however, is that even undifferentiated germ cell tumors, such as embryonal cancer, still are often cured with lymphadenectomy alone. Data recently presented in the New England Journal in the cooperative study of multi-institutional type show that a control group treated with ncde dissection alone had more than half of the patients as long-term survivors without relapse. (Ref. #1)

Fortunately, the relapsers were rescued at the time of relapse, with only a few exceptions. The overall survival in Stage II disease including all levels of involvement (both Stage II-A and II-B) is 97.5%. Naturally, this has been achieved with the use of either adjuvant chemotherapy immediately following RPLND or full course chemotherapy, given only at the time of relapse, in the other half of patients (who relapsed after earlier RPLND and observation only for Stage II disease)

SUMMARY

A general treatment philosophy when considering retorperitoneal node dissections should be as follows:

The surgery should be appropriate (let the punishment fit the crime). Although presently, our position in low-stage low-low-volume disease is divergent from those committed to surveillance only, I see our paths converging. Clearly, no one wants to do staging RPLND for its own sake. If we can get the clinical sensitivity of clinical staging at levels of confidence exceeding the 90% percentile, there will no need to do staging RPLND's. In the meantime, however, a good interim position is the modified RPLND, particularly that employing nerve-sparing techniques. Virtually all patients who have a nerve-sparing modified RPLND will ejaculate. Hence, the patient has not been harmed, and he has also been adequately staged. In fact, those who do have microscopic disease have also been given a therapeutic procedure. At this point, the relapse rate locally in patients with nerve-sparing RPLND is entirely satisfactory in our current small and selected series. This will be a subject of a separate discussion at this meeting. (Ref. #2)

Regarding high-stage disease, our reviews are generally concordant with other groups throughout the world. Disseminated disease requires disseminated treatment first. This implies pre-treatment with systemic chemotherapy, which is platinum-based. Currently, programs employing Platinum, VP-16, with or without Bleomycin are quite popular and effective. Surgery is reserved for those who have residual clinical disease as noted on the CT scan. One of our current challenges is to see if we can develop predictive criteria for those who might have scar tissue and necrosis only in the specimen. There is some analogy with the seminoma data for advanced disease, where it has been found that most patients with a partial remission can be followed because they will have necrosis only in their tissue specimen. However, there are always exceptions to the rule and they must be followed carefully, and relapse treated aggressively when and if it occurs.

Another philosophical point that will impact future management of node dissection in testis cancer is that healthcare providers will want to eliminate qualitative variables in treatment programs as much as possible. Surgery is always a variable in this regard. In order to simplify and codify quantitative aspects of treatment, there will be a move to eliminate initial hospital costs in such things as staging and or treatment for low stage disease. Systemic chemotherapy is more easily standardized and quantified. Surgery for low volume disease, therefore, may be dismantled except in a salvage setting. Unfortunately, this will require many patients with low volume disease limited to the retroperitoneum to undergo a highly toxic program that may well have negative long-term consequences on their fertility. Primary germ cell damage is well-known in our treatment for advanced disease and only about half of our patients regenerate a satisfactory sperm count after two or three years. Hopefully, this will not become a treatment excess for low volume disease patients in the future. It seems a good deal simpler and more direct to treat low volume disease surgically and eliminate the potential of local relapse in an area (retroperitoneum) difficult to monitor and follow.

My own view is that surgery should be more proactive than reactive in the treatment of low stage disease. Surgery can cure it literally in hours. When it does not, a cure is available then, should the patient relapse, almost always in a pulmonary mode, which is easily detectable and treatable. Again, this is the only solid tumor that is curable by surgery alone more than 50% of the time when the regional nodes are positive. So approach to the retroperitoneum is even more feasible and less toxic long-term with the development of anatomical nerve-sparing dissections, which will preserve ejaculation. At least, this gives us an option to surveillance, which seems to be quite effective and reasonable.

Finally, concerning high stage disease, there is general agreement that all persistent tumors after initial chemotherapy should be removed. We have noted certain patients with very favorable response criteria can be followed with expectation of further resolution of their radiographic changes. (Ref #3) Our hope is that we can be more selective in choosing patients for postchemotherapy surgery. But in the meantime, if there is any significant concern about presence of persistent tumor, as a general principle, such patients are more safely managed with exploration and RPLND. Currently, with this approach, in over 300 postchemotherapy RPLND's, we have 44% with necrosis/fibrosis only, 44% with teratoma, and 12% with cancer.

The former two groups are carefully observed postoperatively and the last group with persistent cancer receive two courses of salvage chemotherapy (see Table 1). The overall survival of this group is good (80-90%), but factors predicting for relapse are bulk of tumor, histology, and site (primary mediastinum). (Ref. 4 and 5).

Surgery for massive metastatic disease in testis cancer has become reasonable and appropriate in view of the great advances in chemotherapy for advanced disease. (Ref. #6) The majority of patients will have their bulky disease reduced in volume and also downgraded histologically into a more mature teratomatous or even necrotic form. Of course, some persist with malignant elements as well. (Refs. 4-12)

From a medical oncologic viewpoint, this is critical information because it will guide subsequent medical management. Those with persistent malignant tumor require further salvage chemotherapy. Those with only teratoma or necrosis in the specimen will be managed expectantly. (Table 1)

Often these retroperitoneal tumors are massive. It is of vital importance to resect them completely because local or regional recurrence is quite possible, particularly in the more extensive bulky tumors. Hence, this area represents one of the ultimate surgical challenges. Total tumor extirpation is required with exceptional demands on vascular isolation and preservation. Aggressive ablative purpose must be combined with thoughtful and delicate dissection.

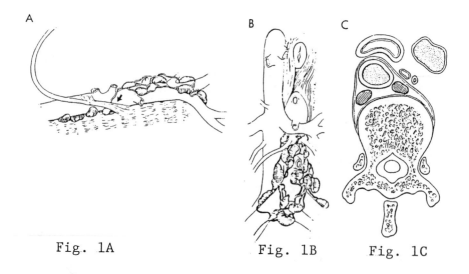

Fig. 1A   Fig. 1B   Fig. 1C

Figure 1A, 1B, 1C:

Schematic representation of the extension of suprahilar nodes from the infrahilar nodal package. In both right and left-sided cases, these run para-aortic and posterior to the renal vessels. They are also retrocrural as they continue to drain up into the posterior mediastinum. Elevating the renal vessels allows examination and clearance of these. The primary zone of spread on the right side is shaded gray in Figure 1A and the primary zone of spread on the left side shaded gray Figure 1B.

Figure 1A:

Lateral view of the lymphatic flow of para-aortic lymphatic drainage into the chest. The drainage passes through the diaphragm in the aortic hiatus bounded on either side by the crus of the diaphragm. It drains posterior and lateral to the aorta into the <u>cyststernachyli</u> and then into the posterior mediastinal nodes.

Figure 1B:

Anterior view of the para-aortic nodes and the relationship with these to the two renal vein. The stippeled nodes above the renal vein are posterior to the aorta, as drainage below the renal vein goes cephalad into the hest below the crura of the diaphragm.

Figure 1C:

Axial view showing the relationship of the crus of the diaphragm, the aorta and the para-aortic nodes which parallel the azygos and hemiazygos venous systems.

TABLE 1.

TREATMENT SCHEME FOR DISSEMINATED TESTIS CANCER
AT INDIANA UNIVERSITY

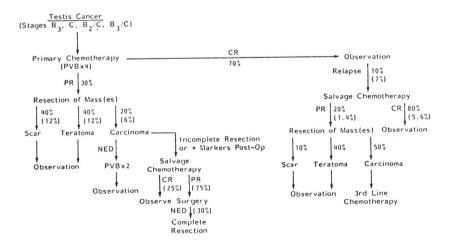

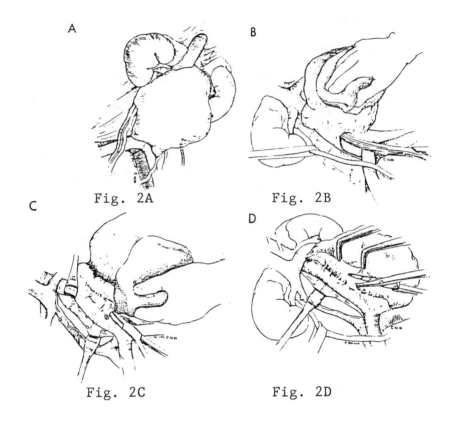

Fig. 2A   Fig. 2B

Fig. 2C   Fig. 2D

Figure 2A, 2B, 2C, 2D:

The principle of the split and roll still applies in bulky disease. The cava in Figure 2A can be split anteriorally through the subadventitial plane. We usually use Bovie cautery over a dissecting clamp. Figures 2C and 2D indicate the dissection of the tumor mass off the aorta which is best done in the adventitial or extra adventitial plane so as to preserve some of the aortic wall. Subadventitial dissection throughout the length of the aorta makes it difficult for suture ligature repair.

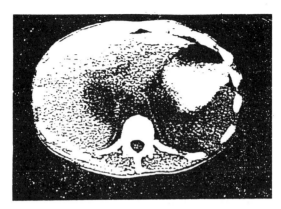

Fig. 3A

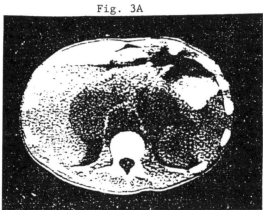

Fig. 3B

Figure 3A, 3B:

CT scans showing retrocrural and nodal disease.
Precrural disease is usually direct extension
retrocrural nodal involvement is the natural
lymphatic pathway of flow from the infrahilar
lymphatics.

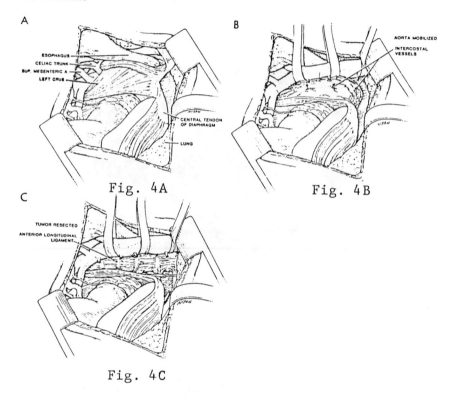

Fig. 4A

Fig. 4B

Fig. 4C

Figure 4A, 4B, 4C:

Posterior mediastinal tumor dissection via left lateral thoracotomy. Note the principle of "split and roll" here as well as in the abdomen. The crus of the diaphragm is divided and the aorta dissected free from tumor. The intercostals are doubly ligated and divided from T8 to T12 so the aorta can be mobilized up and away from the tumor which is then dissected off the anterior spinous ligments and foramen.

BIBLIOGRAPHY

1. Williams, S.D., et al. Immediate adjuvant chemotherapy versus observation with treatment of relapse in pathological stage II testicular cancer. N.E.J.M. 317:1433-1438 (December 3) 1987.

2. Donohue, J.P., et al. Preservation of ejaculation following nerve-sparing retroperitoneal lymphadenectomy. J. Urol. 139: 206A (No. 176), April, 1988. (RPLND)

3. Donohue, J.P., et al. Correlation of CAT changes and histological findings in 80 patients having RPLND after chemotherapy for testis cancer. J. Urol. 137:1176, 1987.

4. Loehrer PJ, Williams SD, Clark SA, et al: Teratoma following chemotherapy for non-seminomatous germ cell tumor (NSGCT): a clinicopathologic correlation. J Urol 135:1183, 1986.

5. Einhorn LH, Williams SD, Mandelbaum I, Donohue JP: Surgical resection in disseminated testicular cancer following chemotherapeutic cytoreduction. Cancer 48:904-908, 1981.

6. Einhorn, LH, Donohue, JP: Cis-diammine-dichloroplatinum, vinblastine and bleomycin combination chemotherapy in disseminated testicular cancer. Ann. Int. Med. 87:293-298, 1977.

7. Donohue JP, Einhorn LH, Williams SD: Cytoreductive surgery for metastatic testis cancer: considerations of timing and extent. J Urol 123:876-880, 1980.

8. Donohue, JP, Rowland RG: The role of surgery in advanced testicular cancer. Cancer 54:2716-2721, 1984.

9. Loehrer PJ, Sledge GW, Einhorn LH: Heterogeneity among germ cell tumors of the testis. Semin Oncol 12:304-316, 1985.

10. Ulbright TM, Loehrer PJ, Roth LM, et al: The development of non-germ cell malignancies within germ cell tumors: a clinicopathologic study of 11 cases. Cancer 54:1824-1833, 1984.

11. Donohue JP, Zachary JM, Maynard BR: Distribution of nodal metastases in nonseminomatous testis cancer. J Urol 128:315-320, 1982.

12. Donohue JP, Rowland RG, Bihrle R. Transabdominal retroperitoneal lymph node dissection. IN DG Skinner and G Leiskovsky (eds), Diagnosis and Management of Genitourinary Cancer. Philadelphia, W. B. Saunders, 1988, p. 802-816.

Uro-Oncology: Current Status
and Future Trends, pages 295–299
© 1990 Wiley-Liss, Inc.

TREATMENT OF LOCOREGIONAL GERM CELL TUMOR

HARRY W. HERR, M.D.

UROLOGIC SERVICE, DEPARTMENT OF SURGERY
MEMORIAL SLOAN-KETTERING CANCER CENTER

NEW YORK, NY 10021

Locoregional germ cell tumor implies neoplasm confined to the testis and scrotum or metastatic only to the retroperitoneal lymphnodes. Management depends on the histology (seminoma vs non-seminoma) and extent (stage) of disease.

Current management of locoregional germ cell tumor of the testis at MSKCC can be summarized as follows:

Non seminomatous germ cell tumor.

Clinical stage I. RPLND remains the standard for diagnosis and treatment. The dissection may be modified in an effort to preserve seminal emission. Surveillance is a permissable alternative for selected patients with T1 tumors without lymphatic or vascular invasion in a patient/physician setting permitting close and careful follow-up.

Clinical stage II, IIA and IIB/bilateral RPLND after sperm banking with patient/physician decision regarding adjuvant chemotherapy pending the pathologic findings.

IIC-initial chemotherapy followed by bilateral RPLND. Disease progression during initial chemotherapy provides an indication for a salvage regimen.

SEMINOMA; Clinical stage I. Retroperitoneal lymph node irradiation. Clinical stage II. Retroperitoneal lymph node irradiation for IIA and IIB. For IIC, initial chemotherapy followed by surgical excision (if feasible) or radiotherapy for a residual mass larger than 3 cm in diameter.

ORCHIECTOMY. Inguinal Orchiectomy is the definitive diagnostic and initial therapeutic step in the management of testicular germ cell tumor. The procedure establishes the histologic diagnosis of the primary tumor and is associated with minimal morbidity and no mortality. The adverse consequences of prior ipsilateral scrotal surgery or suboptimal orchiectomy in the event of a misdiagnosis appears to be small. In such a setting, however, a racket-shaped incision is utilized to encompass the residual spermatic cord and/or ipsilateral scrotum. Even in patients with stage III disease, removal of primary testis germ cell tumor is advised because of the potential persistance of tumor at (30%) that site in spite of apparently complete control of metastatic foci by chemotherapy.

The approximately 2 % risk of a second primary testis tumor and 5 % risk of contralateral in situ carcinoma in patients with a unilateral tumor raises the question of contralateral testis biopsy. No standard policy has yet emerged. An alternative to biopsy is self-examination in conjunction with professional follow-up. Evaluation of semen for tumor cells by cytologic and flow cytometric techniques is under investigation. What courses to follow when testicular biopsy reveals in situ carcinoma is also uncertain. Although disappearance of in situ carcinoma following chemotherapy may occur, the occurence accompanying recovery of spermatogenesis is possible. Irradiation of the testis to abort the possibility of recurrent in situ carcinoma by permanently interrupting spermatogenesis yet preserving Leydig cell function is under investigation.

Non-seminomatous Testis Tumors. RPLND is the standard in management of clinical stage I non-seminomatous tumors of the testis but close and careful surveillane with institution of further treatment only if specifically indicated is an alternative in selected patients. The justification for a surveillance regimen rests with the accuracy of clinical staging and follow-up techniques, the effectiveness of treatment for early failures, and the probability of avoiding treatment beyond orchiectomy. Pathologically, negative nodes at RPLND are associated with an 90-95 % prospect of cure, most of the failures resulting from lung metastases and most being controlled by chemotherapy, yielding overall survival probabilities approaching 100 %. With surveillance regimens about 75 % of patients remain well following orchiectomy. Although the median time to failure is about 5 months, recurrences have been detected more than 3 years post orchiectomy. Such late recurrences at the time of detection with resultant greater burden of therapy and risks of treatment failure, and the psychologic impact of the uncertaintity associated with surveillance are among its disadvantages. The worlds experience with 617 patients entered on surveillance protocol shows a relapse rate of 25 % (154 patients). All but 8 have been salvaged yielding an overall durable survival rate of 98.7 % Surveillance appears to be an alternative to RPLND but should probably be limited to settings in which the volume of experience with testis tumors has sharpened expertise in the staging and follow-up of carefully selected patients.

Surveillance regimens have provided information regarding risk factors which will potentially improve selection of patients. Lymphatic or blood vessel invasion in the primary tumor and embryonal histology appear to be the most significant adverse prognostic risk factors predictive of relapse.

The loss of seminal emission that usually follows conventional bilateral RPLND has provided a major incentive for surveillance regimens as well as stimulated modifications in RPLND. Such modifications more or less involve sparing of the sympathetic nerve ramifications which pass anterior to the aorta and aortic bifurcation below the origin of the inferior mesentary artery. Early experience indicates that such modifications may preserve seminal emission in 50 % of patients, with a meticulous "nerve sparing" dissection of the preganglionic fibers ejaculation may be preserved in over 90 % of patients. Diagnostic accuracy and possible therapeutic efficacy appear comparable to conventional RPLND in patients with clinical stage I tumors, but further prospective experience is required to ascertain whether retroperitoneal recurrences will not prove to be unacceptably high as a result of the shrinking boundaries of dissection.

Patients with clinical stage II NSGCTT are divided into IIA (nodes less than 2 cm in diameter), IIB (nodes 2 cm -5 cm in diameter), and IIC (nodes greater than 5 cm in diameter). For clinical stages IIA and IIB bilateral RPLND is standard with subsequent pathologic classification into NO (negative nodes), N1 (microscopically positive nodes), N2a (grossly positive nodes but less than 5 nodes and none greater than 2 cm in diameter), N2b (5 nodes or > 2 cm in diameter), N3 (positive nodes, gross or microscopic evidence of capsule invasion, completely resected), and N4 (positive nodes, incompletely resected). Although the overall risk of relapse in patients with positive nodes after RPLND is approximately 50 %, the specific risk for nodal subcategories is not well defined. It is approximately less than 10 % for NO, 20 % for N1, 40 % for N2a,

50-60 % for N2b and greater than 75 % for N3 and N4. Whether patients with positive nodes should or should not be given adjuvant chemotherapy remains a matter of patient/physician election, since survival rates overall with either approach are in excess of 90 %. For clinical stage IIC, systemic chemotherapy followed by bi-lateral RPLND is recommended.

Some patients with clinical stage II disease may be controlled by chemotherapy alone. This is suggested from experience with surveillance in clinical stage I disease, from experience with stage III and from clinical investigation in stage II. The cure rates with chemotherapy alone are over 90 %. The disadvantage of primary chemotherapy is the accuracy of staging, perhaps exposing some patients unnecessarily to chemotherapy, 3 or 4 cycles are required therapeutically rather than 2 in an adjuvant setting, the acute and chronic morbidities, the fact that more time is involved which may impact adversely on the quality of life, fertility may or may not be preserved, and more frequent monitoring is required. The risks of persistence and late growth and/or progression of residual mature teratoma remain to be defined better, especially in patients with teratocarcinoma. At present, rather primary RPLND with or without chemotherapy or initial chemotherapy is elected for low volume stage II NSGCTT remains for patient/physician election, depending upon expertise and resources available.

SEMINOMA

Seminoma is one of the most radioresponsive malignancies. These tumors can usually be sterilized by doses of 3000 rad external beam irradiation. 2500 to 3500 rad megavoltage radiation to the retroperitoneal lymph nodes and ipsilateral pelvis over 3-4 weeks results in survival rates in excess of 97 % (91-99 %) for clinical stage I disease and 70-80 % for clinical stage II disease. Mediastinal and supraclavicular radiation is not required since even with clinical stage II disease relapse in this site is uncommon. Such radiation also may prejudice adequate chemotherapy in the event of systemic relapse. Surveillance rather than routine retroperitoneal lymph node irradiation for clinical stage I seminoma is based upon the improbability (10-20 %) of retroperitoneal lymph node metastases with clinical stage I and the high probability of salvage if evidence of disease appears during follow-up. Of 63 stage I seminomas followed for a median of 13 months, 2 have relapsed at 2 and 4 months with non bulky retroperitoneal disease. Both are disease free 5 and 12 months after salvage infradiaphragmatic radiation therapy. The practical argument against surveillance includes the minimal risks and close to 100 % cure of the alternative retroperitoneal irradiation.

For patients with bulky IIB or IIC seminoma, chemotherapy constitutes initial therapy. Indications for surgery thereafter are uncertain. Further treatment seems indicated, however, for patients with a residual mass equal or greater than 3 cm in diameter. If operation identifies residual tumor, additional chemotherapy and/or radiation is indicated; if no residual tumor is found, no further treatment is necessary. In patients with residual tumor masses less than 3 cm or poorly defined fibrotic masses do not contain tumor and such patients require no surgery or irradiation.

Selected References

Fung CY, Garnick MB: Clinical stage I carcinoma of the testis: A review. J Clin Oncol 6: 734-750, 1988.

Herr HW, Whitmore WF, Sogani PC, et al. Selection of testicular tumor patients for omission of retroperitoneal lymph node dissection. J Urol 135: 500-503, 1986.

Hoskin P, Dilly S, Easton D, et al. Prognostic factors in stage I non-seminomatous germ cell testicular tumors managed by orchiectomy and surveillance. J Clin Oncol 4: 1031-1035, 1986.

Williams SD, Stablein DM, Einhorn LH, et al. Immediate adjuvant chemotherapy vs. observation with treatment of relapse in pathological stage II testicular cancer. New Eng. J Med 317: 1433-1438, 1987.

Bosl GJ, Gluckman R, Geller N, et al. VAB-6: An effective chemotherapy regimen for patients with germ cell tumors. J Clin Oncol 4: 1493-1499, 1986.

Motzer RJ, Bosl GJ, Geller N, et al. Advanced seminoma: The role of chemotherapy and adjunctive surgery. Ann Int Med 108: 513-518, 1988.

Herr HW. Quality of life measurement in testicular cancer patients. Cancer 60: 1412-1414, 1987.

Jewett MAS, Kong YSP, Goldberg SD, et al. Retroperitoneal lymphadenectomy for testis tumor with nerve sparing for ejaculation. J Urol 139: 1220, 1988.

Uro-Oncology: Current Status
and Future Trends, pages 301–307
© 1990 Wiley-Liss, Inc.

INTENSIVE CHEMOTHERAPY FOR METASTATIC NONSEMINOMATOUS GERM CELL TUMORS

Christopher J. Logothetis, Clayton Chong, Francisco H., Dexeus, Avishay Sella, and Sheryl Ogden

Department of Medical Oncology, Section of Genitourinary Oncology, The University of Texas M.D. Anderson Cancer Center, 1515 Holcombe Boulevard, Box 13, Houston, Texas 77030, U.S.A.

INTRODUCTION

Intensive chemotherapy with cyclophosphamide, adriamycin, and cisplatin plus vinblastine and bleomycin ($CISCA_{II}/VB_{IV}$) has been used at M. D. Anderson Cancer Center since 1982 (Logothetis et al. 1987). We have gained extensive experience and can now assess long-term disease-free survival rates in adequate numbers of patients. $CISCA_{II}/VB_{IV}$ chemo therapy was initially selected to treat metastatic germ cell tumors because each of these two regimens independently had been proven effective treatment for advanced poor-prognosis extragonadal germ cell tumors (Logothetis et al., 1985). In that experience, the patients had an equal likelihood of achieving a disease-free survival with $CISCA_{II}$ as with VB_{IV}.

$CISCA_{II}/VB_{IV}$

One-hundred sixty-seven patients have been treated with $CISCA_{II}/VB_{IV}$ chemotherapy since the initiation of that protocol. Dosages consist of high-dose cyclophosphamide, adriamycin, and cisplatin delivered intravenously over two days and vinblastine and bleomycin delivered as a simultaneous continuous infusion (Table 1).

TABLE 1. CISCA$_{II}$/VB$_{IV}$ Protocol

Cyclophosphamide	500 mg/m^2 D1 + D2
Adriamycin	45 mg/m^2 D1 + D2
Cisplatin	120 mg/m^2 D1 + D2
Vinblastine	3 mg/m^2 D1 + D2 + D3 + D4 + D5
Bleomycin	30 mg/m^2 D1 + D2 + D3 + D4 + D5

*D, day

Patients were classified by both the Indiana staging system (Table 2) and the modified Samuels' staging system (Table 3).

TABLE 2. Clinical Presentation And Results: Indiana Stage

Stage	Total Patients	Patients No.	Disease-Free Percent
Minimal	87	81	93 %
Moderate	29	26	90 %
Advanced	51	35	69 %
	167	142	85 %

TABLE 3. Samuels' Stage and Results

M.D. Anderson Stage Clinical	Total Pts	% Disease-Free
II	59	93 %
IIIA	3	100 %
IIIB1	3	100 %
IIIB2	23	91 %
IIIB3	16	88 %
IIIB4	28	79 %
IIIB5	22	73 %
Extragonadal	13	62 %
	167	85 %

Clinical stage was assigned on the basis of computerized tomography (CT). The advanced abdominal disease category (clinical stage III-B-4) required the presence of an abdominal mass > 10 cm in maximum diameter. A majority of these patients also had pulmonary metastases. According to the Indiana system, study patients were about evenly divided between moderate/advanced and minimal disease. According to the modified Samuels' system, a large proportion of study patients had either clinically advanced disease (stages III- B-3 to III-B-5) or extragonadal disease.

Patients with Samuels' clinical stage II to clinical stage III-B-3 disease achieved a near-universal cure (Table 3). Significant failure rates were encountered only for those with stages III-B-3 and III-B-4 and III disease and those with advanced extragonadal germ cell tumors.

The distribution of the patients by histologic type is shown in Table 4.

TABLE 4. Histologic Subtype and Results

Dixon-Moore Class	Total Pts	Percent Disease-Free
Seminoma (Dixon-Moore I)	5	100 %
Embryonal (Dixon-Moore II)	59	90 %
Mature T (Dixon-Moore III)	0	
Teratocarcinoma (Dixon-Moore IV)	85	85 %
Choriocarcinoma (Dixon-Moore V)	9	56 %
Pure EST*	6	67 %
Not Determined	3	50 %
	167	85 %

*EST, endodermal sinus tumor.

The most common histologic subtype was mixed teratoma plus embryonal carcinoma. For three patients the cell type was not determined. They had widespread advanced metastatic disease at the time of presentation, and their clinical circumstance did not permit anesthesia and an orchiectomy. The presence of malignancy was confirmed in all patients pathologically by a needle aspiration biopsy, and clinically by physical examination, radiography and measurement of serum biomarkers.

Histologic subtype influenced the frequency of surgery following chemotherapy, but did not greatly affect the long- term disease-free survival except for the rare subgroup of patients who had a pure choriocarcinoma (Dixon-Moore Class V) (Table 4). The majority of these patients had high-volume human chorionic gonadotropin (B-HCG)-secreting tumors of extragonadal origin. The clinical presentation of high- volume germ-cell tumor with diffuse metastases and a serum B-HCG level of greater than 50,000 mIu/ml has been identified previously by us and other investigators as representing a very poor prognosis (Bosl et al., 1983).

TOXICITY

It is our belief that the toxic side effects of chemotherapy should be viewed differently in patients for whom the therapeutic intention is cure than in those for whom the therapeutic intention is palliation. When cure is the intent, acute toxicity may be acceptable but chronic toxicity should be minimal.

Acute toxicity is associated with morbidity and, in inexperienced hands, with occasional mortality. Acute toxicity differs from long-term toxicity in that it is peak-dose dependent and usually reversible. This form of toxicity is usually myelosuppressive or gastrointestinal. In contrast, chronic toxicity is usually attributable to the cumulative dose of each individual drug used. In patients with germ cell tumors, cumulative doses of bleomycin and cisplatin are usually the culprits; in addition, when a clinician uses adriamycin, its cumulative dose may result in cardiac toxicity.

By alternating two high-dose regimens using different agents, the peak dose of each individual drug can be high, yet the total cumulative dose remains low. $CISCA_{II}/VB_{IV}$ therefore, is characterized by formidable acute morbidity that is usually completely reversible and by a low frequency of chronic toxicity. Fatal complications of therapy occurring during myelosuppression are extremely rare at M. D. Anderson Cancer Center (1 of 167 patients). The impact of chronic toxicity on the long-term disease-free survival of patients with germ cell tumors has yet to be totally assessed. Reduced productivity owing to cisplatin neuropathy or nephropathy has not been the subject of quantitative studies thus far, but is likely to occur to the greatest extent in patients whose treatment has included large doses of cisplatin.

The frequency of chronic toxicity in patients receiving $CISCA_{II}/VB_{IV}$ is low. The most threatening forms of chronic toxicity are related to the chronic nephrotoxicity of cisplatin, which is characterized by a reduced creatinine clearance rate and multiple renal tubular defects manifested as hypomagnesemia and other electrolyte abnormalities. Long- term side effects of bleomycin and adriamycin are extremely rare in our experience. None of our patients has suffered persistent cardiac abnormalities owing to adriamycin. Bleomycin, when delivered as a continuous infusion with appropriate monitoring by gallium scans and forced-vital-capacity determinations, results in an extremely low clinical pulmonary toxicity rate and, in our experience, no fatal pulmonary toxicity. Platinum nephrotoxicity (defined as a greater than 0.4 mg/100 ml rise in the serum creatinine level) has been transient and has occured in only 6 % of our patients.

THERAPEUTIC GOALS

Clinical dilemmas persist in the treatment of nonseminomatous germ cell tumors of the testis, both for patients with minimal disease and for those with far advanced disease. Attempts have recently been made to reduce the intensity and the amount of treatment required for the former group. These attempts reflect the belief that a reduced amount of chemotherapy combined with surgery may maintain a similarly high response rate with exposure to less cytotoxic and potentially morbid drugs. The first randomized trials have been performed by the Indiana group. They have demonstrated that patients with Indiana- stage moderate or minimal tumor volumes can maintain a high- complete-remission rate (88 % and 92 % disease-free survivals). Such trials are very difficult to perform, however, partly because the small differences in the two treatment arms require the enrollment of a large number of patients. Unless the new reduced-intensity approach has significantly worse results than the standard therapy, the probable result is that the trials will show no difference in therapeutic outcome.

It is our belief that the therapeutic goal in the 1980s for patients with minimal- and moderate-stage disease is a 100 % disease-free survival. A near-universal survival rate for patients in these categories is currently achieved with $CISCA_{II}/VB_{IV}$. A recent prospective randomized trial performed at our institution compared two cyclic chemotherapy regimens, $CISCA_{II}/VB_{IV}$ and a combination of vincristine, bleomycin, and cisplatin alternating with VP-16 and cisplatin; the outcome for those patients treated with the alternate (non-CISCA) chemotherapy regimen was significantly inferior (Logothetis et al., 1987). Only patients whose serum B-HCG levels were less than 50,000 mIu/ml at presentation were involved in this study. Patients were observed closely, and therapy was altered immediately if tumor recurred or failed to respond after two consecutive courses of chemotherapy. Despite this close attention, 4 of 16 patients in the less-intense arm eventually succumbed to their disease, whereas only 1 of the 16 patients treated with $CISCA_{II}/VB_{IV}$ has subsequently died.

The results of this clinical trial cautioned us against further attempts at reducing the intensity of treatment for patients with minimal disease. Nevertheless, we believe the goal of reducing the intensity of chemotherapy while maintaining a high complete-remission rate must be pursued for patients with minimal or moderate disease by the Indiana staging system or with a serum B-HCG level less than 50,000 mIu/ml. A novel clinical trial of individualized therapy employing the slope of the drop of the serum B-HCG level as a predictor of response may permit a reduction in the intensity of chemotherapy in patients who respond, while the intensity of therapy is maintained or increased for those patients for whom the slope of the drop of serum B-HCG level is adequate. Patients with inadequate slopes of decreasing serum B-HCG levels were most likely to relapse.

Although controversy remains over the treatment of patients with minimal disease, little controversy exists for patients with truly advanced disease. The degree of elevation of the serum B-HCG is an important predictor of adverse outcome in a number of clinical studies. In our own study, patients with a serum B-HCG level of greater 50,000 mIu/ml at presentation had a reduced likelihood of achieving a long-term disease-free survival. Such patients typically present with a choriocarcinoma syndrome, and high-volume hemorrhagic metastases and are clinically acutely ill. The B-HCG level represents an ideal tumor marker for individualized therapy. Our initial attempt at response-directed therapy revealed that we could cure a significant portion of these patients with extremely high-volume disease (Chong et al., 1988). Such continued intensity, determined by the slope of the drop of the B-HCG, is a therapeutic approach that needs to be explored further and refined.

We conclude that $CISCA_{II}/VB_{IV}$ chemotherapy results in a near-universal long-term disease-free survival in patients with less than 50,000 mIu/ml of serum B-HCG at presentation. This regimen is acutely toxic, but long-term morbidity and acute mortality are low. Despite the excellent survival rates achieved in patients with clinically advanced (III-B- 4, III-B-5, and extragonadal) germ cell tumors, we believe that such patients may benefit from more intensive therapy directed by response in the drop of serum B-HCG. In order to achieve the therapeutic goal of reduced intensity of therapy with near universal survival for patients with minimal disease, we believe that clinical trials employing response- directed therapy for both minimal and advanced disease need to be performed.

REFERENCES

Bosl GJ, Geller N, Cirrincione C, Scher H, Whitmore W, Golbey R (1983). A multivariate analysis of prognostic variables in patients (pts.) with metastatic germ cell tumors of the testis (GCT). Cancer Res 43: 3403-3406.

Chong C, Logothetis C, Dexeus F, Sella A (1988). Response directed chemotherapy (CT) for high beta HCG producing nonseminomatous germ cell tumors (NSGCT) (Abstract). Pro ceedings of the American Association for Cancer Research 29: 204.

Logothetis C, Dexeus F, Chong C, Ogden S, Sella A (1987). A prospective randomized trial comparing two cyclic chemotherapy regimens for the treatment of patients (pts) with favorable prognostic nonseminomatous germ cell tumors of the testes (NSGCTT) (Abstract). Proceedings of the American Society of Clinical Oncology 6: 103.

Logothetis CJ, Samuels ML, Selig DE, Ogden S, Dexeus FH, Swanson D, Johnson D, and von Eschenbach A (1986). Cyclic chemotherapy with cyclophosphamide, doxorubicin, and cisplatin plus vinblastine and bleomycin in advanced germinal tumors. Am J Med 81: 219-228.

Uro-Oncology: Current Status
and Future Trends, pages 309–318
© 1990 Wiley-Liss, Inc.

ACTIVE SURVEILLANCE FOR STAGE I NON-SEMINOMATOUS
GERM CELL TESTIS TUMORS: PRACTICE AND PITFALLS.

Derek Raghavan and Michael Boyer

Urological Cancer Research Unit & Dept.
Clinical Oncology, Royal Prince Alfred
Hospital, Sydney, N.S.W., Australia.

INTRODUCTION:

The cure rate for stage I non-seminomatous
germ cell tumors (NSGCT) of the testis is
greater than 90%, whether treated by inguinal
orchidectomy and adjuvant radiotherapy (Peckham
et al, 1981; van der Werf Messing and Hop, 1982)
or subsequent retroperitoneal lymph node
dissection (Donohue et al, 1978; Lieskovsky and
Skinner, 1984). As discussed elsewhere,
radiotherapy and lymph node dissection have
significant attendant morbidity, and may not
contribute to the cure rate for most patients
with stage I testicular NSGCT (Peckham et al,
1982; Raghavan, 1984). As a result, Peckham and
colleagues at the Royal Marsden Hospital,
London, introduced an innovative approach to the
management of such patients, in which a policy
of close non-invasive follow-up was introduced
after careful initial staging ("active
surveillance"), with early salvage chemotherapy
for patients who relapsed (Peckham et al, 1982).
The intention of this approach has been to
minimize unnecessary treatment for the majority
of patients with stage I NSGCT, while preserving
a high chance of cure by ensuring early
diagnosis and appropriate management for
patients who relapse. As this policy has been
implemented for a decade, with experience
reported from several centers, it is timely to

assess its impact on morbidity and survival, and to address the problems that have been encountered.

METHODOLOGY OF ACTIVE SURVEILLANCE PROTOCOLS

Although a common rationale is implicit in all of the policies of active surveillance, there has been substantial variation in the implementation of this approach to management (Table 1). Hence there is a substantial risk that the reported efficacy and morbidity may reflect the broad range in the details of these protocols with differing margins of safety for risk of relapse and for its early diagnosis and management.

Criteria for Inclusion:

In the published series, most patients have had biopsy-proven NSGCT, with clinical stage I disease on the basis of extensive non-invasive investigations. However, the confidence intervals for the prediction of "true" stage I disease are likely to have been broad, because of variations in the characteristics of the tumors (T stage, histology, prior scrotal violation, vascular or lymphatic invasion), the staging protocols (lymphography versus computerized tomography of abdomen and pelvis; chest radiography versus whole lung tomography versus computerized tomography of chest; review of investigations from referring institutions versus acceptance of "external" reporting of these tests) and of the patients (age, education, the nature of the explanation and the patients' comprehension of the protocol, informed consent). As a result, there is likely to have been substantial variation in the risk of occult dissemination (and hence of relapse) and in the speed of diagnosis.

With respect to the tumor characterics, there has not yet been agreement with respect to the prognostic implications of factors such as histological subtype, vascular invasion and T

TABLE 1: PARAMETERS OF ACTIVE SURVEILLANCE:

SERIES 1st Author	TUMOR MARKERS	CXR	CAT ABDO	CAT CHEST	LG	WLT
Crawford	yes	yes	once	no	±	no
Gelderman	yes	yes	yes	yes	no	no
Jewett	yes	yes	yes	no	yes	yes
Peckham	yes	yes	yes	yes	yes	no
Pizzocarro	yes	yes	yes	no	yes	no
Raghavan	yes	yes	yes	yes	no	no
Read	yes	yes	yes	±	±	±
Rorth	yes	yes	yes	±	±	no
Sogani	yes	yes	yes	no	yes	no
Swanson	yes	yes	yes	no	yes	no

KEY: CXR chest X-ray; CAT computerized axial
     tomography; abdo abomen; LG lymphography;
     WLT whole lung tomography.
     ± variable use

TABLE 2: PROGNOSTIC FACTORS FOR STAGE I NSGCT:

SERIES	FACTOR					
	TUMOR SIZE	T STAGE	V-L INVAS.	SCROT. VIOL.	ECC	TM
Raghavan	no	yes	?	?	no	yes
Peckham	no	yes	yes	?	yes	yes
Pizzocarro	?	yes	yes	yes	yes	?
Sandeman	?	yes	yes	?	yes	?

KEY:
V-L INVAS: Vascular/lymphatic invasion;
SCROT.VIOL.: Scrotal violation at operation;
ECC: embryonal carcinoma;
TM: persistently elevated tumor markers after
     orchidectomy
?: factor not addressed in study
yes: factor influences prognosis
no: factor does not influence prognosis

stage (Table 2).   As a result, in some centres, patients with embryonal carcinoma, with lymphatic or vascular invasion, or with advanced T stage have been excluded from surveillance programmes.

At Royal Prince Alfred Hospital, patients undergo a CT scan of chest, abdomen and pelvis and assessment of tumor markers, routine biochemistry and hematology at presentation. Lymphography, whole lung tomography and radionucleide scans are not routinely employed (Raghavan et al, 1988).   Despite our previous experience that advanced T stage constitutes an adverse prognosticator for stage I NSGCT (Raghavan et al, 1982a, 1982b), the relapse rate has not been 100% and thus patients with T2-T4 tumors have been included in the series. Similarly, all histological subtypes and tumors with vascular or lymphatic invasion have been included   The rationale for this is that effective chemotherapy can be administered with a high probability of cure, provided that the schedule of follow up is meticulously followed. Thus some patients with adverse histological prognostic factors, who are not destined to relapse, will be saved unnecessary surgery or chemotherapy; those who do relapse will be identified promptly (with low volume recurrence) and can be treated effectively.   It is emphasized that this approach remains investigational, and further assessment will be required to prove its safety.

Diagnosis of Relapse:

Few of the published protocols have identical follow up schedules, with respect to frequency and nature of investigations, and the need for biopsy proof of relapse. In our institution, biopsy proof (at least by fine needle aspiration cytology) is obtained for all tumors that appear clinically to have relapsed, unless repeated assays of human chorionic gonadotrophin or alphafetoprotein are definitely abnormal.

TABLE 3: RESULTS OF ACTIVE SURVEILLANCE PROGRAMS

STUDY 1st Author	NO.	% FREE DISEASE	DEAD	ALIVE	MEDIAN FOLLOW UP (months)
Crawford	46	69	0	46	?
Gelderman	54	80	1	53	29
Jewett	30	60	0	30	16
Peckham	132	73	1	131	43
Pizzocarro	85	73	1	84	42
Raghavan	46	72	2	44	40
Read	45	76	0	45	>18
Rorth	79	70	0*	77	41
Sogani	102	75	3	99	40
Swanson	82	71	1	81	?
	701	72.4	9	692(98.7%)	

*plus 2 deaths from intercurrent disease

Treatment of Relapse:

Most programs of active surveillance define cytotoxic chemotherapy as the treatment of choice for relapse, although in some institutions, retroperitoneal lymph node dissection has been effected for patients with relapse only in the lymph nodes. At Royal Prince Alfred Hospital, chemotherapy is used routinely, with surgery being reserved for occasional patients with apparent residual disease after the completion of chemotherapy.

Another variable has been the nature of chemotherapy employed. In our institution, a standard protocol of cisplatin (delivered as a single dose of 100 mg/m2), vinblastine and bleomycin has been used since 1979, in accordance with the policy of the Australasian Germ Cell Trial Group (Levi et al, 1988). More recently, vinblastine has been replaced by etoposide in the management of relapsed stage I testicular cancer. However, a wide range of chemotherapy regimens have been reported in the literature.

RESULTS:

In our review of 10 series reported in the past decade (Table 3), 9 deaths (1.3%) have been recorded from a denominator of 701 patients, although the median duration of follow up has varied widely. Most deaths have been reported from series with longer periods of surveillance (median greater than 3 years). The total relapse rate has been 28% (range 20-40%), with most relapses occurring within the first 9 months, but occasionally being documented after 3 years.

DISCUSSION:

The intention in effecting the policy of active surveillance was to preserve high cure rates while reducing morbidity from unnecessary treatment. After 10 years, it appears that this approach is relatively safe when used by experienced urological oncologists with a specific interest in stage I testis cancer. However, an obsessional commitment to the implementation of the protocol has been required by clinicians and patients alike. With the increased passage of time from the commencement of a surveillance program or from entry of an individual patient, the patient and the clinician may tend to be less meticulous in adherence to the details of the protocol.

The death rate of less than 2% is comparable to that found in the larger series of patients treated by lymph node dissection or adjuvant radiotherapy, although it must be emphasized that the follow up period in some of the published series is relatively short. The broad range of relapse rates is a function of the differences in the criteria of eligibility for surveillance, the nature and extent of initial staging procedures, and in the duration of follow up. Higher relapse rates have been documented in series in which on-study review of outside investigations has not been a requirement (Jewett et al, 1984).

Whether this approach is safe for use in the general medical or oncological community is not yet known. However, we believe this to be unlikely because of several important problems in its implementation that have emerged:

a) inexperienced clinicians have come to regard surveillance as an "easy option", without a clear understanding of the rationale of meticulous follow up or of the hazards of protocol violation;

b) there is no current mechanism for the registration of cases, nor for the reporting of morbidity and mortality – this applies especially to cases treated by isolated clinicians away from specialist units; hence there is a risk that a substantial increase in the death rate from early stage NSGCT could occur before being recognized by the medical community;

c) some clinicians regard this approach as the treatment of choice, and do not offer their patients the alternative of lymph node dissection, nor a discussion of the relative benefits and hazards of each treatment option; this may lead to dissatisfaction among the patient population or even to increased litigation;

d) no optimal protocol has been defined, and clinicians have already begun to implement modifications in an unstructured and unevaluated fashion – for example, reduction of frequency of follow up visits, changes in the schedule of investigations;

e) the level of biological hazard of repeated radiological investigations in this context has not yet been documented with certainty; while there is no evidence that active surveillance creates a biological hazard in young men, it is premature to regard a program that requires monthly radio-logical tests as "standard".

f)   the late toxicity of cisplatin-based chemo-therapy has not yet been defined with certainty. Although we have shown a paucity of late side effects by objective testing of 4-12 year survivors after PVB chemotherapy (Boyer and Raghavan, in press), longer periods of follow up will be required to confirm this. Thus the possible increase in the numbers of patients requiring chemo-therapy could theoretically offset the benefits of avoiding the morbidity of unnecessary node dissection or radiotherapy.

Having achieved high cure rates for all stages of NSGCT, the emphasis of management has now shifted to the reduction of toxicity. In the quest to reduce the acute morbidity of treatment, we must not sacrifice the chance of cure. Active surveillance is not yet the gold standard of management and remains an investigational approach. We recommend that an international registry of active surveillance programs be established to monitor the impact of this new approach to the management of early stage testicular cancer. Finally, changes to this program may be beneficial, but should only be introduced in carefully structured and evaluated clinical trials.

REFERENCES:

Boyer, M. and Raghavan, D. (in press). Intensive late toxicity assessment program (LTAP) for patients (pts) treated for metastatic germ cell tumors (MGCT) with cisplatin-containing combination chemotherapy. Proc. Amer. Soc. Clin. Oncol., 1989, in press.
Crawford, S.M., Rustin, G.J.S., Begent, R.H.J., Newlands, E.S. and Bagshawe, K.D. (1988). Safety of surveillance in the management of stage I anaplastic germ celltumours of the testis. Br. J. Urol., 61: 250-253.
Donohue, J.P., Einhorn, L.E. and Perez, J.M. (1978). Improved management of non-

seminomatous testis tumors.   Cancer, 42: 2903-
2908.
Gelderman,   W.A., Koops, H.S., Sleijfer, D.T. et
al (1987).   Orchidectomy alone in stage I
non-seminomatous testicular germ cell tumours.
Cancer, 59: 578-580.
Jewett,   M.A.S.,   Herman, J.G., Sturgeon, J.F.G.
et al (1984).   Expectant therapy for clinical
stage A non-seminomatous germ cell testicular
cancer? Maybe.   World J. Urol., 2: 57-58.
Levi,   J.A.,   Thomson,   D.,   Sandeman,   T.,
Tattersall,   M.,   Raghavan,   D. (1988). A
prospective   study   of   cisplatin-based
combination chemotherapy in   advanced   germ
cell malignancy: Role of   maintenance and
long-term follow up.   J. Clin. Oncol., 6: 1154-
1160.
Lieskovsky,   G.   and   Skinner,   D.G.   (1984).
Expectant   therapy for clinical stage A non-
seminomatous germ-cell tumors of the testis?
World J. Urol., 2:   53-56.
Peckham,   M.J.   and   Brada,   M.   (1987).
Surveillance   following orchidectomy for
stage I testicular   cancer.   Int. J.
Androl., 10: 247-254.
Peckham, M.J., Barrett, A., McElwain, T.J.,
Hendry, W. and Raghavan, D. (1981). Non-
seminoma germ cell tumours (malignant
teratoma) of the testis: Results of
treatment and an analysis of prognostic
factors. Br. J. Urol., 53: 162-172.
Peckham, M.J., Barrett, A., Husband, J.E. et al
(1982). Orchidectomy alone in testicular stage
I non-seminomatous germ-cell tumours.   Lancet,
2: 678-680.
Pizzocarro,   G.,   Zanoni, F., Salvioni, R. et al
(1987).   Difficulties of a surveillance study
omitting   retroperitoneal lymphadenectomy in
clinical stage I nonseminomatous germ cell
tumours of the testis. J. Urol. 138: 1393-
1395.
Raghavan,   D.   (1984).   Expectant   therapy for
clinical   stage A nonseminomatous germ-cell
cancers of the testis? A qualified "yes".
World J. Urol., 2: 59-63.

Raghavan, D., Peckham, M.J., Heyderman, E.,
Tobias, J. and Austin, D.E. (1982a).
Prognostic factors in clinical stage I NSGCT
of the testis. Br. J. Cancer, 45: 167-173.
Raghavan, D., Vogelzang, N.J., Bosl, G. et al
(1982b). Tumor classification and size in
germ-cell testicular cancer: influence on the
occurrence of metastases. Cancer, 50: 1591-
1595.
Raghavan, D., Colls, B., Levi, J. et al (1988).
Surveillance for stage I non-seminomatous germ
cell tumours of the testis: the optimal
protocol has not yet been defined. Br. J.
Urol., 61: 522-526.
Read, G., Johnson, R.J., Wilkinson, P.M. and
Eddleston, B. (1983). Prospective study of
follow-up alone in stage I teratoma of the
testis. Br. Med. J., 287: 1503-1505.
Rorth, M., Van Der Maases, H., Nielsen, E.S. et
al. (1987). Orchidectomy alone versus orchidectomy plus radiotherapy in stage I non-
seminomatous testicular cancer. A randomized
study by the Danish Testicular Carcinoma Study
Group. Int. J. Androl., 10: 255-262.
Sandeman, T.F. and Matthews, J.P. (1979). The
staging of testicular tumors. Cancer, 43:
2514-2525.
Sogani, P.C. and Fair, W.R. (1988). Surveillance
alone in the treatment of clinical stage I non-
seminomatous germ cell tumor of the testis.
Semin. Urol., 6: 53-56.
Swanson, D., Johnson, D., von Eschenbach, A. et
al. (1987). Five years experience with
orchiectomy (surveillance) for clinical stage I
nonseminomatous germ cell testicular tumors.
J. Urol., 137: 211A.
Van der Werf Messing, B. and Hop, W.C.J. (1982).
Radiation therapy of testicular non-seminomas.
Int. J. Radiat. Oncol. Biol. Phys., 8: 175-178.

Uro-Oncology: Current Status
and Future Trends, pages 319–329
© 1990 Wiley-Liss, Inc.

STUDIES OF THE AUSTRALASIAN GERM CELL TRIAL
GROUP: THE MANAGEMENT OF ADVANCED TESTIS CANCER

D. Raghavan, J. Levi, D. Thomson, and
V. Harvey for the AUSTRALASIAN GERM CELL
TRIAL GROUP.

Reprints: D. Raghavan, Dept. of Clinical
Oncology, Royal Prince Alfred Hospital,
Sydney, Australia.

INTRODUCTION:

In the past decade, the management of
advanced testicular cancer has improved
substantially, with an increase in cure rates
for patients with metastatic or recurrent
disease from 20% to more than 60% (Einhorn,
1981; Peckham et al, 1981). The major factor in
this improvement in prognosis has been the
introduction of cisplatin into combination
chemotherapy regimens (Einhorn, 1981). With the
development of the "PVB" combination regimen
(cisplatin, vinblastine, bleomycin), overall
response rates have increased to 70%, depending
upon the extent of the tumor, and a cure rate of
more than 80% has been reported for patients
with small volume metastatic disease (Einhorn,
1981; Peckham et al, 1981). Several other
investigators have used the same or similar
regimens, with comparable results.

The Australasian Germ Cell Trial (AGCT)
Group has carried out a series of clinical
trials with the aim of rationalizing the use of
cytotoxic chemotherapy for advanced testicular
cancer by improving the cost effectiveness of
schedules of delivery and by reducing the
toxicity of the treatment. To this end, a
series of trials has been carried out since
1979.

PATIENTS AND METHODS:

Patients with biopsy proven germ cell tumors were entered into the first AGCT between 1979 and 1983 (Levi et al, 1988). In this study, patients were treated with the following regimen:

cisplatin, 100 mg/m2 IV, day 1;
vinblastine, 6 mg/m2 IV, days 1&2;
bleomycin, 30 U IV/IM day 1 and then weekly.

All patients had inoperable stage II or III tumors, classified according to the system of Samuels et al (1976). Histological review was obtained, with tumors classified according to the system of the World Health Organisation (Mostofi and Sobin, 1976). Each patient underwent detailed clinical staging, including a complete history and physical examination, chest X-ray, full blood count, biochemical profile (including renal and liver function), and measurement of tumor markers (alphafetoprotein and human chorionic gonadotrophin). Tumor mass was assessed clinically and by computerized axial tomographic (CAT) scanning or chest X-ray, or occasionally by lymphography or radionucleide scanning. Baseline audiometry and pulmonary function tests were obtained for most patients.

In most patients, 4-6 cycles of chemotherapy were administered, based on the rationale of "maximum remission plus two cycles". Tumor response was monitored clinically, by serial measurement of tumor markers and by CAT scanning or other objective tests, as required. When apparent partial remission was achieved and was not converted into complete remission by further chemotherapy, most patients underwent surgery to resect the residual abnormality. If viable cancer was found in the specimen, but had been completely removed, the patient was classified as having "no residual evidence of disease" (NED) and received two further courses of PVB chemotherapy; if resection of viable cancer was incomplete, or if the blood levels of tumor markers remained elevated, the patient was regarded as having a failure of treatment. Most of these patients were treated on salvage protocols, at the discretion of the investigators. Patients achieving complete remission (CR) were randomized to receive maintenance vinblastine or to have no further treatment.

In the second AGCT, patients with "bad prognosis" GCT, classified on the basis of the results of the first AGCT (Levi et al, 1988), were treated in a phase II study with cisplatin (70 mg/m2/day IV, days 1 and 2) and etoposide (120 mg/m2/day IV, days 1-3). Patients were ented in 1984 and 1985. The aim of this study was to assess the feasibility of delivering a higher dose of cisplatin (ie. 140 mg/m2) in a 2-day schedule, and to define its anti-tumor activity in bad prognosis GCT. The assessment of response and toxicity were the same as in the first AGCT. In the second trial, tumors that failed to respond were treated at the discretion of the investigators with the PVB (Levi et al, 1988) or POMBACE (Newlands et al, 1983) regimens). No maintenance chemo-therapy was given.

In the third AGCT, patients with "good prognosis" GCT, as defined elsewhere (Levi et al, 1988), were treated with cisplatin (100 mg/m2 IV, day 1), vinblastine (6 mg/m2 IV, days 1 and 2) and were randomly allocated to receive bleomycin (30 U IV/IM weekly) or not to receive bleomycin. The aim of this study was to assess the contribution of bleomycin to anti-tumor efficacy and to toxicity of the PVB regimen, as it had been a major cause of side effects in the first AGCT. The assessment of response and toxicity was similar to that described above. No maintenance chemotherapy was given. Patients were entered into this study between 1985 and 1988.

TABLE 1: DETAILS OF PATIENTS:

DETAIL	TRIAL		
	AGCT1	AGCT2	AGCT3 *
Number registered	260	29	184+
Number assessed	253	28	152+
Median age (years)	29	30	29
Age range (years)	15-65	16-59	14-67
ECOG performance status			
0-1	215	22	143+
2-3	32	6	41+
4	6	0	0
Primary tumor			
Testicular	223	23	152+
Ovarian	7	0	0
Extragonadal	23	5	0
Prognostic group	any	bad	good
HCG>1000IU/L	53	12	21+
AFP>1000ng/ml	47	7	13+
Prior treatment			
Radiotherapy	33	4	10+
Chemotherapy	3	5	0

KEY:

    AFP alphafetoprotein
    HCG human chorionic gonadotrophin
    ECOG Eastern Cooperative Oncology Group
    AGCT Australasian Germ Cell Trial
    * details of final accrual not yet available

RESULTS:

First AGCT:

The results of the first AGCT have been reported in detail elsewhere (Levi et al, 1988). Treatment with the PVB regimen yielded a complete response rate of 72% among 253 evaluable patients. Complete surgical resection of residual masses was carried out in 63 of these patients, revealing necrosis/fibrosis in 37 and differentiated teratoma in 26; in addition, viable cancer was fully resected in 8 patients, yielding an overall CR/NED rate of 76%. The eight-year actuarial survival of the whole group was 68%; 84% of the CR/NED group are long term survivors. Maintenance therapy with vinblastine had no effect on survival. Although most relapses occurred within two years, isolated late relapses were noted between three and five years.

As reported in detail elsewhere, univariate analysis yielded the following prognostic factors for "bad prognosis" disease: extent of tumor, poor performance status, an extragonadal origin, and circulating levels of alphafetoprotein or human chorionic gonadotrophin (HCG) greater than 1000 ng/ml or 1000 IU/L, respectively (Levi et al, 1988). Multivariate regression analysis showed that only the extent of tumor and a level of HCG greater than 1000 IU/L constituted adverse independent prognostic factors.

Substantial toxicity was encountered with this program of treatment. Leukopenia was the major hematological side effect, with 23% of patients having nadir leukocyte counts of <1000/uL; 7 deaths from sepsis occurred in leukopenic patients. Chronic normocytic, normochromic anemia (Hb < 10g/dL) was noted in 49% of patients, especially those receiving more than 4 courses of PVB. Thrombocytopenia occurred in 32% of patients, but no significant hemorrhagic episodes were recorded. Hematological toxicity was significantly worse in

TABLE 2: NON-HEMATOLOGICAL TOXICITY*:

SIDE EFFECT	NUMBER OF PATIENTS ASSESSED	TOXICITY GRADE**	
		0 - 2	3 - 4
Nausea/vomiting	229	71%	29%
Alopecia	240	74%	26%
Stomatitis	236	94%	6%
Pulmonary	239	95%	5%
Auditory	217	97%	3%
Renal dysfunction	240	97%	3%
Cutaneous	245	98%	2%
Neuropathy	235	99%	1%

*   Modified from Levi et al (1988)
** Criteria of World Health Organisation

patients who had received prior radiotherapy, compared to those who had only surgery for their primary tumors (p<0.01). The pattern of severe non-hematological toxicity is summarized in Table 2. Of particular importance, bleomycin-related lung toxicity was noted in 46% of patients, was severe in 4%, and was the direct cause of death in 8 patients (7 among the first 100 patients treated before DLCO monitoring was routine in all centers).

Second AGCT:

In this study, 12 of 28 patients with "bad prognosis" tumors achieved CR/NED, with an overall long term survival rate of 54%. The regimen of etoposide and cisplatin (140 mg/m2) was associated with modest toxicity. Although nausea and vomiting were severe in 53%, there were no severe cases of lung, auditory or neurological side effects. Severe (grade 3) renal dysfunction was reported in 11% of patients; 11% also had leukocyte nadirs less than 1000/uL, but 40% had grade 4 thrombocytopenia. No treatment-related deaths occurred.

Third AGCT:

Although accrual to this study has closed, the final results are not yet available. In an interim analysis, no significant difference in response rates or survival had emerged, although the three-drug combination was significantly more toxic than the two drugs (Levi et al, 1986).

DISCUSSION:

Although cisplatin-containing chemotherapy regimens now have an established place in the curative management of advanced germ cell tumors, attention is being focused increasingly on the financial cost and possible late toxicity of such treatment. The use of a 5-day schedule of delivery of PVB frequently requires continuous inpatient care, with considerable financial expense to health care systems. Furthermore, chronic toxicity of cisplatin-containing chemotherapy has been demonstrated in several studies: pulmonary damage (Weiss and Muggia, 1980; Levi et al, 1988); reno-vascular complications (Rothberg, 1978; Sundstrup, 1978; Edwards et al, 1979; Vogelzang et al, 1980; Bosl et al, 1988); and occasional second malignancies (Mead et al, 1983). Hence an increasing emphasis is being placed on the reduction of toxicity of these approaches to treatment (Bosl et al, 1980; Wettlaufer et al, 1984; Stoter et al, 1986; Levi et al, 1986). However, it is of crucial importance that such attempts should not compromise the chance of cure.

The first AGCT showed that a PVB regimen with a one-day schedule of administration of cisplatin apparently has comparable efficacy and toxicity to the conventional 5-day regimen, based on a comparison with published data (Einhorn, 1981; Peckham et al, 1981; Stoter et al, 1986); however, it is emphasized that this was not a randomized trial of these two regimens. This study also confirmed the earlier report (Einhorn, 1981) that maintenance vinblastine does not improve the resultrs of chemotherapy for advanced germ cell tumors.

The demonstration by multivariate analysis that the extent of disease and a high pre-treatment blood level of HCG constitute independent adverse prognostic determinants is consistent with results from other series (Einhorn, 1981; Bosl et al, 1983; Birch et al, 1986; Stoter et al, 1986). Lactic acid dehydrogenase (LDH), a major prognostic factor in the series of Bosl et al (1983), was not measured routinely in any of the AGCT Group studies and could not be assessed in this context. Patients for the second and third AGCT were divided on the basis of the prognostic determinants defined in the first Trial.

High dose (200 mg/m^2) cisplatin has substantial activity against bad prognosis GCT, but at the expense of major toxicity (Ozols et al, 1983). The moderate escalation of cisplatin dose to 140 mg/m2 was quite well tolerated, apart from grade 4 thrombocytopenia, but did not yield any obvious improvement in response rates when compared with prior experience with the PVB regimen. Further development of this approach was deferred pending late follow up. The recent observation that the complete remissions achieved with this schedule have been sustained may lead to its incorporation into future studies.

The third AGCT has now completed accrual. Although an interim analysis did not reveal significant differences in response rates or survival between the two arms (Levi et al, 1986), a higher relapse rate has been noted after treatment with the two-drug regimen; this is not statistically significant, and may siimply represent an artefact of interim analysis. Nevertheless, the outcome of this study will be of considerable importance, and both arms will continue to be monitored closely for several years for differences in overall survival. Whatever the outcome with regard to anti-tumor efficacy, a statistically significant reduction in toxicity has already been demonstrated with the two-drug regimen (Levi et al, 1986).

Future randomized trials have not yet been defined, pending the analysis of current studies. Interim studies are addressing the efficacy and toxicity of the POMBACE regimen (Newlands et al, 1983) and the incorporation of carboplatin into the management of advanced germ cell tumors. The maintenance of a high cure rate, with attempted reduction of toxicity of treatment, remains an important emphasis of the Australasian Germ Cell Trial Group.

ACKNOWLEDGEMENTS:

We thank our colleagues in the AGCT for their active participation in our clinical trials and for allowing us to present this report on their behalf: R. Abbott, Royal Adelaide Hospital; J. Bishop, Peter MacCallum Cancer Institute, Melbourne; W.I. Burns, St. Vincent's Hospital, Melbourne; M. Byrne, Sir Charles Gairdner Hospital, Perth; A. Coates, Royal Prince Alfred Hospital, Sydney; D. Dalley, St. Vincent's Hospital, Sydney; R. Fox, Royal Melbourne Hospital; P.G. Gill, Royal Adelaide Hospital; A. Gray, Wellington Hospital, Wellington, N.Z.; R. Kefford, Westmead Hospital, Sydney; R. Lowenthal, Royal Hobart Hospital; K. MacMillan, Peter MacCallum Clinic, Launceston; M. Schwarz, Alfred Hospital, Melbourne; K. Phadke, St. George Hospital, Sydney; R. Snyder, St Vincent's Hospital, Melbourne; B. Sundstrup, Peter MacCallum Clinic, Launceston; M. Tattersall, Royal Prince Alfred Hospital, Sydney; and R. Woods, Repatriation General Hospital, Sydney.

REFERENCES:

Birch, R., Williams, S., Cone, A. et al (1986). Prognostic factors for favorable outcome in disseminated germ cell tumors. J. Clin. Oncol., 4: 400-407.

Bosl, G.J., Geller, N., Cirrincione, C. et al (1983). Multivariate anlaysis of prognostic variables in patients with metastatic testicular cancer. Cancer Res., 43:3403-3407.

Bosl, G.J., Kwong, R., Lange, P.H. et al (1980). Vinblastine, intermittent bleomycin and single-dose cisdichlorodiammineplatinum (II) in the management of stage III testicular cancer. Cancer Treat. Rep., 63: 331-334.

Bosl, G.J., Leitner, S.P., Atlas, S.A. et al (1986). Increased plasma renin and aldosterone in patients treated with cisplatin-based chemotherapy for metastatic germ cell tumors. J. Clin. Oncol., 4: 1684-1689.

Edwards, G.S., Lane, M., Smith, F.E. (1979). Long-term treatment with cis-dichlorodiammino-platinum (II)-vinblastine-bleomycin: Possible association with severe coronary artery disease. Cancer Treat. Rep., 63: 551-552.

Einhorn, L.H. (1981). Testicular cancer as a model for a curable neoplasm. The Richard and Hinda Rosenthal Foundation Award Lecture. Cancer Res., 41: 3275-3280.

Levi, J., Raghavan, D., Harvey, V. et al (1986). Deletion of bleomycin from therapy for good prognosis advanced testicular cancer: A prospective randomized study. Proc. Amer. Soc. Clin. Oncol., 5: 97.

Levi, J.A., Thomson, D., Sandeman, T. et al (1988). A prospective study of cisplatin-based combination chemotherapy in advanced germ cell malignancy: Role of maintenance and long-term follow up. J. Clin. Oncol., 6: 1154-1160.

Mead, G.M., Green, J.A., Macbeth, F.R. et al (1983). Second malignancy after cisplatin, vinblastine, and bleomycin (PVB) chemotherapy. A case report. Cancer Treat. Rep., 67: 410.

Mostofi, F.K. and Sobin, L.S. (1976). Histological Typing of Testicular Tumours - World Health Organization Report. Geneva, World Health Organization.

Newlands, E.S., Bagshawe, K.D., Begent, R.H.J. et al (1983). Further advances in the management of malignant teratomas of the testis and other sites. Lancet, i: 948-951.

Ozols, R.F., Deisseroth, A.B., Javadpour, N. et al (1983). Treatment of poor prognosis non-seminomatous testciular cancer with "high dose" platinum combination chemotherapy regimen. Cancer, 51: 1803-1807.

Peckham, M.J., Barrett, A., McElwain, T.J., Hendry, W.F and Raghavan, D. (1981). Non-seminoma germ cell tumours (malignant teratoma) of the testis: Results of treatment and an analysis of prognostic factors. Br. J. Urol., 53: 162-172.

Rothberg, H. (1978). Raynaud's phenomenon after vinblastine-bleomycin chemotherapy. Cancer Treat. Rep., 62: 569-570.

Stoter, G., Sleyfer, D.T., Ten Bokkel Huinink, W. et al (1986). High-dose versus low-dose vinblastine in cisplatin-vinblastine-bleomycin combination chemotherapy for non-seminomatous testicular cancer. A randomized study of the EORTC Genitourinary Tract Cancer Cooperative Group. J. Clin. Oncol., 4: 1199-1206.

Sundstrup, B. (1978). Raynaud's phenomenon after bleomycin treatment. Med. J. Aust., 2: 266.

Vogelzang, N.J., Frenning, D.H., Kennedy, B.J. (1980). Coronary artery disease after treatment with bleomycin and vinblastine. Cancer Treat. Rep., 64: 1159-1160.

Weiss, R.B., Muggia, F.M. (1980). Cytotoxic drug-induced pulmonary disease. Update 1980. Am J. Med., 68: 259-266.

Wettlaufer, J.N., Feiner, A.S., Robinson, W.A. (1984). Vincristine, cisplatin, and bleomycin with surgery in the management of advanced metastatic nonseminomatous testis tumors. Cancer, 53: 203-209.

Index